What Radiology Residents Need to Know

Series Editor
Ronald L. Eisenberg, Harvard University, Boston, MA, USA

AF148483

The books in the *What Radiology Residents Need to Know* series act as an introduction to radiology, specifically designed for the needs of residents on their first rotation in a specific subspecialty. Radiology residents are asked to learn significant amounts of information at a fast and unrelenting space. The current available literature for residents, though, is dense and includes more information than they can easily digest, while the number, variety, and quality of images is often limited. This forces residents to turn to quick searches on the internet to seek out information that often is not at their exact level of knowledge and leaves gaps in their learning. *What Radiology Residents Need to Know* answers resident needs for each radiology rotation, presenting the material in bullet fashion and dividing it into convenient sub-units, such as introductory clinical information followed by "imaging findings" and, when appropriate, "management." In most cases, an individual pathological condition is presented in one page or less, allowing residents to quickly review the essential information on a specific pattern or disease. Books in the *What Radiology Residents Need to Know* series contain a large number of high-quality images, as well as a downloadable set of additional images that give readers a comprehensive library of illustrations. With both readable text and a broad spectrum of images, the books in the *What Radiology Residents Need to Know* series serve as an ideal guide for radiology residents.

Priscilla J. Slanetz · Vandana Dialani
Editors

What Radiology Residents Need to Know: Breast Imaging

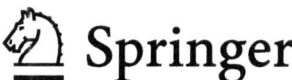 Springer

Editors
Priscilla J. Slanetz
Division of Breast Imaging,
Department of Radiology
Boston University Medical Center
Boston, MA, USA

Vandana Dialani
Division of Breast Imaging,
Department of Radiology
Beth Israel Deaconess Medical Center
Boston, MA, USA

ISSN 2662-9569   ISSN 2662-9577   (electronic)
What Radiology Residents Need to Know
ISBN 978-3-031-66273-7   ISBN 978-3-031-66274-4   (eBook)
https://doi.org/10.1007/978-3-031-66274-4

This Springer imprint is published by the registered company Springer Nature Switzerland AG
The registered company address is: Gewerbestrasse 11, 6330 Cham, Switzerland

If disposing of this product, please recycle the paper.

Contents

Contributors

Kimberly Dao Division of Breast Imaging, Department of Radiology, Boston University Medical Center, Boston, MA, USA

Danielle Del Re Division of Breast Imaging, Department of Radiology, Boston University Medical Center, Boston, MA, USA

Vandana Dialani Division of Breast Imaging, Department of Radiology, Beth Israel Deaconess Medical Center, Boston, MA, USA

Michael D. C. Fishman Division of Breast Imaging, Department of Radiology, Boston University Medical Center, Boston, MA, USA

Bernadette Jakomin Division of Breast Imaging, Department of Radiology, Boston University Medical Center, Boston, MA, USA

Anna Rives Division of Breast Imaging, Department of Radiology, Boston University Medical Center, Boston, MA, USA

Leah Schafer Division of Breast Imaging, Department of Radiology, Boston University Medical Center, Boston, MA, USA

Donna Lee Selland Division of Breast Imaging, Department of Radiology, Boston University Medical Center, Boston, MA, USA

Kitt Shaffer Division of Breast Imaging, Department of Radiology, Boston University Medical Center, Boston, MA, USA

Priscilla J. Slanetz Division of Breast Imaging, Department of Radiology, Boston University Medical Center, Boston, MA, USA

Tom Soker Division of Breast Imaging, Department of Radiology, Boston University Medical Center, Boston, MA, USA

Patrick Tivnan Division of Breast Imaging, Department of Radiology, Boston University Medical Center, Boston, MA, USA

Introduction

Michael D. C. Fishman, Patrick Tivnan,
and Priscilla J. Slanetz

Breast cancer is the second leading cause of death in women and the most common cancer globally surpassing lung cancer in 2021[1]

- 1 in 8 women will develop breast cancer in lifetime
  - Incidence increases with age (1:1000 age 40 to 5:1000 by age 80)
- Approximately 310,720 invasive carcinomas and 56,500 DCIS diagnosed annually in the USA (2024 estimate); men account for 1% of these diagnoses
  - Overall 5-year survival 93–98%; varies by race with non-Hispanic Blacks having lowest and non-Hispanic Whites having highest
  - Survival decreases with increasing stage at diagnosis; late stage 5-year survival only 21–34%
  - Blacks and Hispanics more often diagnosed at later stage
- Greatest risk factors are female gender and increasing age; others include family history of breast cancer (especially premenopausal first-degree relative), prior benign biopsy revealing atypia, BRCA mutation carrier, early menarche, late menopause, dense breast tissue, Black race, late child-bearing (first child after age 30 years), nulliparity, obesity (high BMI), excessive alcohol intake

Imaging is performed for both screening (asymptomatic) and diagnostic (symptomatic) indications.

No imaging test can 100% exclude cancer so if clinically suspicious, biopsy may still be indicated even if imaging is normal.

M. D. C. Fishman · P. Tivnan · P. J. Slanetz (✉)
Division of Breast Imaging, Department of Radiology, Boston University Medical Center, Boston, MA, USA
e-mail: mdfishman@mgb.org; priscilla.slanetz@bmc.org

Breast Imaging Reporting and Data System (BIRADS)

Standardized reporting and communication system used by radiologists in interpretation of mammography, ultrasound, and breast MRI implemented in April 1999

- Report structure—clinical indication, comparisons, breast composition, important findings, impression/assessment, management recommendation
  - Separate paragraph per modality
  - Specify mammographic views obtained
  - Breast density and assessment category mandated by Mammography Quality Standards Act (MQSA)
  - Assessment
    - **BIRADS 0**: Incomplete: Needs Additional Imaging Evaluation **OR** Incomplete: Need Prior Mammograms for Comparison
      - Used for abnormal screening exam, technical recall, incomplete diagnostic workup, or awaiting outside imaging
    - **BIRADS 1**: Negative (nearly 0% chance of malignancy)
      - Routine screening recommended
    - **BIRADS 2**: Benign findings (Nearly 0% chance of malignancy)
      - Routine screening recommended
    - **BIRADS 3**: Probable benign finding (<2% chance of malignancy)
      - Follow up imaging in 3–12 months
    - **BIRADS 4**: Suspicious abnormality
      - 4A: Low suspicion (2–10% chance of malignancy)
      - 4B: Moderate suspicion (11–50% chance of malignancy)
      - 4C: High suspicion (51–94% chance of malignancy)
      - Image-guided biopsy to obtain definitive diagnosis
    - **BIRADS 5**: Highly suggestive of malignancy (>95% chance of malignancy)
      - Image-guided biopsy to obtain definitive diagnosis
    - **BIRADS 6**: Known biopsy-proven malignancy
      - Surgical excision when clinically appropriate

BIRADS abnormality hierarchy—5, 4, 0, 6 , 3, 2, 1; e.g. in patient undergoing chemo for known malignancy, if the post chemo images show a suspicious finding other than known malignancy, the BIRADS 4 or 5 trumps the BIRADS 6 assessment.

Screening—Goal is to save lives; early detection maximizes survival; only options BIRADS 0, 1, or 2

- Recall rate (percentage asked to return for additional imaging) 5–14% (ideally <10%)
- Routine mammographic screening reduces mortality by 22–45% in randomized controlled trials and observational studies
- Supplemental screening (whole breast ultrasound(US), breast MRI) for women with dense breast tissue or those with ≥20% elevated lifetime risk for breast cancer
  - Incremental cancer detection of 1–4 cancers/1000 screened (US) and 7–27 cancers/1000 screened (MRI)

- US performed hand-held or using automated device
- MRI performed using dedicated breast coil and administration of IV gadolinium

- Screening guidelines—ongoing controversy regarding optimal time to start, optimal interval, and when to stop
  - Why? Concern about overdiagnosis (estimated to be 1–10%, primarily DCIS), increased patient anxiety due to false positives, and radiation exposure
    - Analysis based on multiple prospective randomized controlled and observational studies in the USA and Europe showing 30–45% reduction in mortality in women ages 40–74 years
    - Flawed studies:
      - Canadian National Breast Screening Study—improper randomization and poor-quality images invalidate results
      - United States Preventive Services Task Force (USPSTF)—lack of experts in breast cancer diagnosis or care; included Canadian study in analysis; recommendations based on presumed anxiety not based on evidence
  - CURRENT SCREENING RECOMMENDATIONS
    - Guidelines based on existing evidence and individual risk as determined by established risk model (Gail, BRCAPRO, BOADICEA, Tyrer-Cuzick)
    - Average risk—annual mammography starting at age 40 years
    - Intermediate risk (15–20%)—annual mammography starting at age 40 years, if not sooner based on risk factors; possibly whole breast US or MRI screening (but not necessarily covered by insurance in all states)
      - Includes women with personal history of breast cancer or prior benign biopsy revealing atypia and women with dense breast tissue
    - High risk (≥20%)—annual mammography and MRI, often alternating at 6-month intervals annually at age 40 years if not sooner based on risk factors
      - Includes women with BRCA-1/2 mutation, other known genetic predisposition, history of chest irradiation between age 10 and 30 years, and strong family history of breast cancer
    - Stop screening when life expectancy ≤ 7–10 years

Diagnostic evaluation—Goal is to confirm or rule out breast cancer

- Mammography (Full field digital mammography (FFDM) and Digital breast tomosynthesis (DBT)) and US are primary modalities; MRI used selectively
  - Additional mammographic views include true lateral, rolled views, spot compression, and/or magnified views as needed
  - Ultrasound (US) targeted to area of concern
  - MRI for integrity of silicone implants, staging newly diagnosed cancer, finding occult malignancy, problem-solving
- Common indications—recall for abnormal screening exam, symptoms (e.g. lump, nipple discharge, focal pain), imaging follow-up for probable benign finding, monitoring response to treatment
- Imaging workup—(1) Find it. (2) Is it real? (3) What is it? (4) What to do about it?

- ○ If symptomatic, note laterality, clock-face position, distance from nipple
- ○ Mammographic views vary depending on presentation

  - • Screening—CC and MLO views of both breasts (Fig. 1.1)
  - • Spot compression—small paddle to determine if finding is real (Figs. 1.2 and 1.3)
  - • Magnification—characterize mass margins or morphology of calcifications (Fig. 1.4)
  - • Tangential—displace palpable finding into subcutaneous fat or to confirm dermal location (Fig. 1.5)

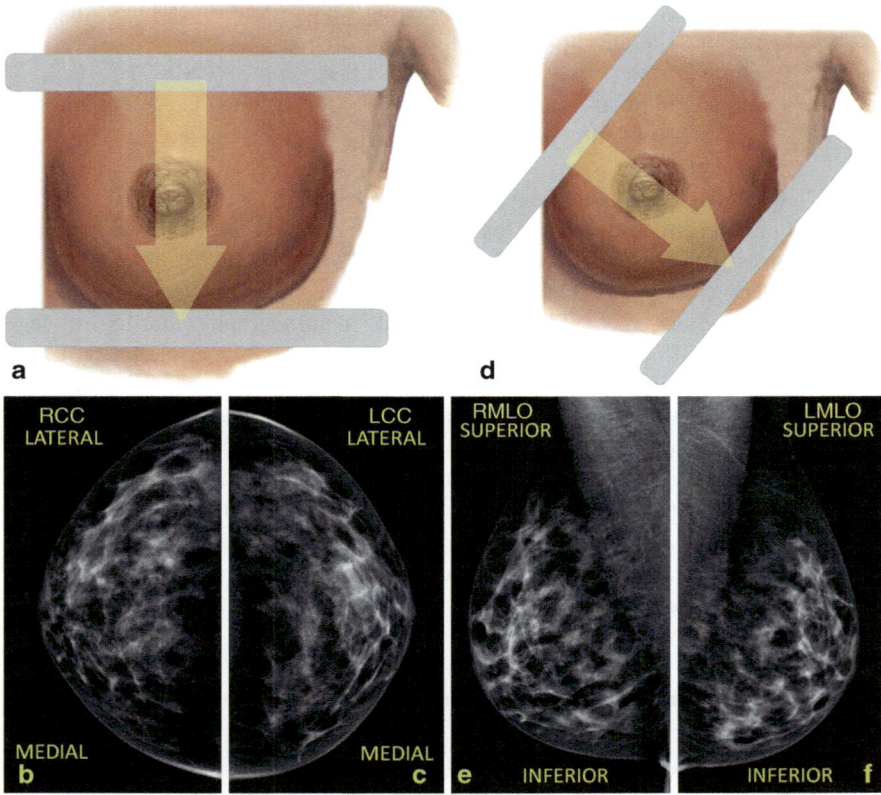

Fig. 1.1 48-year-old asymptomatic woman for screening. Craniocaudal compression (**a**), bilateral craniocaudal or CC views (**b, c**), mediolateral oblique compression (**d**), and bilateral MLO (**e, f**) views show heterogeneously dense breast tissues. The location of a finding on the mammogram can be determined by combining its location on the CC and MLO views thereby guiding subsequent diagnostic imaging, such as ultrasound

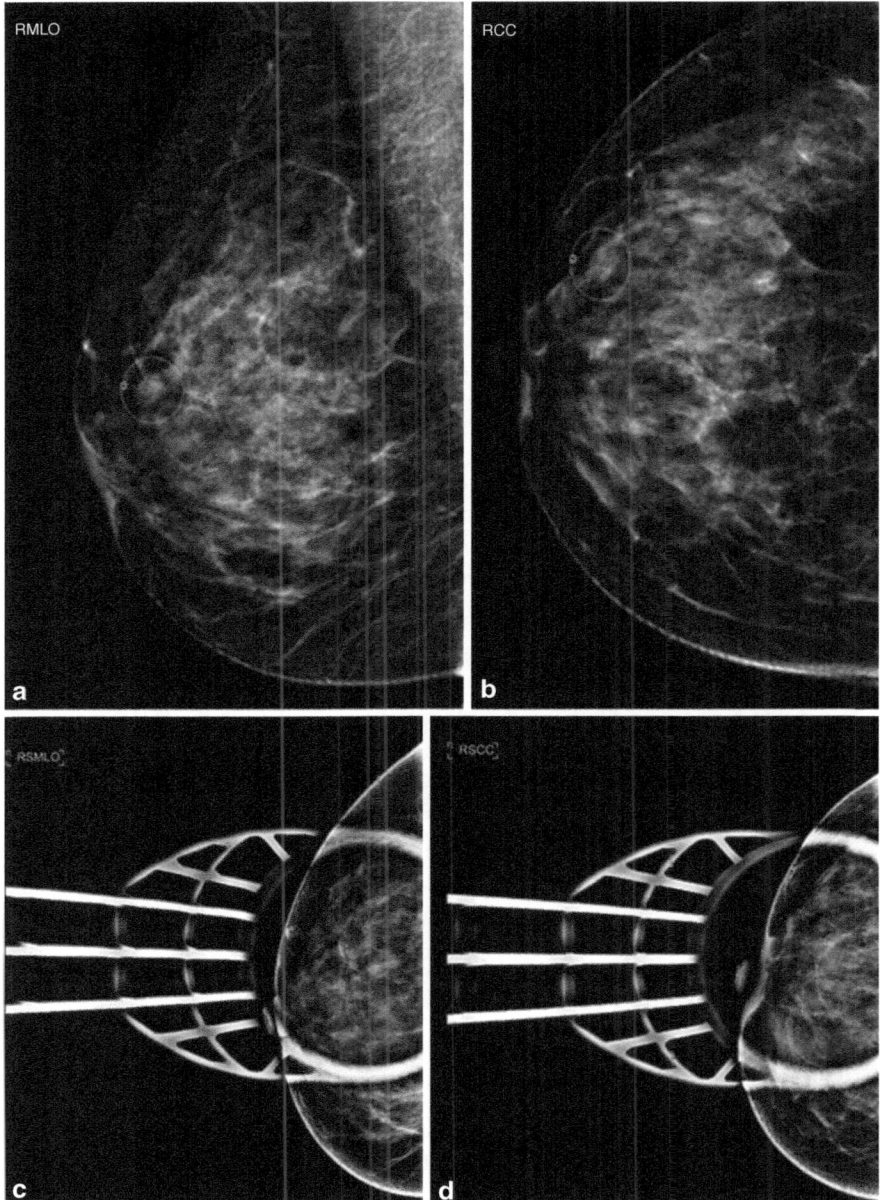

Fig. 1.2 **42-year-old woman with possible upper outer right breast mass (circle) on MLO and CC screening views (a, b)**. Diagnostic imaging with spot compression MLO and CC views (c, d) show that the mass did not persist and therefore represented superimposed breast tissue (BIRADS 1). The patient resumed routine screening

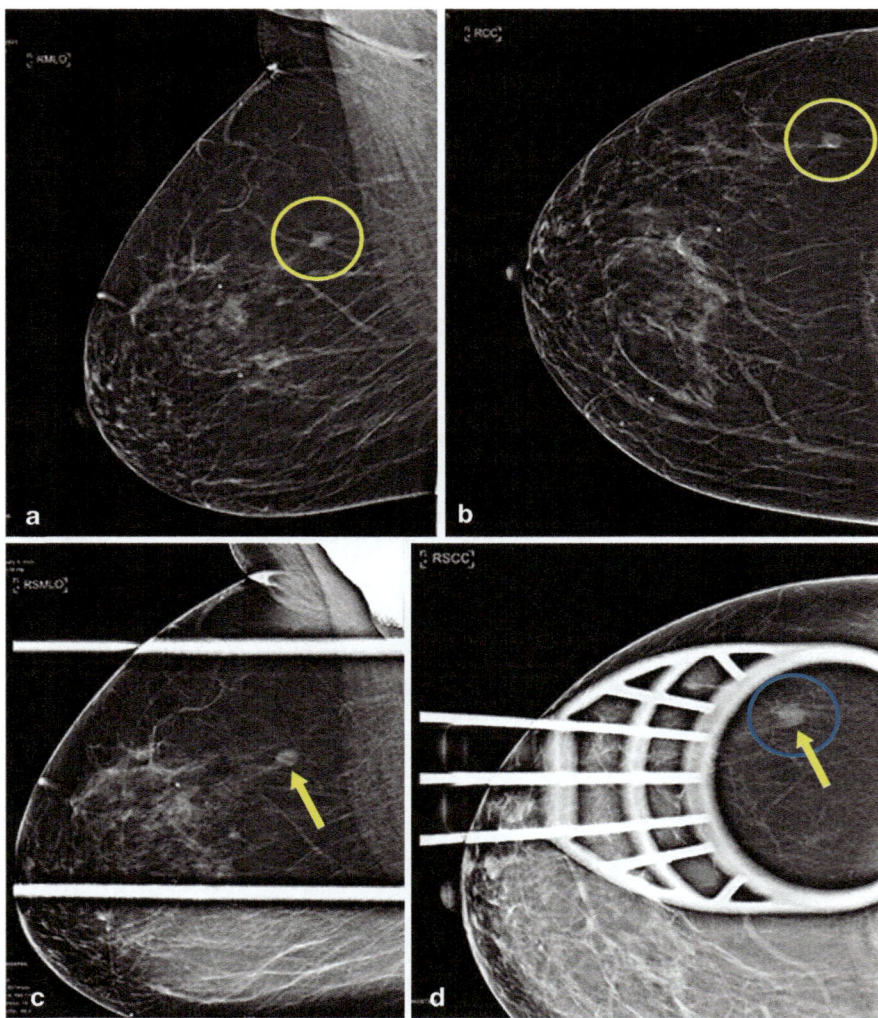

Fig. 1.3 **64-year-old woman with history of prior lung cancer recalled from screening for possible upper outer right breast mass (circle; a, b).** Spot MLO (**c**) view using the larger rectangular paddle and spot compression CC view (**d**) using the smaller round paddle both confirm a persistent mass (arrows). Note that with spot compression, the goal is to acquire at least 0.5 cm more of compression than the initial view, and optimally ≥ 1 cm. For this patient, ultrasound-guided biopsy confirmed invasive ductal cancer

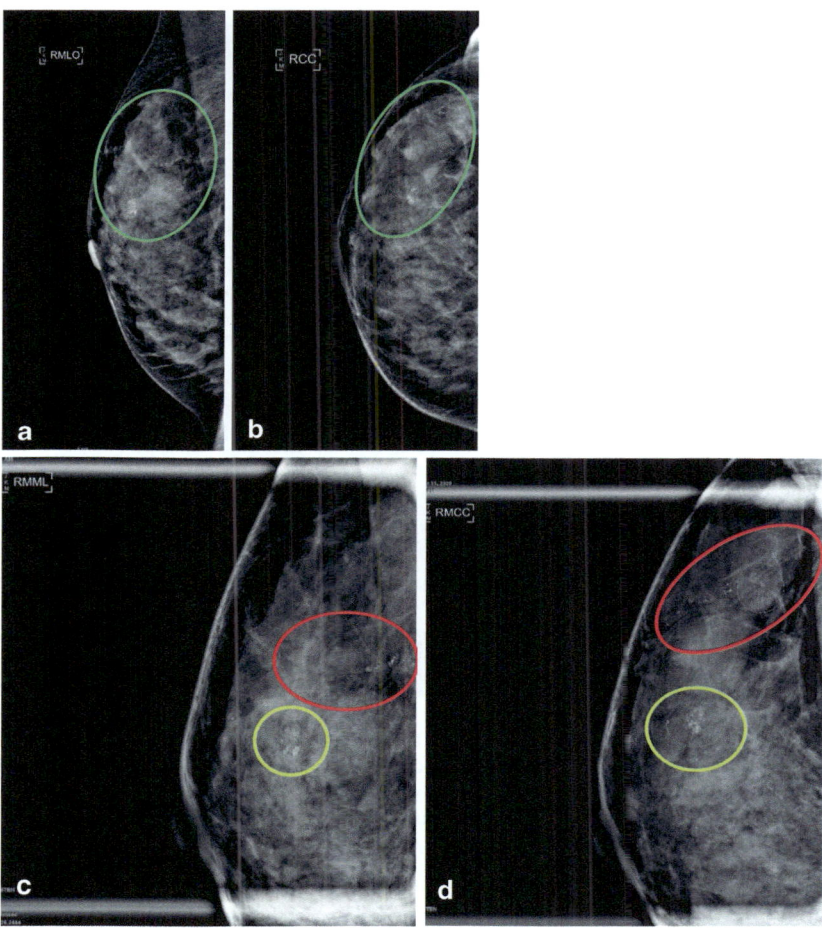

Fig. 1.4 **49-year-old woman with grouped upper outer right breast calcifications (green circle) on RMLO (a) and CC (b) views** Magnification views ML (**c**) and CC (**d**) confirm grouped pleomorphic (yellow circle) and pleomorphic branching segmental calcifications (red oval). Magnification imaging allows characterization of both the morphology and distribution of calcifications thereby guiding management. In this case, stereotactic core biopsy confirmed high-grade ductal carcinoma in situ (DCIS)

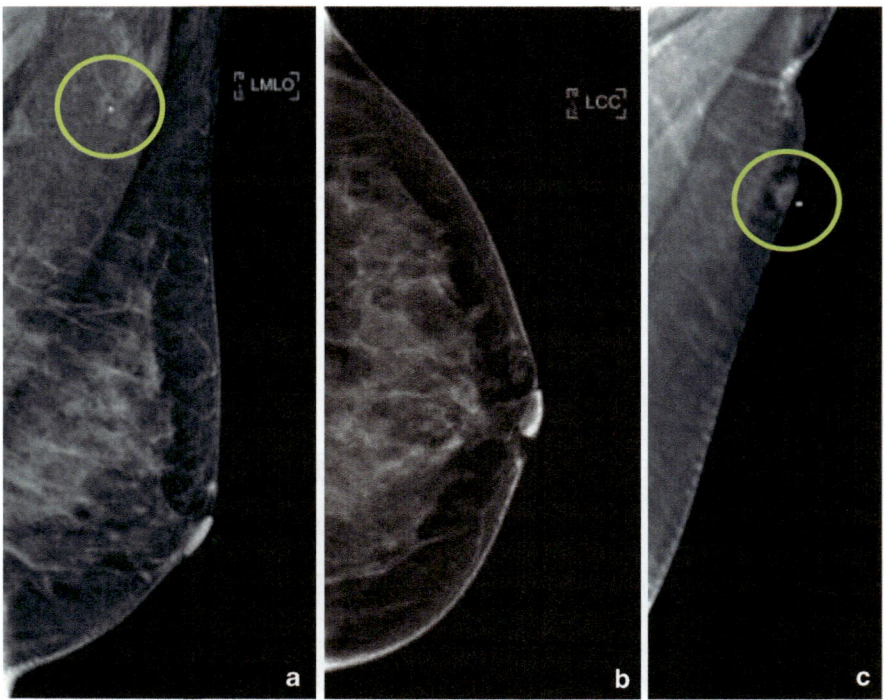

Fig. 1.5 41-year-old woman with palpable left axillary lump. A metallic BB placed on the skin shows the area of concern on the MLO view (**a**; circle). No finding is seen on the CC view (**b**) due to the axillary location. A tangential view clearly shows the finding and localizes the mass to the skin (**c**). Imaging was consistent with a sebaceous or epidermoid inclusion cyst

- ACR Appropriateness Criteria—evidence-based guidelines to assist radiologists and referring providers
  - Abnormal screening/BIRADS 0
    - Technical recall—repeat screening view due to suboptimal positioning, technical parameters, or artifact (e.g. motion)
    - Possible finding, diagnostic mammographic views ± US
      - If circumscribed mass on DBT screen, often can start with US if > 1cm; otherwise, spot compression CC and MLO and 90° lateral followed by US
      - If calcifications on screen, magnified CC and 90° lateral
      - If single view asymmetry, spot compression on that single view and 90° lateral; rolled views for some cases
      - If architectural distortion, spot compression CC and MLO followed by US
  - Palpable lump—majority are benign, but can be cancer
    - < 30 years—targeted ultrasound
    - ≥ 30 years—diagnostic mammogram and ultrasound
      - BB placed on lump and CC/MLO/90° lateral/tangential views obtained
    - Negative imaging in setting of palpable lump carries 0–3% chance of malignancy

○ Breast pain—prevalence 70–80%
  • Diffuse breast pain—no imaging indicated beyond annual screening mammogram (if applicable); likely hormonal or dietary
  • Focal breast pain (localized to <1 quadrant) or non-cyclical breast pain—0–3% associated with cancer
  • <30 years—targeted ultrasound
  • ≥ 30 years—diagnostic mammogram and ultrasound
    ▪ Radiolucent triangle placed in area of pain
• Nipple discharge—experienced by > 80% premenopausal women
  • Physiologic—bilateral; from multiple duct orifices; often white, green, or yellow; may be non-spontaneous
    ▪ Screening mammography, if not up to date
  • Pathologic—unilateral; single duct orifice; spontaneous; often serous or bloody
    ▪ < 30 years—retroareolar US
    ▪ ≥ 30 years—diagnostic mammogram and retroareolar US
    ▪ Ductography or breast MRI if diagnostic imaging negative and patient symptomatic
○ BIRADS 3—imaging follow-up of probable benign finding (<2% chance of malignancy)
  • Follow-up protocols include every 6 months for 2 years or 6mo–1 year–2 year–3 year; some stop followup at 2 years if patient compliant with screening
  • Views depend on what is being followed

Mammography Quality Standards Act (MQSA)

• Federal law setting minimum quality standards for facility accreditation including technologist and radiologist qualifications, inspection of equipment, mammographic positioning, and practice outcomes analysis
• Annual practice inspections by state and federal government
• Separate ACR accreditation for stereotactic and US-guided breast intervention and breast MRI
• Goal—provide group and individual performance metrics as compared to national benchmarks as means to promote high quality imaging
  ○ Total number of screening and diagnostic exams in audit period
  ○ Frequency of initial BIRADS 3 assessments and percentage that resulted in breast cancer diagnosis
  ○ Number of recommendations for further imaging evaluations (BIRADS 0)
  ○ Number of recommendations for biopsy or surgical consultation (BIRADS 4/5)
  ○ Biopsy results
  ○ Tumor staging (histologic type, size, grade, nodal status); positive lesions include DCIS, pleomorphic LCIS, florid LCIS, and invasive cancers

- Derived data:
  - True positives (TP), False positives (FP), True negatives (TN), and False negatives (FN)
  - Positive predictive value (PPV) = TP/(TP + FP)
    - PPV_1 based on abnormal screening = # cancer/all recalls
    - PPV_2 based on recommendations for biopsy = # cancer/biopsy recommendation
    - PPV_3 based on biopsy results = # cancer/biopsies performed
  - Recall rate (% recalled from screening for diagnostic imaging) = TP + FP/all screens cancer detection rate (CDR) = TP/all screens
  - Percentage of minimal cancers (defined as ≤ 1 cm or in situ)
  - Percentage of node-positive cancers
  - Mammography goals:
    - Recall rate < 5–12% (screening)
    - PPV_1 3–8% (screening); 8–25% (diagnostic)
    - PPV_2 20–40% (screening); 20–55% (diagnostic)
    - CDR 2–8/1000 (screening); 20–40/1000 (diagnostic)
    - % minimal cancer: > 50%
- Audit performed for screening and diagnostic mammography, whole breast US screening, and screening and diagnostic MRI; for screening, BIRADS 0, 3, 4, and 5 are considered positive whereas for diagnostic imaging, BIRADS 4 and 5 are considered positive

Further Readings

1. Breast Cancer Facts & Figures 2019–2020—American Cancer Society. https://www.cancer. org/content/dam/cancer-org/research/cancer-facts-and-statistics/breast-cancer-facts-and-figures/breast-cancer-facts-and-figures-2019-2020.pdf.
2. ACR Appropriateness Criteria Breast Imaging. https://www.acr.org/Clinical-Resources/ACR-Appropriateness-Criteria.

Breast Anatomy, Physiology, and Development

2

Kitt Shaffer and Priscilla J. Slanetz

Modified sweat gland is comprised of skin, fat, glandular tissue (milk-producing lobules and ducts), and stroma (fibrous connective tissue).

Anatomy is key to understanding the spread of breast malignancy (hematogenous through venous drainage and lymphatic) and surgical approaches to cancer management and breast reconstruction.

Most breast diseases, including cancer, develop in terminal duct lobular unit (TDLU) (Fig. 2.1a, b).

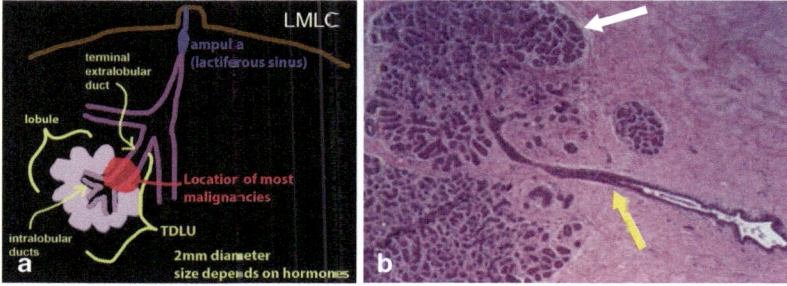

Fig. 2.1 (a) **Schematic diagram of terminal duct lobular unit (TDLU).** (b) Histopathologic image of the TDLU. Ductal cancers develop in the terminal duct (yellow arrow) whereas lobular cancers occur in the lobule (white arrow). When the cancer is confined by an intact basement membrane, the term carcinoma in situ is applied. Once the basement membrane is disrupted, the cancer can spread into the surrounding stroma and connective tissue and is considered invasive

Supplementary Information The online version contains supplementary material available at https://doi.org/10.1007/978-3-031-66274-4_2.

K. Shaffer · P. J. Slanetz (✉)
Division of Breast Imaging, Department of Radiology, Boston University Medical Center, Boston, MA, USA
e-mail: kitt.shaffer@bmc.org; priscilla.slanetz@bmc.org

BREAST ANATOMY (Fig. 2.2a, b)

Fascial Layers

• Muscles—pectoralis major and minor, serratus anterior, intercostal upper external oblique
• Deep fascia covering surface of muscles
• Retromammary space—fat and loose connective tissue
  ○ Deep layer of superficial fascia (Scarpa's fascia)
  ○ Retromammary fat
• Breast stroma—interspersed ductal and glandular elements with fat between lobules
• Pre-mammary fat
• Superficial layer of superficial fascia (Camper's fascia)
• Subcutaneous fat
• Dermis and epidermis

Glandular Tissue

• 15–20 lobes containing smaller lobules—milk-producing, functional component of breast
• Ducts connect lobules to the nipple (Fig. 2.3a, b)
• Terminal duct lobular unit (TDLU) = lobule (10–100 acini) + terminal duct
  ○ Lobule—simple cuboidal to columnar cells with outer layer of myoepithelial cells
  ○ Terminal duct—stratified cuboidal layer with outer layer of myoepithelial cells

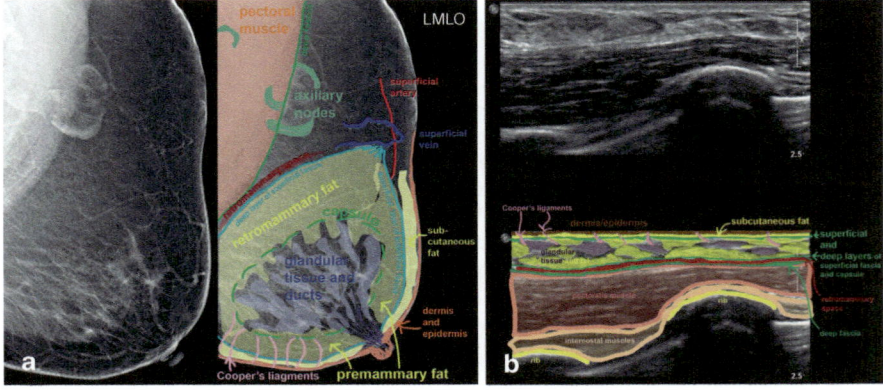

Fig. 2.2 (a) **Schematic of breast anatomy as seen on the mediolateral oblique (MLO) view of a mammogram**. (b) Schematic of breast anatomy as seen on an ultrasound image

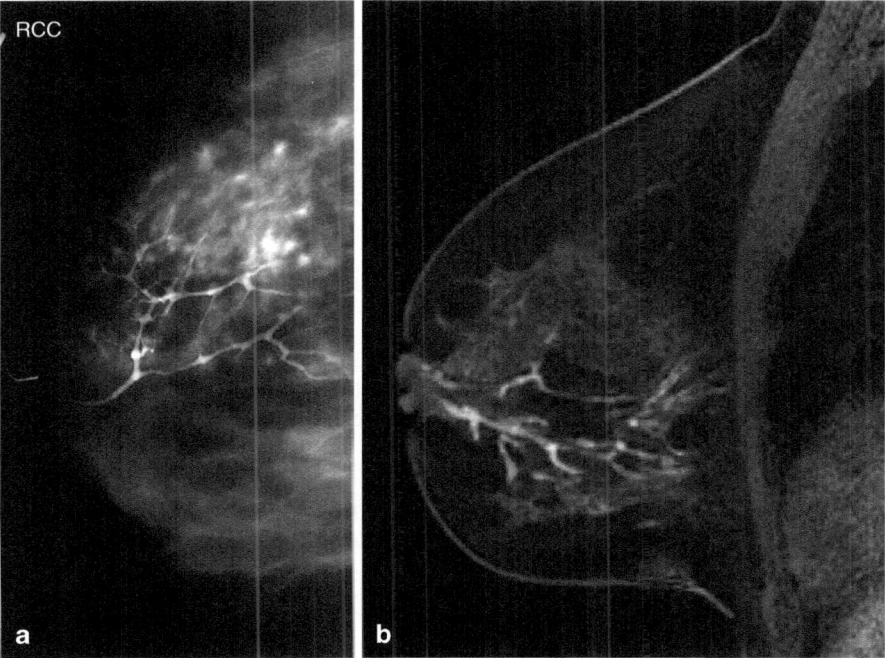

Fig. 2.3 (a) **Ductogram in a 44-year-old who presented with spontaneous nipple discharge.** No abnormalities were detected. Notice the branching ductal system with a blush more distally which represents contrast filling the lobules. (b) T2-weighted sagittal image from a diagnostic breast MRI shows high signal from proteinaceous debris within a dilated ductal system

Stroma

- Fibrous connective tissue surrounding and supporting glandular tissue, ducts, nerves, and vessels between superficial and deep pectoral fascia
- Cooper's ligaments—fibrous bands connecting the two fascial layers

Nipple

- 5–20 ducts converge on retroareolar lactiferous sinus
- Terminal duct lined by stratified squamous epithelium
- Smooth muscle results in erection of nipple due to sensory stimuli

Areola

- Pigmented skin surrounding the nipple
- Montgomery glands secrete lubricating fluid during lactation

Vasculature

- Arterial supply from internal thoracic (mammary) artery (60%), lateral thoracic artery (30%) and thoracoacromial and posterior intercostal arteries (10%) (Fig. 2.4a, b)
- Venous drainage primarily through axillary vein, and lesser extent, internal mammary vein into superior vena cava (Fig. 2.4c)
  - Limited drainage via posterior intercostal veins into azygos/hemiazygos veins

Lymphatics

- Breast cancers are most likely to spread through the lymphatic system
- ≥95% drainage from subareolar lymphatic plexus to axillary nodes (Fig. 2.4a):
  - Level 1—lateral to pectoralis minor
  - Level 2—deep to pectoralis minor
  - Level 3—medial and superior to pectoralis minor
- Rotter's nodes—between pectoralis minor and major
- < 5% drainage to internal mammary lymph nodes and contralateral breast

Innervation

- Fourth to sixth intercostal nerves provide anterior and lateral cutaneous branches providing sensory and sympathetic fibers to vessels and smooth muscle in nipple-areolar region

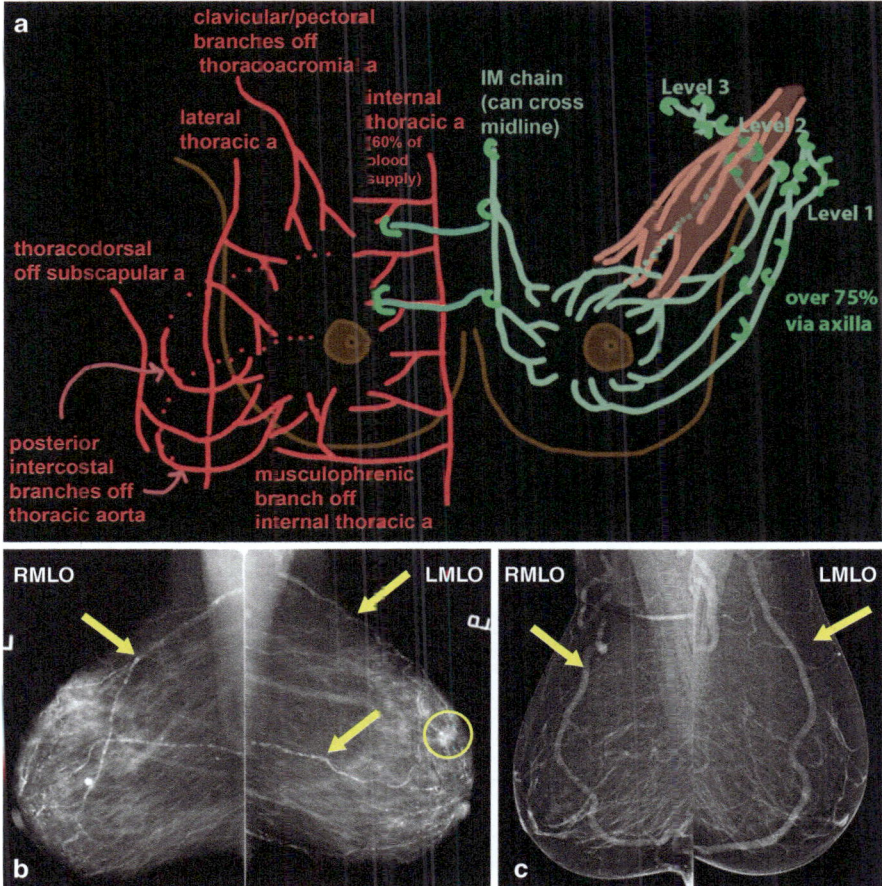

Labels in figure:

(a)
clavicular/pectoral branches off thoracoacromial a

lateral thoracic a

internal thoracic a (60% of blood supply)

IM chain (can cross midline)

Level 3
Level 2
Level 1

thoracodorsal off subscapular a

over 75% via axilla

posterior intercostal branches off thoracic aorta

musculophrenic branch off internal thoracic a

(b) RMLO   LMLO

(c) RMLO   LMLO

Fig. 2.4 (**a**) **Schematic of the vascular supply and lymphatic drainage to the breasts**. (**b**) Mammogram shows extensive vascular calcifications of arteries in the breast (arrows). These tubular calcifications are often seen in patients with diabetes. Incidental note is made of an irregular mass in the anterior upper left breast (circle). This finding was subsequently shown to be an invasive ductal carcinoma. (**c**) MLO views shows dilated veins bilaterally (arrows) due to central occlusion of both brachiocephalic veins from prior radiation treatment for lymphoma

BREAST EMBRYOLOGY AND DEVELOPMENT

- Develops from ectodermal infolding (mammary ridge) during fifth to sixth gestational week which extends from axilla to groin
- Mammary ridge involutes nearly completely with exception of primary breast bud
  - Lack of involution results in accessory axillary breast tissue (2–6%) (Figs. 2.5 and e2.1), accessory breasts (< 1%; polymastia), and supernumerary nipples (2–5%; polythelia)
- Secondary epithelial breast buds grow vertically around primary bud during second and third trimester to form lactiferous ducts, glandular tissue, stromal connective tissue, and Cooper's ligaments
  - At birth, 15–20 lobes of glandular tissue containing ducts and stroma
  - From birth–2 years, nipple everts and areolar pigmentation develops
- During puberty, epithelial and connective tissue proliferate to form lobules and fat accumulates
  - Male breast is nearly all fat and has only ducts, very rarely lobules

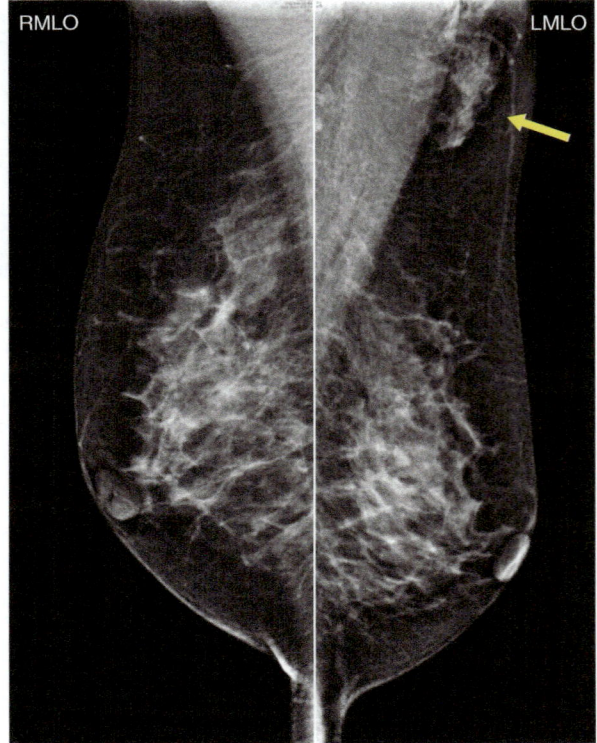

Fig. 2.5 MLO views in a 45-year-old woman show glandular tissue in the left axilla (arrow) consistent with accessory breast tissue. Most often, these patients are asymptomatic; however, during pregnancy and lactation, accessory breast tissue may enlarge and produce milk, although the ductal units are not necessarily connected to the rest of the breast resulting in substantial discomfort

- Most common embryological variants include:
  - Sternalis muscle—vestigial parasternal muscle extending from manubrium to inferior sternal edge occurring in about 8%; twice as common in males than females (Figs. 2.6 and e2.2)
  - Poland's syndrome—congenital hypoplasia or absence of pectoralis muscle, most often unilateral; 3X more common in men; 75% right-sided (Fig. 2.7)

Fig. 2.6 Unilateral sternalis muscle. 40-year-old woman found to have left posterior medial triangular asymmetry only seen on the CC view (**a**, **b**; arrow). Findings are consistent with a sternalis muscle

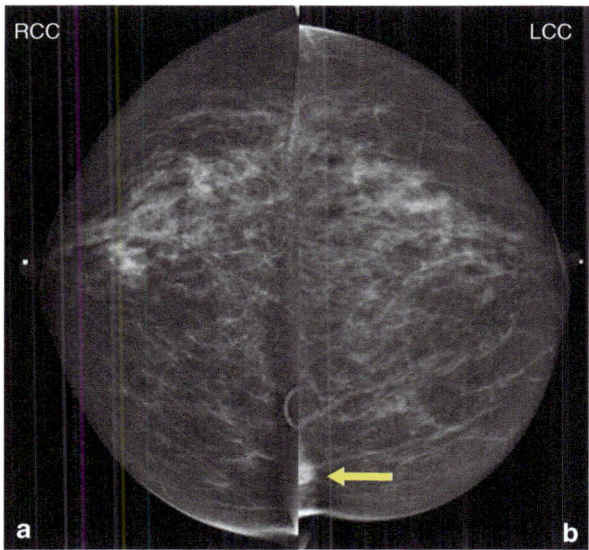

Fig. 2.7 45-year-old asymptomatic woman presented for screening. Bilateral MLO views (**a**, **b**) show markedly smaller right breast and absence of the pectoralis muscle on the right as compared to the left (arrow) consistent with Poland's syndrome

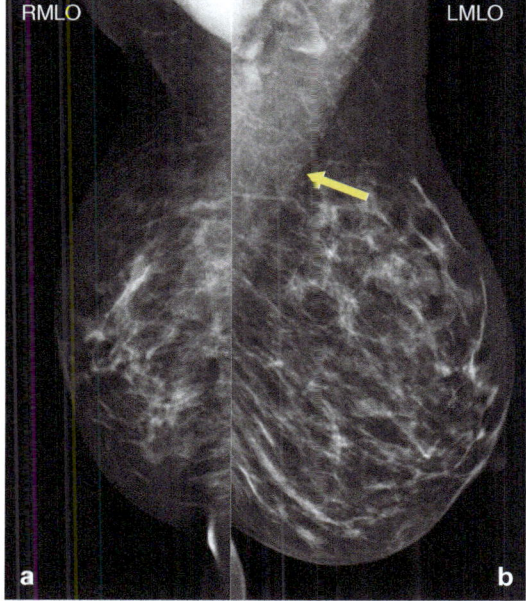

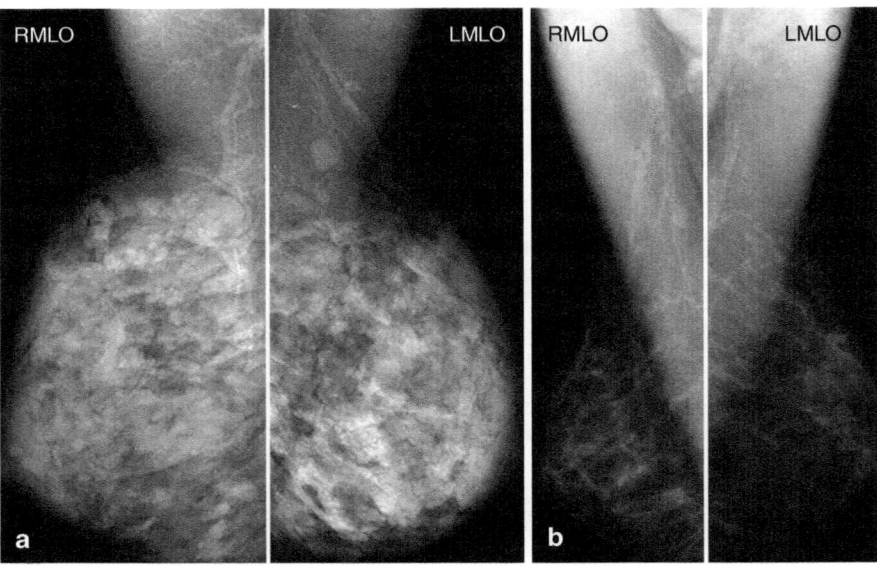

Fig. 2.8 **33-year-old currently lactating woman presenting with a palpable lump**. Bilateral MLO views reveal enlarged breasts with dense breast tissue (**a**) consistent with lactational state. After cessation of lactation, routine screening MLO views show resolution of the lactational findings as demonstrated by markedly smaller and less dense breast tissues (**b**)

BREAST CHANGES IN PREGNANCY, LACTATION, AND MENOPAUSE

- Hormonal stimulation of pregnancy causes proliferation of both ducts and lobules resulting in overall breast enlargement (Fig. 2.8a, b)
  - ○ Lobular epithelium becomes fully differentiated for milk production
  - ○ Drop in estrogen and progesterone at delivery induces lactation
  - ○ At cessation of lactation, involution returns breast to resting state
- After menopause, glandular tissue atrophies, fibrous stroma decreases, and fat accumulates

Further Readings

1. Sadler TW. Langman's medical embryology. 12th ed. New York: Lippincott, Wilkins & Williams; 2012.
2. AUR Core Curriculum. https://radiologyresidentcorelectures.com/breast-imaging-courses/.

Mammography

3

Anna Rives and Priscilla J. Slanetz

A low-dose X-ray of the breast is used to detect breast cancer.

It is performed for screening of asymptomatic women and diagnostic evaluation of symptomatic patients (palpable lump, focal pain, nipple discharge).

Types of Mammograms

- *Analog* (screen-film mammography) (Fig. 3.1a)
  - ○ Film exposed, processed in dark room, and displayed on viewbox
    - Older technology, no longer commonly used

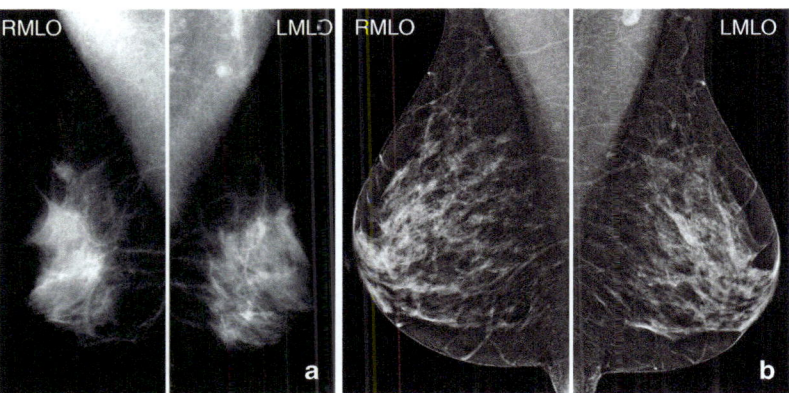

Fig. 3.1 **Analog vs. FFDM.** (a) Analog mammogram. (b) Full-field digital mammogram. Note how skin surface and subcutaneous fat is better visualized on the digital images

A. Rives · P. J. Slanetz (✉)

Division of Breast Imaging, Department of Radiology, Boston University Medical Center, Boston, MA, USA

e-mail: anna.rives@bmc.org; priscilla.slanetz@bmc.org

- *Full-field digital mammography* (FFDM) (Fig. 3.1b)
  - ○ Digital detector converts absorbed X-rays into pixels viewed on high resolution monitor
    - Lower spatial resolution, lower or comparable dose to analog
    - Easier image archiving, faster interpretation time
    - Digital Mammographic Imaging Screening Trial (DMIST) showed overall similar cancer detection to analog but increased detection in women with dense breast tissue and women ≤ 50 years
- *Digital breast tomosynthesis* (DBT)) (Fig. 3.2)
  - ○ Multiple images acquired along 15–50° arc reconstructed into scrollable 1 mm thick slices eliminating superimposition of breast tissue
    - "Combo" imaging (FFDM and DBT) commonly performed—2–8× radiation dose of FFDM alone; higher doses seen with increasing compression thickness
    - Synthetic 2D image created from DBT stack (i.e. synthesized)—dose equivalent to FFDM
    - Increased cancer detection rate and decreased recall rate compared to FFDM
    - Benefit in both dense and fatty breasts
- *Contrast-enhanced mammography* (CEM) (Fig. 3.3)
  - ○ Combines digital mammography with IV water-soluble iodinated contrast administration
    - Dual energy imaging technique above (high energy) and below (low energy) the k-edge of iodine performed after IV contrast administration (0.1 mmol/kg injected at 3 cc/s); low-energy image equivalent to

Fig. 3.2 Tomosynthesis. Digital breast tomosynthesis (DBT) decreases the effect of superimposed breast tissue, allowing for better lesion visualization. (**a**) FFDM and (**b**) DBT image, right MLO view. The malignant architectural distortion (arrows) is visualized on tomosynthesis (**b**) and not well appreciated on the 2D image (**a**)

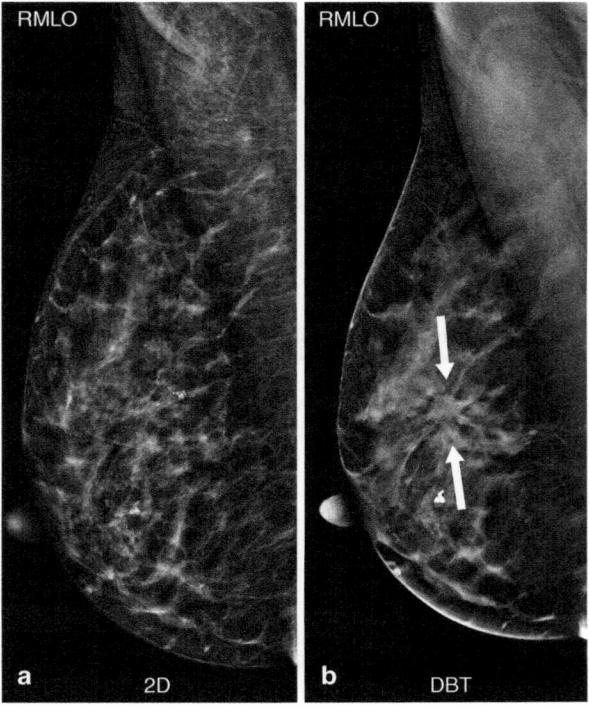

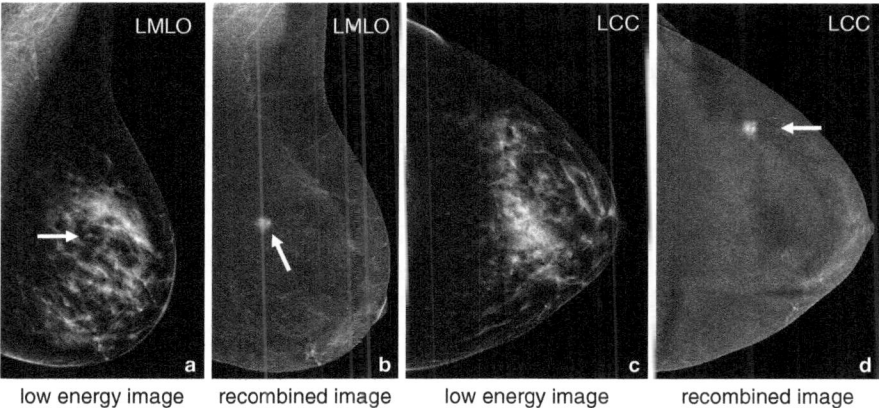

low energy image   recombined image   low energy image   recombined image

Fig. 3.3 Contrast-enhanced mammography (CEM). Contrast-enhanced mammography (CEM) uses intravenous injection of iodinated contrast to visualize tumor neovascularity, similar to MRI. Dual-energy mammography is performed after injection, including low-energy (**a, c**) and recombined images (**b, d**), showing any enhancing lesions. Images from a CEM of the left breast show an enhancing mass in the upper outer quadrant (arrow) corresponding to screen-detected asymmetry on the MLO view (arrow)

conventional mammogram; subtract low-energy and high-energy acquisitions to get recombined image that shows enhancement
- Sensitivity similar to breast MRI
- FDA approved for diagnostic imaging
- Indications similar to breast MRI (disease extent, problem-solving, monitoring response to chemotherapy) but may have role in high risk screening
- Specialized lexicon for interpretation—findings on low energy only, recombined only, or both images
  - Background enhancement (minimal, mild, moderate, marked; symmetric vs. asymmetric)
  - Low energy (LE) finding—describe using mammographic lexicon
  - Recombined finding—describe enhancing mass (shape, margin, internal enhancement), non-mass enhancement (distribution, internal enhancement pattern), or enhancing asymmetry (only on one projection) and lesion conspicuity (degree of visibility over background; low, moderate, high)
  - If on both LE and recombined—also describe enhancement extent (enhances partially, completely, beyond mammographic finding, or around mammographic finding)

Mammography Physics

- Breast compression decreases breast thickness thereby improving contrast and reducing X-ray scatter, patient dose, motion artifact, and geometric magnification
- Lower energy (16–23 keV) compared to conventional radiography enhances attenuation difference between cancers and normal breast tissue—achieved using 25–30 kVp

- Smaller focal spot (0.1–0.3 mm) compared to conventional radiography increases spatial resolution
  - Spatial resolution: 11–15 lp/mm analog; 5–10 lp/mm FFDM
- Must use lower mA for small focal spot (50–100 mA) but longer exposure time (up to 2 s) to limit heat accumulation; otherwise, anode could melt
- Anode/filter:
  - Target anodes (Molybdenum (Mo) or Rhodium (Rh)) generate lower k-characteristic X-rays with resultant energy around 18 keV
  - K-edge filter (Mo or Rh) creates nearly mono-energetic beam of 16–23 keV as filter blocks both lower and higher energy X-rays
  - Anode/filter combinations: Mo/Mo, Rh/Mo, Rh/Rh, Tungsten (W)/Rh
    - Mo/Mo most common combination
    - Rh/Rh used for larger or denser breasts
    - W/Rh has highest energy and thus greater penetration with lower dose but lower contrast
- Average glandular dose per view not to exceed 3 mGy (300 mrads)
- Oscillating grid removes scattered X-rays but results in increased dose
- Automated exposure control (AES) determines factors for image acquisition for each patient
- Magnification views—breast moved closer to focal spot and further from detector resulting in 1.5–1.8× magnification of image; no grid due to air gap (increased distance between breast and detector)
  - To increase spatial resolution, uses 0.1 mm focal spot, 25–50 mA, and longer exposure time than standard view (approx. 3 s)

Digital Mammography Physics

- Detector: X-ray film is replaced by a solid-state detector that converts absorbed X-rays into electrical signals
  - Indirect: scintillator absorbs X-rays and generates light detected by photodiode or charge-coupled device
  - Direct: X-rays captured by photoconductor which converts them to digital signal
- Post-processing allows image manipulation after acquisition by adjusting brightness, contrast, magnification, etc.
- Lower spatial resolution and approximately 15% less dose than analog
- Wider dynamic range than analog

Quality Control (QC)

Technical procedures that ensure high level image quality

- Responsibility of all radiologists and technologists
- QC team: lead radiologist (i.e. LIP - lead interpreting physician), QC technologist, and medical physicist
- Facilities undergo annual inspection by state and federal government
- Any new mammography unit must pass QC defined by ACR Manual prior to clinical use

Fig. 3.4 Phantom.
Phantom image. The
phantom is designed to
assess the mammography
unit for its ability to detect
small structures. 2 fibers, 3
speck groups, and 2 masses
must be seen (digital
system)

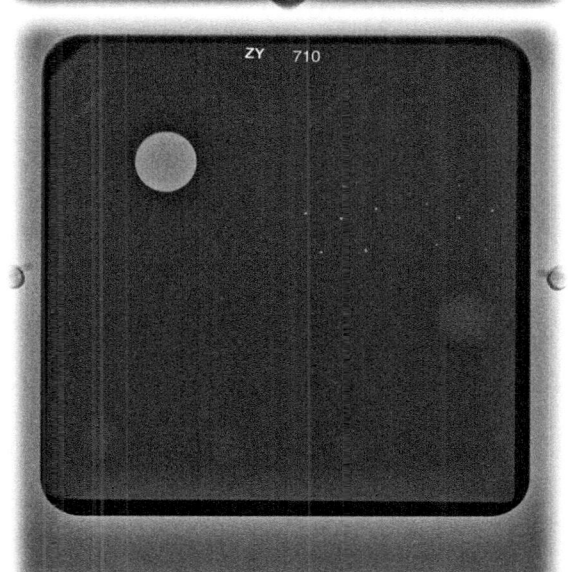

- Common QC tests:
  - Daily—Processor QC (if printing images); Darkroom Cleanliness (analog only)
  - Weekly—Phantom Image Quality on each mammographic unit including contrast-to-noise ratio and signal-to-noise ratio (Fig. 3.4); Workstation monitor QC (radiologist)
    - ACR Phantom simulates average breast (4.2 cm compressed breast with 50:50 fat:glandular composition)
    - Must see 4 fibers, 3 specks and 3 masses for analog and 2 fibers, 3 specks and 2 masses for digital
  - Monthly—Workstation Monitor QC (radiologist and technologist); Compression Thickness Indicator; Visual Checklist; View Box Cleanliness (analog only); Film Printer QC (analog only)
  - Quarterly—Repeat/Reject Analysis; Facility QC review
  - Semi-annually—Compression Force; Geometry Calibration; Darkroom Fog (analog only); Screen-film Contrast (analog only)
  - Additional digital QC as specified by manufacturer

Mammographic Technique and Image Quality

- Breast compressed between image detector and compression paddle
- Two standard views used primarily in screening—CC (craniocaudal) and MLO (mediolateral oblique)
- Additional projections obtained for diagnostic imaging (small paddle spot compression, magnification, 90° lateral, rolled CC, tangential views)
- Labels (side, view, technologist initials) mark axillary side of image

Assessing Image Quality

- Technical factors—exposure, contrast, sharpness, noise
- Positioning (Fig. 3.5)
    - Nipple in profile on at least one of two projections
    - No skin folds
    - MLO positioning—breast pulled "up and out"
        - Pectoralis muscle visualized down to *posterior nipple line* (line drawn from nipple perpendicular to pectoralis muscle)
        - Pectoralis convex or straight
        - Inframammary fold visible
    - CC positioning
        - Pectoralis visualized on 30%
        - Nipple centered
        - Length of posterior nipple line on CC view within 1 cm of that on MLO view

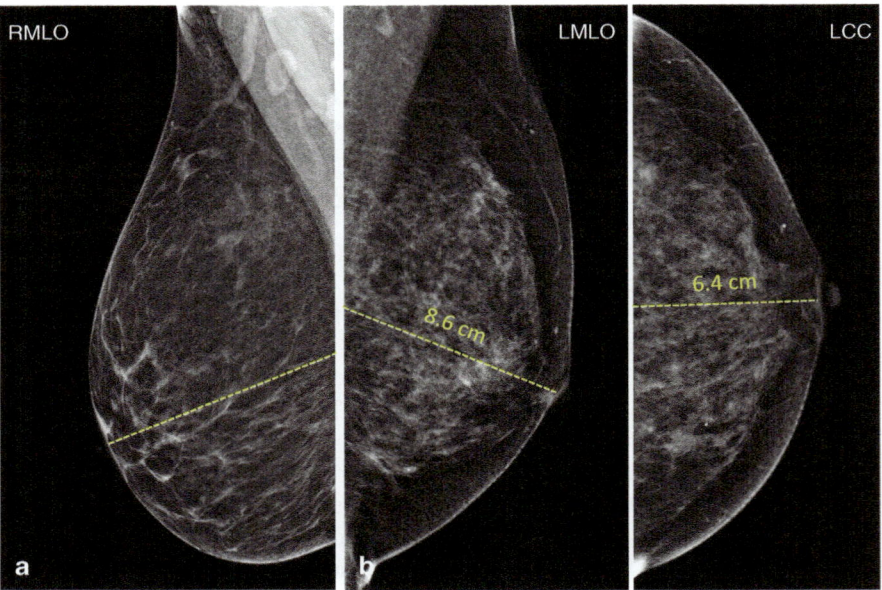

Fig. 3.5 Positioning problems. Common positioning problems. (**a**) The pectoralis muscle is not visualized to the level of the posterior nipple line (dotted line). The inframammary fold is not visible. (**b**) The length of the posterior nipple line on the CC view is more than 1 cm shorter than that on the MLO view

- Artifacts (Fig. 3.6a–k)—can be related to patient, hardware, or software
  - Motion (a, b)—patient movement causing blurring of image
  - Foreign objects—hair (c), other body parts (d), patient gown, bed sheets (e), medicine patch (f)
  - Antiperspirant (g)—radiopaque material overlying axillary region; on first slice if DBT. Note: deodorants do not contain metal so are not visible on mammography
  - Collimator misalignment (h)—white line on edge of image
  - Grid lines (i)—criss-crossing lines due to halted or slower grid oscillation during exposure
  - Pixel defects (j)—defective pixels (lost data) as black, less often white, dots
  - Ghosting (k)—prior exposure superimposed on current image; only with selenium systems

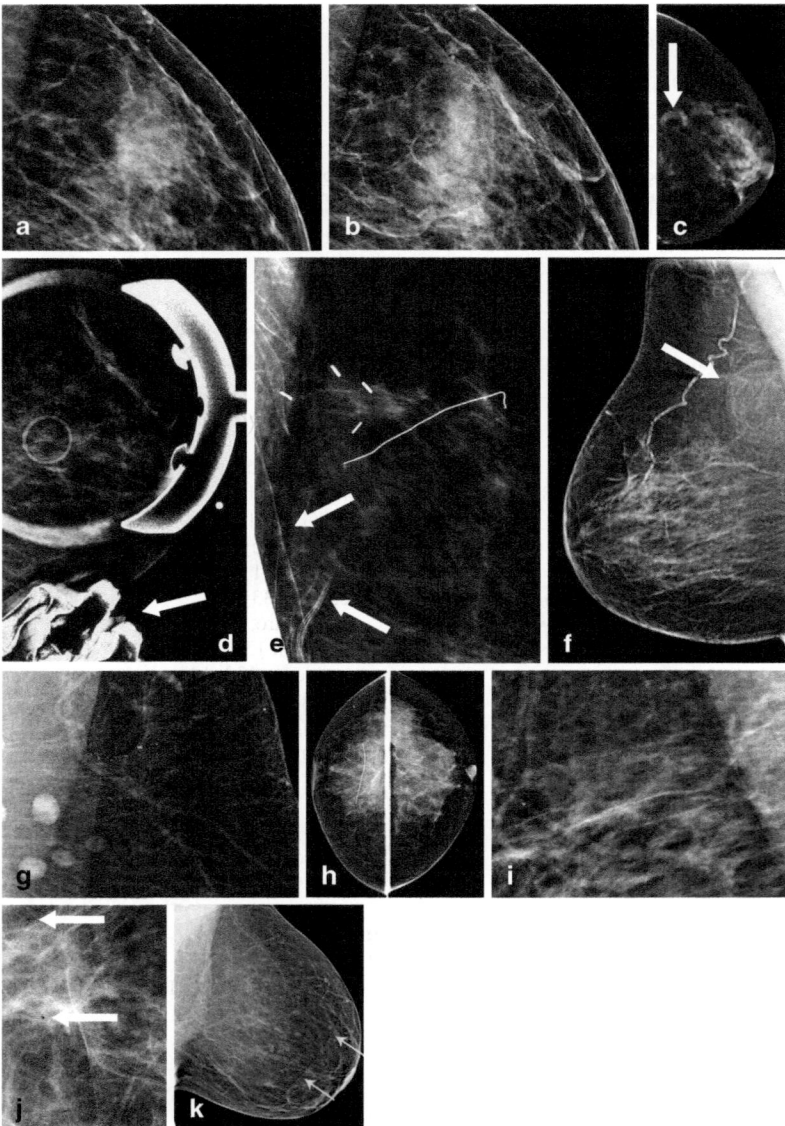

Fig. 3.6 Digital mammography artifacts. Common digital mammography artifacts. (**a**) Blur caused by patient motion during image acquisition. (**b**) After repeat mammogram, the blur is gone. (**c**) The patient's hair causes dense curvilinear lines overlying the image (arrow). (**d**) Patient's hand is included in the image. (**e**) Bed sheets on the edge of the image. (**f**) Nitroglycerin patch projecting over the upper posterior right breast. (**g**) Anti-perspirant artifact appears as radiopaque densities in the axillary region, often following skin folds. (**h**) Collimator misalignment visible as white line at edge of image. (**i**) Grid lines are visible as diagonal criss-crossing lines. (**j**) Pixel defects as black dots scattered on the image. (**k**) Ghosting visible as a prior exposure superimposed on the current mammogram as the selenium plate was not fully recharged prior to the next acquisition

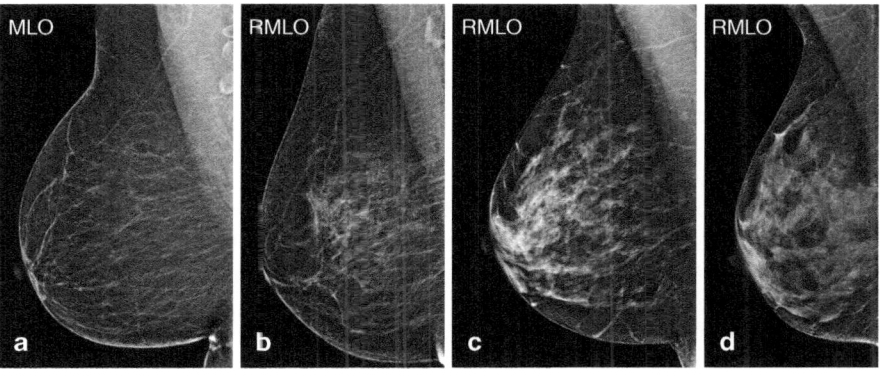

Fig. 3.7 Mammographic breast density (composition). The four breast density categories. (**a**) The breasts are almost entirely fatty. (**b**) There are scattered areas of fibroglandular density. (**c**) The breasts are heterogeneously dense which may obscure small masses. (**d**) The breasts are extremely dense, which lowers the sensitivity of mammography

Breast Density

Ratio of glandular tissue (white or radiopaque) to fatty tissue (gray or radiolucent) as seen on mammogram; category assigned based on densest area

- Does not correlate with clinical breast exam
- BI-RADS density categories (Fig. 3.7)
    - (a) The breasts are almost entirely fatty (10% of women)
    - (b) There are scattered areas of fibroglandular density (40% of women)
    - (c) The breasts are heterogeneously dense, which may obscure small masses (40% of women)
    - (d) The breasts are extremely dense, which lowers the sensitivity of mammography (10% of women)
    - ○ Not dense = Categories (a) and (b); Dense = Categories (c) and (d)
- Independent risk factor for breast cancer (relative risk (RR) 1.2 for heterogeneously dense and 2.1 for extremely dense)
- Dense tissue can "mask" cancers lowering mammographic sensitivity
- FDA now requires facilities to notify patients about breast density, although supplemental screening (MRI, US) not always covered by insurance

Approach to Interpretation

- Review breast intake sheet for symptoms, prior breast history (surgery, biopsies), risk factors for breast cancer
- Assess image quality—if technically inadequate, recall for repeat imaging
- Assess breast density
- Look for findings using systematic search pattern
  - General overview looking for gross abnormalities and change from priors
  - View MLO and CC views back-to-back to assess for symmetry of fibroglandular tissue
  - Look for asymmetries, masses, calcifications, architectural distortion, pulling or tethering of tissue at fat-glandular interfaces, skin or trabecular thickening, nipple retraction, lymphadenopathy; use BIRADS lexicon to describe all findings
  - Assess retroglandular fat—should be all fat, no masses or asymmetries
  - Compare to prior mammograms
  - Review computer-aided detection (CAD/AI) findings
- Record MOD (method of detection) of any malignancy in report (e.g. identified by patient or provider, by screening 2D or DBT mammogram, US, MRI, CEM, MBI or other screening modality (i.e. CT, PET/CT), at surgery); add to report for any lesion recommended for biopsy

Further Readings

1. Mahesh M. AAPM/RSNA physics tutorial for residents, digital mammography: an overview. Radiographics. 2004;24:1747–60.
2. ACR Quality Control Manual. https://www.acr.org/-/media/ACR/NOINDEX/QC-Manuals/Mammo_QCManual.pdf.

Patterns on Mammography

4

Anna Rives and Priscilla J. Slanetz

Mass

A three-dimensional lesion is seen on at least two mammographic views; space-occupying with convex-outward border; if seen only on one DBT, if margin is clear, can describe as a mass rather than asymmetry

Breast cancer most often presents as an irregular mass with spiculated or indistinct margin

BI-RADS characterizes masses by shape, margin, and density.

A. Rives · P. J. Slanetz (✉)
Division of Breast Imaging, Department of Radiology, Boston University Medical Center, Boston, MA, USA
e-mail: anna.rives@bmc.org; priscilla.slanetz@bmc.org

© The Author(s), under exclusive license to Springer Nature Switzerland AG 2025
P. J. Slanetz, V. Dialani (eds.), *What Radiology Residents Need to Know: Breast Imaging*, What Radiology Residents Need to Know,
https://doi.org/10.1007/978-3-031-66274-4_4

- **Shape** (Fig. 4.1)
  - ○ **Oval**—elliptical or egg-shaped, up to three undulations
  - ○ **Round**—spherical, ball-shaped
  - ○ **Lobulated**—undulating contour
  - ○ **Irregular**—not round or oval
  - ○ Irregular shape suspicious for malignancy; oval and round favors benign

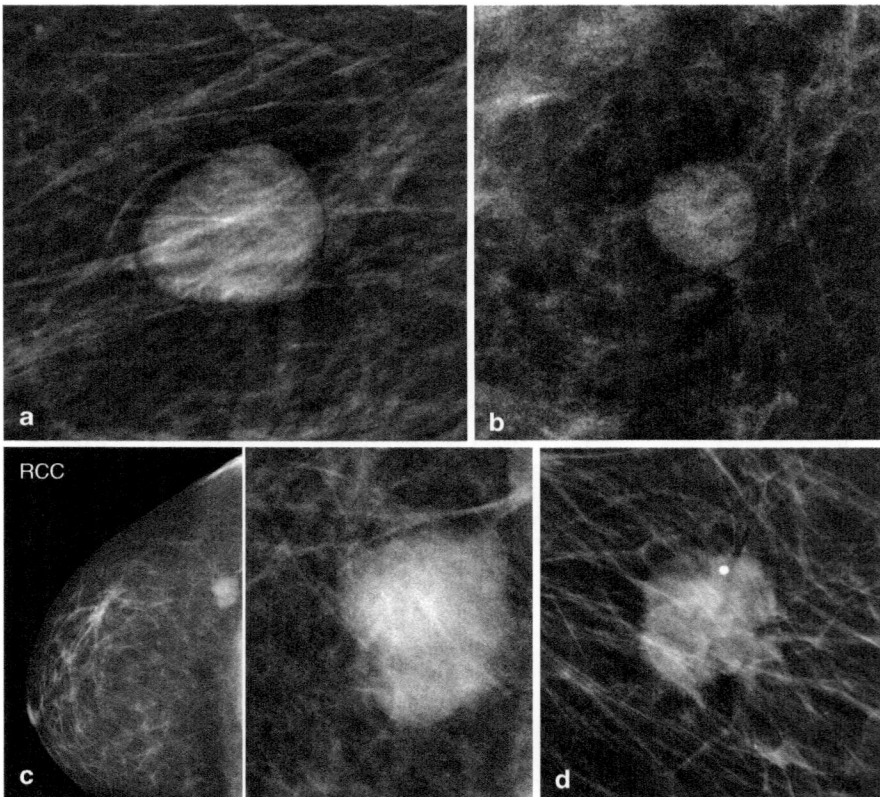

Fig. 4.1 **Mass shape**. BI-RADS descriptors for mass shape. (**a**) Oval (**b**) Round (**c**) Lobulated (**d**) Irregular

- **Margin** (Fig. 4.2)
  - The margin describes the border of the mass; readily assessed on magnified views or DBT
    - **Circumscribed**—well-defined border between mass and surrounding tissue
      - At least 75% must be well-defined to qualify (not obscured)
    - **Obscured**—hidden by superimposed tissue
      - Used when the visible margin is circumscribed, but > 25% is hidden
    - **Indistinct**—blends in with surrounding tissue
    - **Spiculated**—lines radiating from the mass
  - Indistinct and spiculated margins are suspicious for malignancy; circumscribed favors benign

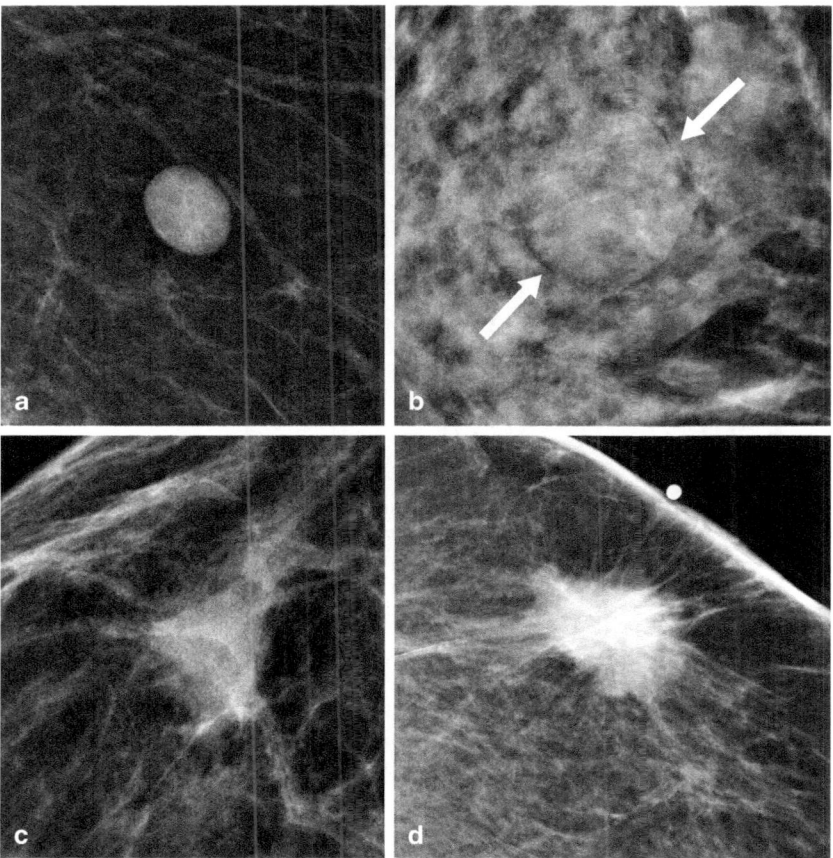

Fig. 4.2 **Mass margin**. BI-RADS descriptors for mass margin. (**a**) Circumscribed. (**b**) Obscured (arrows). (**c**) Indistinct. (**d**) Spiculated

- **Density** (Fig. 4.3)
  - Defined as X-ray attenuation relative to fibroglandular tissue; dense tissue in any region is considered dense; if asymmetric, the densest pattern prevails
    - Fat-containing—includes oil cyst, hamartoma, lipoma, lymph node, galactocele
    - Low density—x-ray attenuation less than glandular tissue
    - Equal density—x-ray attenuation similar to glandular tissue
    - High density—higher x-ray attenuation than glandular tissue
  - Cancers are more likely to be high or equal density; fat-containing almost always benign

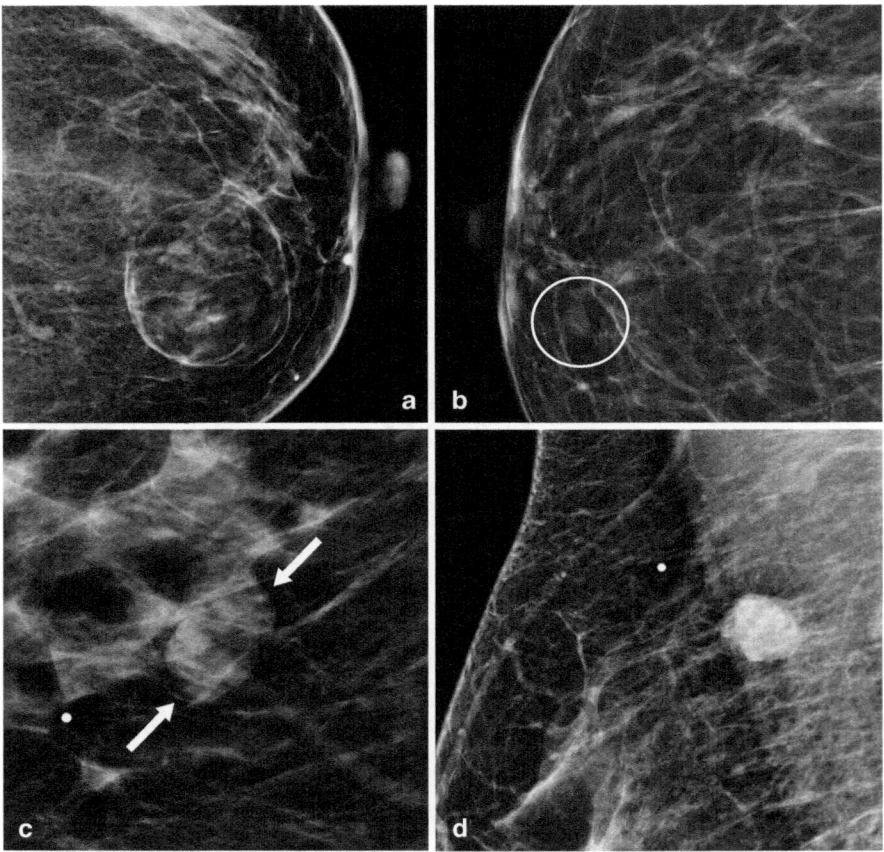

Fig. 4.3 **Mass density**. BI-RADS descriptors for mass density. (**a**) Fat-containing. This is a classic hamartoma. (**b**) Low density (circle). (**c**) Equal density (arrows). (**d**) High density

Calcifications

- Seen on up to 85% of mammograms with majority being benign; composed of calcium hydroxyapatite and calcium oxalate
- Microcalcifications (< 0.5 mm size) worrisome for malignancy
- Macrocalcifications (> 2 mm) almost certainly benign
- BI-RADS characterizes calcifications by morphology and distribution

- **Morphology**
  - ○ **Typically benign**—usually do not require any additional imaging (Fig. 4.4)
    - **Skin**—small, often lucent centered, often tight grouping of 3–5 calcifications
      - Most commonly seen along inframammary fold, parasternal region, or periareolar
      - Tangential view or tomosynthesis confirms dermal location or seen on first slice of DBT image
    - **Vascular**—tubular or linear calcifications (tram-track) associated with blood vessel
      - Related to medial sclerosis
      - Associated with diabetes, coronary artery disease, metabolic disorders
    - **Coarse**—large calcifications associated with involuting fibroadenoma or seen secondary to breast trauma, surgery, or irradiation (dystrophic)
    - **Large rod-like**—coarse smooth intact rods in intraductal or periductal location; associated with duct ectasia; often called secretory or plasma cell mastitis
      - Seen in women over 60
    - **Round**—often in lobular acini
      - Benign when diffuse
      - Isolated group on baseline safe to follow; new group or calcifications in linear or segmental distribution warrant biopsy
    - **Rim**—calcified rim with radiolucent center, usually fat necrosis or calcified cyst wall
    - **Layering**—sedimented calcifications within cysts, "smudgy" on CC view, curvilinear or "layering" on lateral view; previously called "milk of calcium"
    - **Suture**—calcified suture material, may look like "knots"
  - ○ **Suspicious**—usually necessitate biopsy (Fig. 4.5)
    - **Amorphous**—hazy microcalcifications with PPV of biopsy 20%; DDx fibrocystic change, sclerosing adenosis, DCIS
    - **Coarse heterogeneous**—coarse irregular calcifications with PPV of biopsy 15%; DDx calcified fibroadenoma, early dystrophic, DCIS
    - **Fine pleomorphic**—microcalcifications of variable shape and size with PPV of biopsy 29%
    - **Fine linear or fine-linear branching**—thin, linear, irregular microcalcifications often intraductal with PPV of biopsy 70%

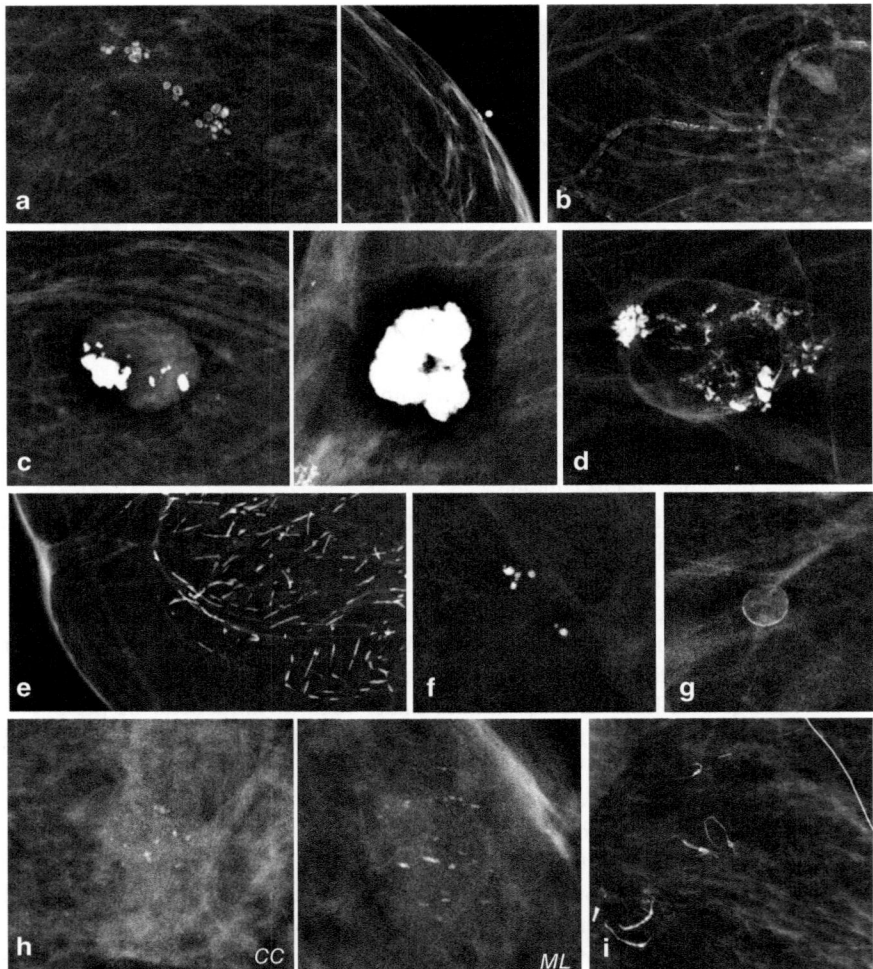

Fig. 4.4 Calcification morphology: typically benign. BI-RADS descriptors for typically benign calcifications. (**a**) Skin. Typical lucent-centered calcifications (left). Tangential view showing calcifications in the skin (right). (**b**) Vascular. (**c**) Coarse. These calcifications are associated with an involuting fibroadenoma. A circumscribed mass may be visible (left) or replaced by the calcifications (right). (**d**) Coarse Dystrophic. Large calcifications which form in response to trauma, surgery, or radiation, often associated with an area of fat necrosis. (**e**) Large rod-like. (**f**) Round. While these calcifications are typically benign, an isolated group on a baseline mammogram should be assessed as BI-RADS 3 and followed. A new group or round calcifications in a linear or segmental distribution should be biopsied. (**g**) Rim. Most commonly fat necrosis (oil cysts) or calcified cysts. (**h**) Layering. Sedimented calcifications within cysts appear "smudgy" on the CC view (left), and curvilinear or layering on the lateral view (right). (**i**) Suture. Often can see "knots"

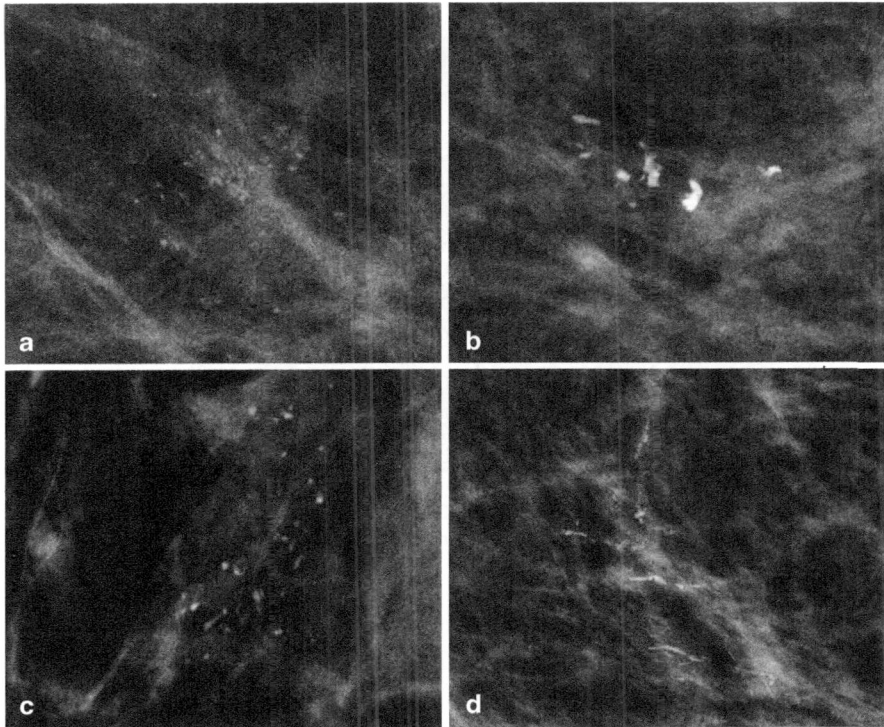

Fig. 4.5 Calcification morphology: suspicious. BI-RADS descriptors for suspicious calcifications. (**a**) Amorphous. (**b**) Coarse heterogeneous. (**c**) Fine pleomorphic. (**d**) Fine linear/fine-linear branching

- **Distribution** (Fig. 4.6)
  - **Diffuse**—distributed randomly in breast; almost always benign
  - **Regional**—occupying > 2 cm breast tissue but not in ductal distribution
  - **Grouped**—five or more calcifications within 1 cm^3
  - **Linear**—distributed in a line suggesting ductal origin; suspicious for malignancy
  - **Segmental**—triangular region concerning for involvement of ductal system; suspicious (approx. 60% malignant)

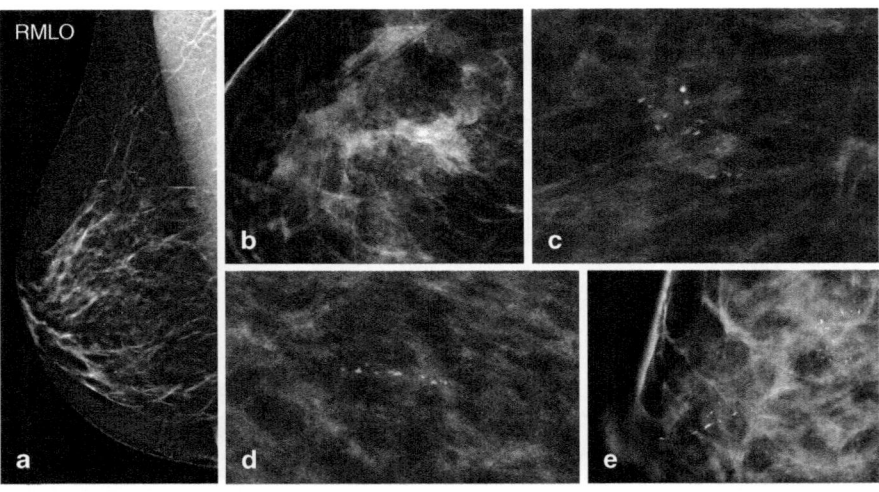

Fig. 4.6 Calcification distribution. BI-RADS descriptors for calcification distribution. (**a**) Diffuse. (**b**) Regional. (**c**) Grouped. (**d**) Linear. (**e**) Segmental

Asymmetries

Unilateral non-mass forming area of tissue unmatched in mirror image location of contralateral breast

Characterized by concave borders and interspersed fat

BI-RADS describes three types: asymmetry, focal asymmetry, global asymmetry

- **Asymmetry** (Fig. 4.7)
  - ○ Visible on only one mammographic view
  - ○ Most often superimposed breast tissue or asymmetric island of tissue

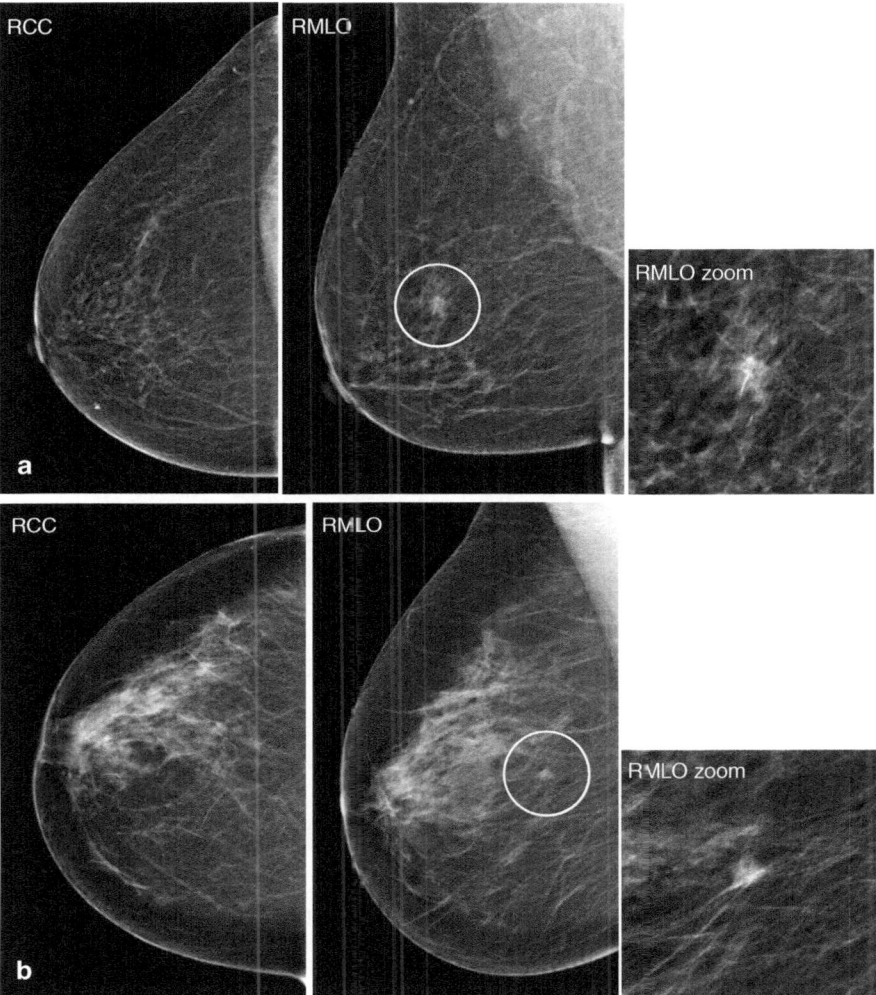

Fig. 4.7 Asymmetry. (**a**) Benign asymmetry. An asymmetry (circle) is present only on the MLO view of a screening mammogram. It did not persist at the time of diagnostic imaging consistent with superimposed fibroglandular tissue. (**b**) Malignant asymmetry. An asymmetry on the MLO view of a screening mammogram (circle) was confirmed to be a mass at diagnostic work-up. The mass is obscured by fibroglandular tissue on the CC view. Biopsy revealed invasive ductal carcinoma

- **Focal asymmetry** (Fig. 4.8)
  - ○ Visible on two orthogonal views with concave outward borders and interspersed fat occupying less than one quadrant
  - ○ May be a mass or two separate asymmetries at diagnostic work-up
  - ○ New or increasing focal asymmetry (formally referred to as developing asymmetry) warrants biopsy as often malignant (PPV 7.4-12.8% on screening and 19.7-26.7% on diagnostic evaluation)
- **Global asymmetry** (Fig. 4.9)
  - ○ Large focal asymmetry occupying at least one quadrant asymmetric to opposite breast
  - ○ Most often asymmetric breast tissue but suspicious if palpable
- **New or increasing asymmetry** (Fig. 4.10)
  - ○ New or increasing focal asymmetry (formerly referred to as developing asymmetry)

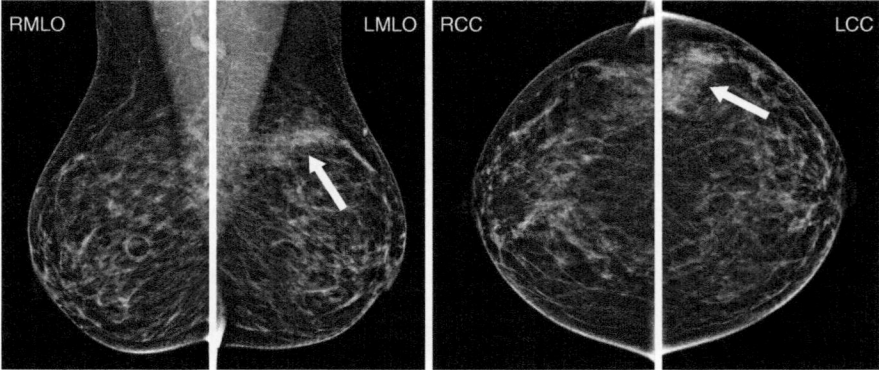

Fig. 4.8 Focal asymmetry. Focal asymmetry. Baseline screening mammogram shows a focal asymmetry in the upper outer left breast (arrows), assessed as BI-RADS 3 at the time of diagnostic imaging. Note the concave-outward borders and interspersed fat. The focal asymmetry remained stable during the surveillance period, presumed asymmetric fibroglandular tissue

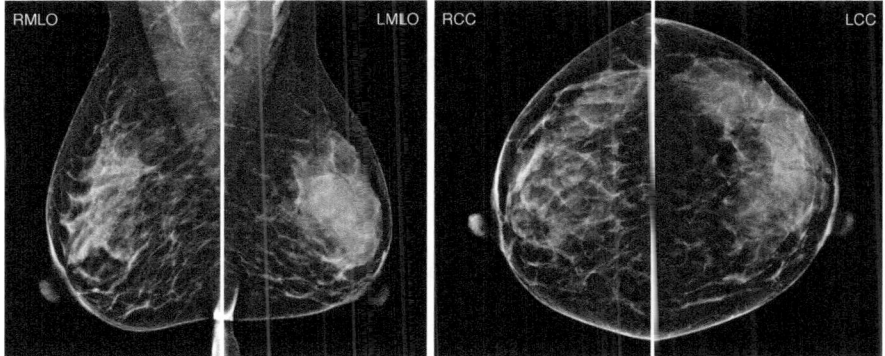

Fig. 4.9 Global asymmetry. A global asymmetry occupies much of the left upper outer quadrant on this baseline screening mammogram, assessed as BI-RADS 3 at the time of diagnostic imaging. It remained stable during the surveillance period, presumed asymmetric fibroglandular tissue

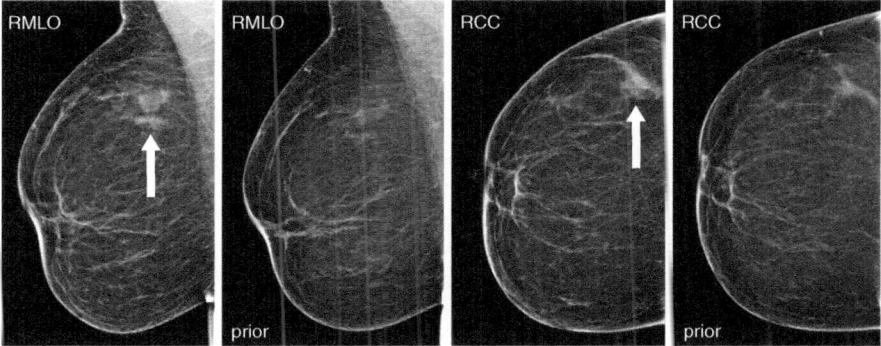

Fig. 4.10 New or Increasing asymmetry. The focal asymmetry (arrows) in the upper outer quadrant is larger compared to prior, making it a concerning finding. Biopsy revealed pseudoangiomatous stromal hyperplasia (PASH). Biopsy of a new or increasing focal asymmetry is indicated unless shown to be benign at diagnostic imaging

Architectural Distortion (Fig. 4.11)

Pulling-in or apparent tethering of tissue, often seen as straight lines radiating from central point with or without a mass

- DDx: prior surgery, radial scar/complex sclerosing lesion, fat necrosis, sclerosing adenosis, fibrosis, granular cell tumor, malignancy
- If no surgical history or history of prior trauma, biopsy indicated as 25% malignant; lack of sonographic correlate should not preclude biopsy

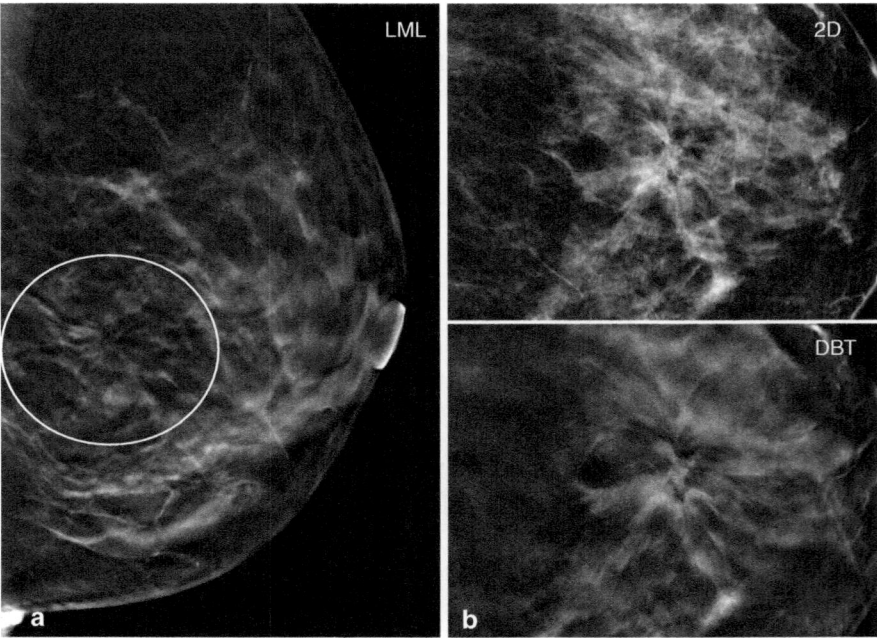

Fig. 4.11 Architectural distortion. Benign (**a**) and malignant (**b**) examples of architectural distortion. (**a**) Left ML tomosynthesis slice shows screen-detected architectural distortion (circle). In the absence of surgical history, biopsy is indicated. Tomosynthesis-guided biopsy showed radial scar. (**b**) Digital zoom images demonstrate the increased conspicuity of architectural distortion on DBT versus FFDM (2D) imaging. Biopsy showed invasive ductal carcinoma.

Miscellaneous Findings

- **Intramammary lymph node** (Fig. 4.12)
  - ○ Reniform circumscribed mass with central fat most commonly seen in upper outer quadrant; generally < 1cm in long axis; often adjacent to vessel; if > 1cm, considered abnormal and may warrant biopsy
- **Skin lesion** (Fig. 4.13)
  - ○ Circumscribed mass with radiolucent halo or air within crevices of mass
    - Technologist should mark lesion with radiopaque "mole" marker
    - Triangulates to skin on first few DBT slices

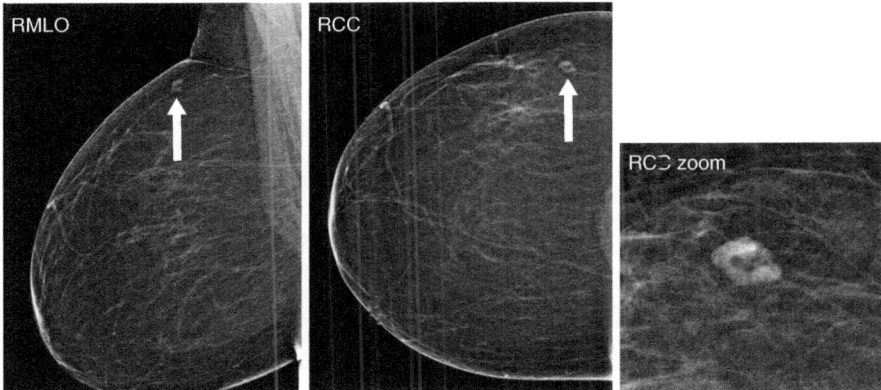

Fig. 4.12 Intramammary lymph node. Normal intramammary lymph node. MLO and CC views from a screening mammogram show a normal intramammary lymph node in the upper outer quadrant measuring under 1 cm (arrows) Note the circumscribed margin radiolucent fatty hilum and denser cortex on the zoomed image

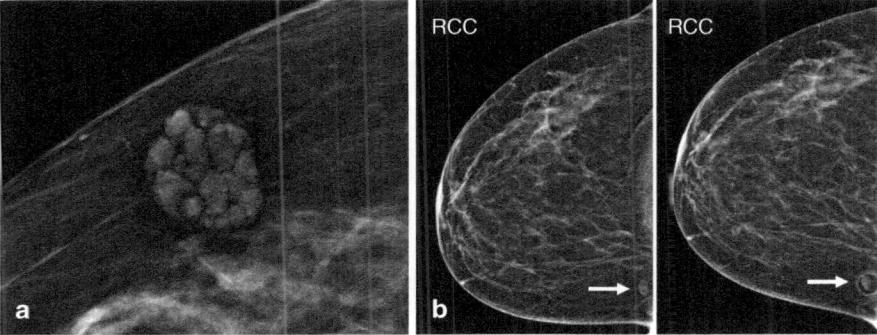

Fig. 4.13 Skin lesion. Skin lesions. (**a**) Typical appearance of a raised skin lesion (seborrheic keratosis) with radiolucent air trapped around and within the lesion. (**b**) A skin lesion in the medial breast (arrows) marked by the technologist with a radiopaque "mole marker".

- **Skin thickening** (Fig. 4.14)
  - ○ Up to 0.2 cm thickness considered normal; near areola, up to 0.4 cm may be normal
    - • If > 0.2 cm, differential includes mastitis, heart/renal failure, radiation therapy, malignancy (locally advanced or inflammatory breast cancer)
      - ▪ Unilateral thickening should be viewed with suspicion
- **Trabecular thickening** (Fig. 4.14)
  - ○ Thickening of fibrous stroma indicating edema, often occurring with skin thickening; seen with both benign (mastitis, heart failure, radiation) and malignant diseases
- **Nipple retraction** (Fig. 4.15)
  - ○ Pulling-in of nipple
    - • New nipple inversion worrisome for malignancy; look for associated subareolar mass

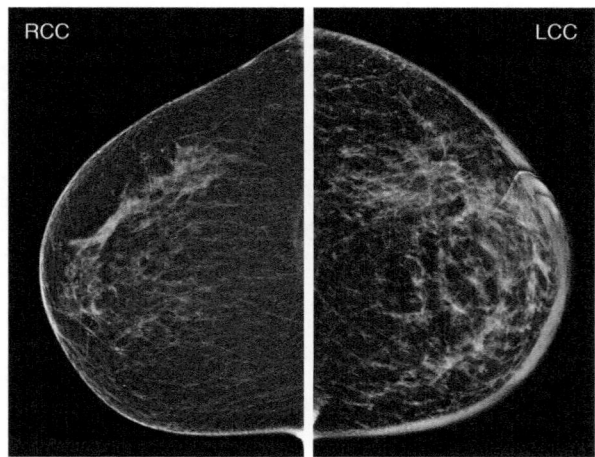

Fig. 4.14 Skin and trabecular thickening. Diffuse left breast skin and trabecular thickening of the left breast as compared to the right would be an expected finding following radiation therapy for breast cancer. In this clinical context, the findings are benign

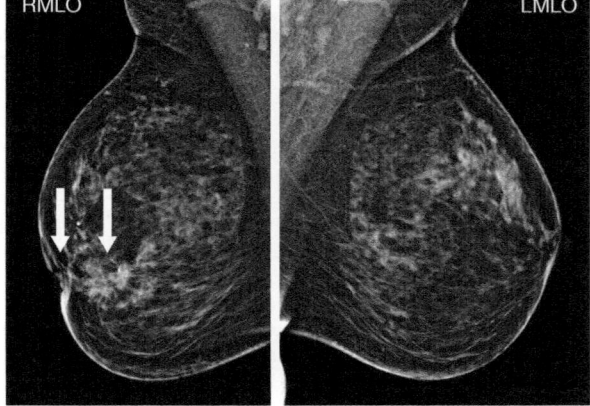

Fig. 4.15 Nipple retraction. The right nipple is retracted (front white arrow), and there is an adjacent irregular mass (back white arrow) with associated skin thickening and distortion. Biopsy showed invasive ductal carcinoma. New nipple retraction should raise suspicion for malignancy

Fig. 4.16 Axillary
lymphadenopathy.
Axillary lymphadenopathy.
Bilateral MLO views from
a screening mammogram
show unilateral left axillary
lymphadenopathy. Biopsy
revealed sarcoidosis

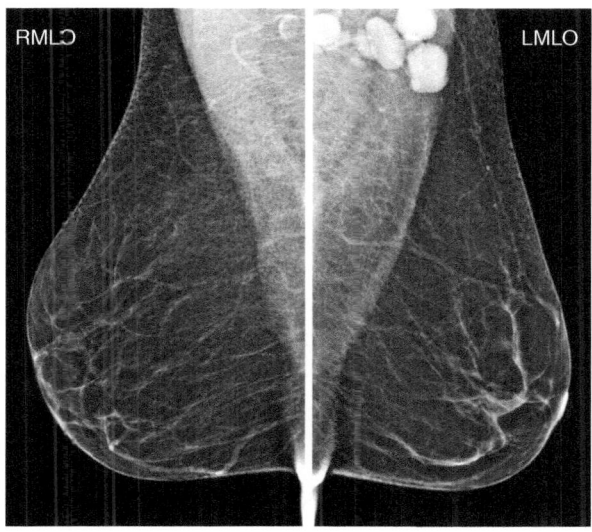

- **Axillary lymphadenopathy** (Fig. 4.16)
  - ○ Normal level 1 nodes up to 2.5 cm in size with fatty hilum; often seen on MLO view
  - ○ Unilateral or bilateral lymphadenopathy warrants correlation with clinical history; if abnormal, report location and approximate number
    - Unilateral DDx: reactive hyperplasia, recent vaccination (esp. COVID), metastatic cancer, infectious (e.g. Cat-scratch, HIV), inflammatory (e.g. silicone, sarcoid, rheumatoid), lymphoma/leukemia
    - Bilateral DDx: reactive hyperplasia, infectious (e.g. HIV, TB), inflammatory (e.g. silicone, rheumatoid, sarcoid, SLE), lymphoma/leukemia, metastatic disease
  - ○ Suspicious features include large size/enlarging, round shape, and high density
- **Dilated ducts**
  - ○ Retroareolar duct ectasia is common and benign (Fig. 9.25); often seen incidentally on screening mammogram
  - ○ Solitary dilated duct—warrants additional imaging, but if no suspicious findings on diagnostic imaging, consider benign; may be seen with intraductal papilloma (Fig. 9.28)
  - ○ Solitary dilated duct warrants diagnostic imaging; most often benign, but if suspicious features, biopsy indicated
  - ○ Segmental ductal dilatation—warrants additional imaging, as can indicate malignancy

Further Reading

1. BIRADS atlas. 5th ed. American College of Radiology; 2013. https://www.acr.org/Clinical-Resources/Reporting-and-Data-Systems/Bi-Rads.

Breast Ultrasound

5

Leah Schafer, Bernadette Jakomin, Vandana Dialani, and Priscilla J. Slanetz

INDICATIONS

- Targeted
  - Characterization of abnormality on mammography, MRI or other modality (CT, PET/CT), such as mass, asymmetry, or calcifications (Figs. 5.1, 5.2, and 5.3)
  - Evaluation of palpable finding or other clinical symptoms (focal pain, discharge, abscess) (Figs. 5.4, 5.5, and e5.1)
- Whole breast screening of high risk patients or those with dense breasts
  - Performed via hand-held or automated device; assess as BIRAD 0, 1 or 2; if normal, document single image from each quadrant and behind nipple; if finding, document two orthogonal images with and without calipers in three dimensions, distance from nipple, o'clock, and location (skin, subcutaneous, fibroglandular, retroglandular, chest wall, axilla)
  - Detects additional 2–4 additional cancers/1000 screened at cost of PPV of biopsy < 10%

Supplementary Information The online version contains supplementary material available at https://doi.org/10.1007/978-3-031-66274-4_5.

L. Schafer · B. Jakomin · P. J. Slanetz (✉)
Division of Breast Imaging, Department of Radiology, Boston University Medical Center, Boston, MA, USA
e-mail: Bernadette.jakomin@bmc.org; priscilla.slanetz@bmc.org

V. Dialani
Division of Breast Imaging, Department of Radiology, Beth Israel Deaconess Medical Center, Boston, MA, USA
e-mail: vdialani@bidmc.harvard.edu

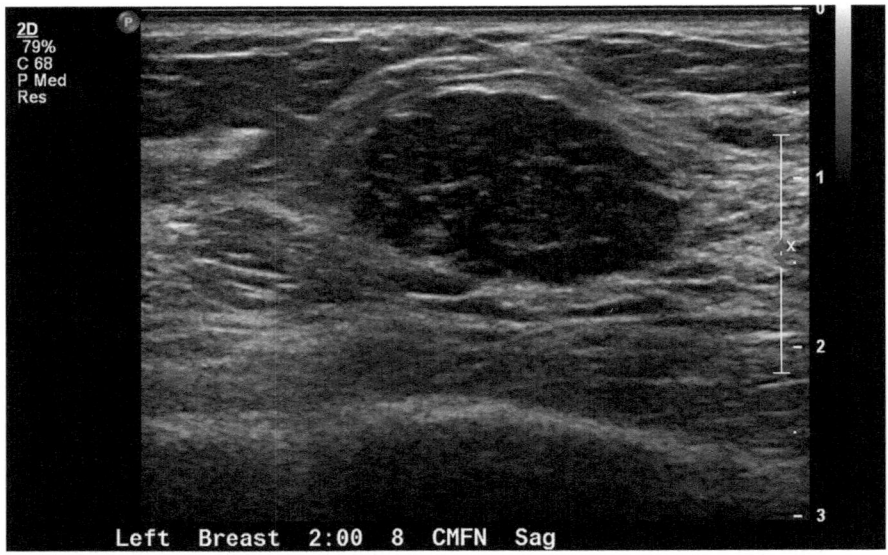

Fig. 5.1 Screening mammogram showed a well-circumscribed mass in the left breast (not shown). Ultrasound was performed for further evaluation. An oval hypoechoic mass with an echogenic pseudocapsule is consistent with a fibroadenoma (biopsy proven)

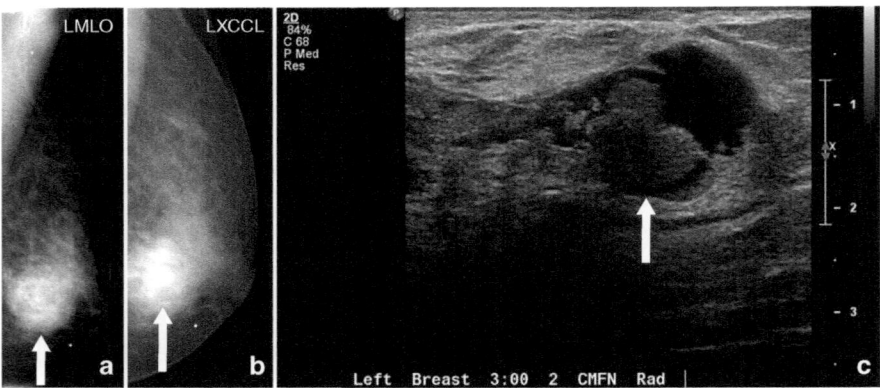

Fig. 5.2 (a) MLO and (b) XCCL views shows an ill-defined mass (arrow) underlying a palpable lump marked by a BB. (c) Ultrasound shows an irregular mixed solid and cystic mass (arrow), highly suspicious for malignancy. Biopsy showed invasive papillary cancer

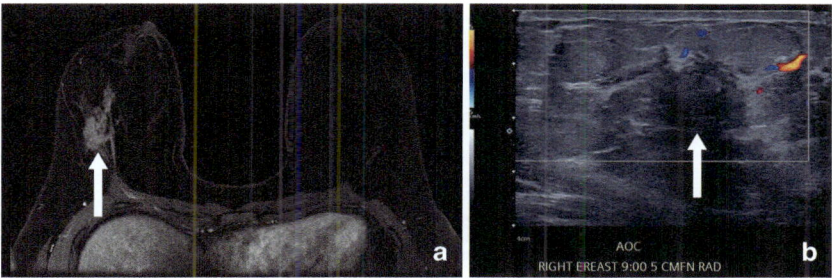

Fig. 5.3 (a) **Screening MRI shows an irregular enhancing mass (arrow).** (b) Targeted ultrasound was performed to identify the MRI-identified mass (arrow). Biopsy of the irregular hypoechoic mass with posterior acoustic shadowing and peripheral vascularity confirmed invasive ductal carcinoma

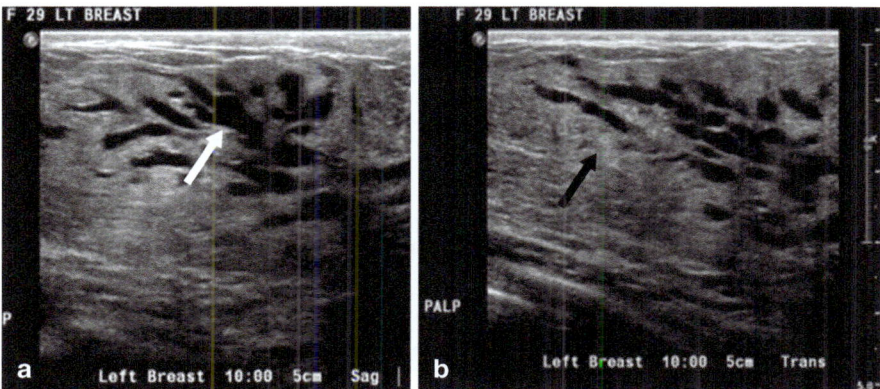

Fig. 5.4 **29-year-old lactating woman presents with a palpable mass.** (a, b) Note the prominent fluid-filled branching ducts (white arrow) and overall hyper echogenicity of the tissue (black arrow), typical of lactational state

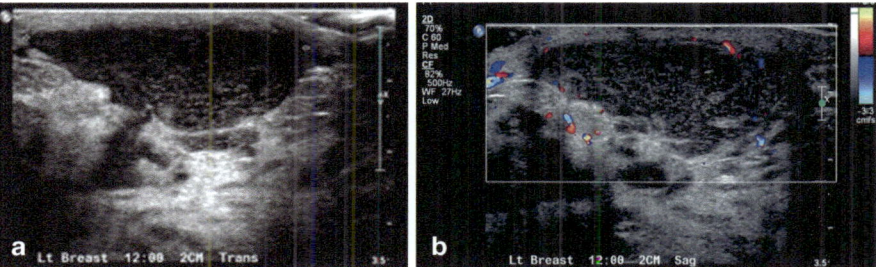

Fig. 5.5 **28-year-old lactating patient with 3-day history of focal breast tenderness and redness, fever, and chills and little response to antibiotics.** (a) Note the complicated hypoechoic mass which has (b) peripheral but no internal vascularity and overlying skin thickening. On realtime imaging, the debris could be seen moving. The collection was drained and sent to microbiology for Gram stain and culture. Culture grew *Staphylococcus aureus*

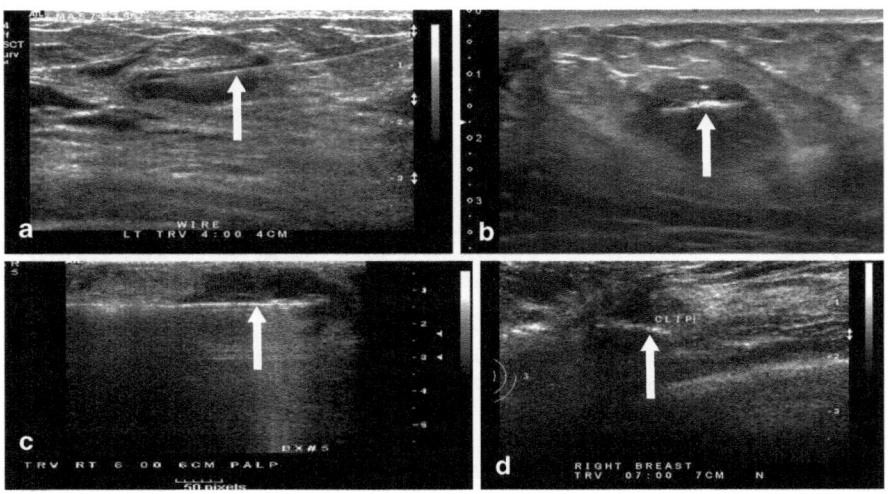

Fig. 5.6 **Ultrasound (US)-guided procedures**. (**a**) US-guided wire localization (arrow shows wire)), (**b**) US-guided Savi Scout placement (arrow shows reflector), (**c**) US-guided core biopsy (arrow shows needle), and (**d**) US-guided clip placement (arrow shows clip)

- Ultrasound guidance for procedures (Fig. 5.6)
  - Image-guided core biopsy, fine needle aspiration, and hook wire or seed/reflector localization

ADVANTAGES

- No radiation, lesion characterization (differentiates cystic from solid lesion) (Fig. 5.7), more comfortable than mammography
- Can be challenging in large or treated breast

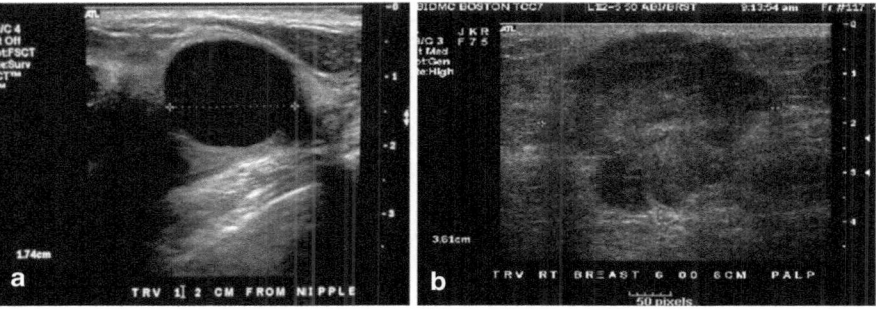

Fig. 5.7 (a) Cystic mass (anechoic with thin imperceptible wall and posterior acoustic enhancement) and (b) solid mass (hypoechoic irregular and lobulated mass with circumscribed margin)

PHYSICS

- Probe emits and detects sound wave
    - Variable reflection of beam based on tissue density and architecture creates image
    - Doppler detects directional flow in vasculature
- 12–18 MHz linear phased array probe
    - Higher frequency = greater spatial resolution but lower penetration

SCANNING TECHNIQUE

- Transducer parallel and beam perpendicular to breast surface
- Gel to eliminate air gap allowing beam to penetrate breast tissue
- Patient supine ± oblique with arm above head
- Focal zone centered between subcutaneous fat and pectoralis muscle; subcutaneous fat should be medium gray
- Stand-off pad or extra gel for improved visualization of superficial structures
- Rolled-nipple technique for improved visualization of subareolar tissue
- Document focal lesion (mass, non-mass finding) with and without calipers in two orthogonal planes (sagittal/transverse or radial/anti-radial); also document largest dimension
- Elastography—assess tissue stiffness using manual compression with probe or using shear wave generated by ultrasound probe
    - Presented as color map
    - Normal breast tissue less stiff than either benign or malignant mass
    - Increased stiffness in geographic area larger than on gray scale image = suspicious for malignancy

ANATOMY ON ULTRASOUND (Fig. 5.8)

- Skin—echogenic most superficial layer; up to 2 mm considered normal (up to 4 mm near areola)
- Subcutaneous and retromammary fat—isoechoic (medium shade of gray)
- Fibroglandular tissue/mammary layer—heterogeneous echogenicity depending on amount of glandular tissue
- Lactiferous ducts—anechoic tubular structures radiating out from nipple; < 3 mm retroareolar, < 2 mm peripheral
- Pectoralis muscle—posterior striated tissue layers
- Ribs/costochondral cartilage—peripherally echogenic with dense posterior acoustic shadowing
- Pleura—echogenic line deep to ribs moving with respiration

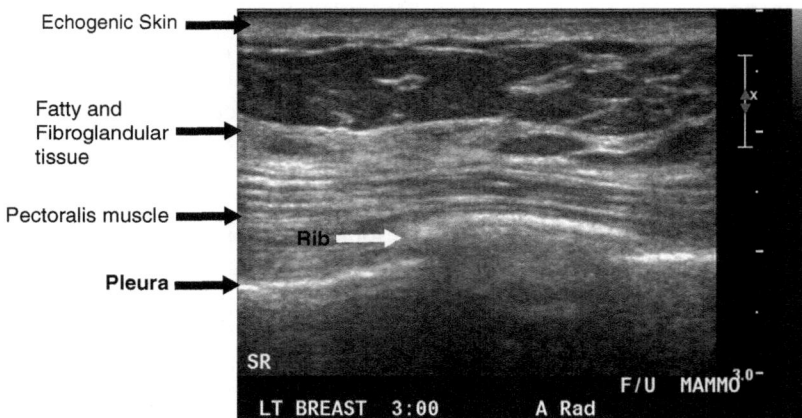

Fig. 5.8 Normal breast ultrasound

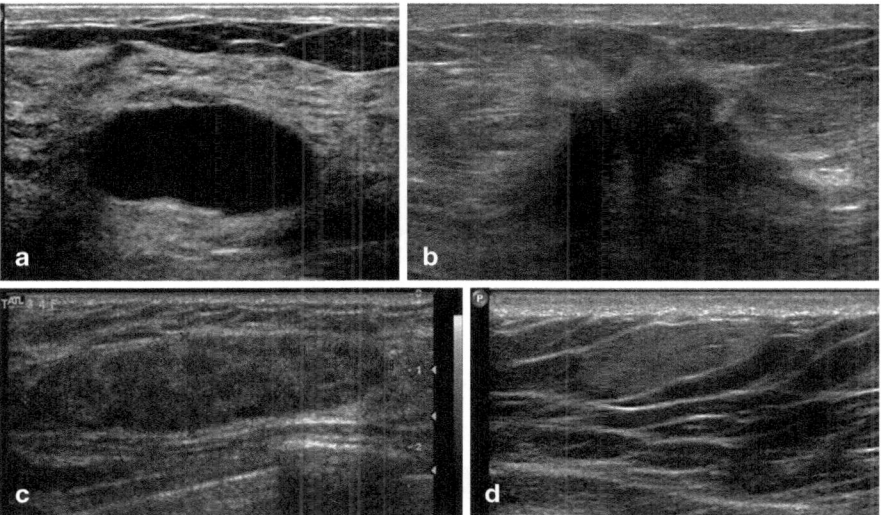

Fig. 5.9 Echogenicity of the mass relative to breast parenchyma: (a) anechoic, (b) hypoechoic, (c) isoechoic, and (d) hyperechoic

TERMINOLOGY (Fig. 5.9)

- Anechoic = entirely black with no internal echoes
- Hypoechoic = decreased echotexture relative to fat
- Isoechoic = equal echogenicity to fat
- Hyperechoic (echogenic) = increased echotexture relative to fat or equal to fibro-glandular tissue

ARTIFACTS

- Noise
- Reverberation artifact (Fig. 5.10a)
- Ring down vs comet tail (Fig. 5.10b)
    - Ultrasound beam reflects back and forth between two strong reflectors
- Posterior acoustic enhancement (Fig. 5.11a)
    - Increased whiteness posterior to imaged object
- Posterior acoustic shadowing (Fig. 5.11b)
    - Lack of sound penetration or "shadowing" posterior to imaged object

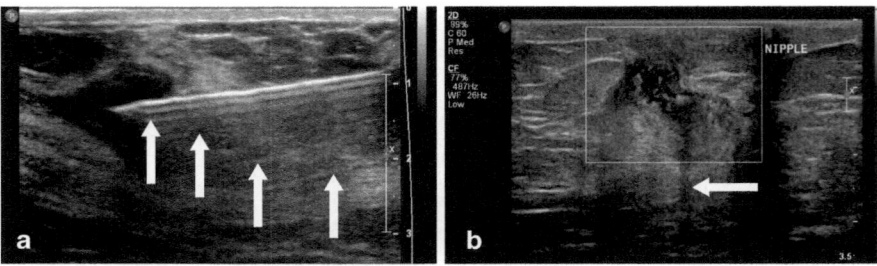

Fig. 5.10 Ultrasound artifacts: (a) reverberation artifact and (b) ring down/comet tail artifact

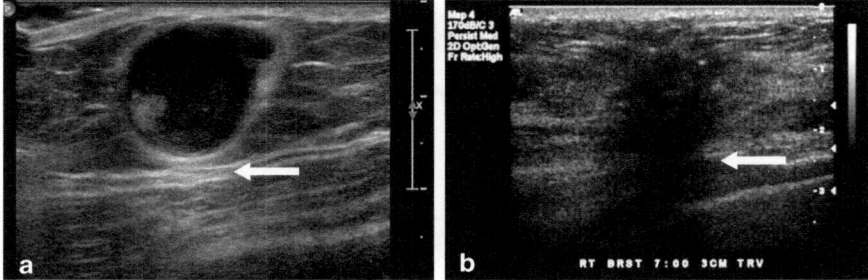

Fig. 5.11 (a) Posterior acoustic enhancement and (b) posterior acoustic shadowing

Further Readings

1. American College of Radiology Practice Parameter for the performance of a breast ultrasound examination. 2016. https://www.acr.org/-/media/ACR/Files/Practice-Parameters/US-Breast.pdf.
2. Baker JA, Soo MS, Rosen EL. Artifacts and pitfalls in sonographic imaging of the breast. Am J Roentgenol. 2001;176:1261–6.

Patterns on Ultrasound

6

Leah Schafer, Bernadette Jakomin, Vandana Dialani,
and Priscilla J. Slanetz

BIRADS ULTRASOUND LEXICON

- Tissue composition
  - ○ Tissue pattern - homogeneous background echotexture-fat; homogeneous background echotexture - fibroglandular; heterogeneous background echotexture
  - ○ Glandular tissue component (GTC) - amount of glandular tissue (hypoechoic) to fibrous stroma (hyperechoic); four categories - minimal (< 25%), mild (25-49%), moderate (50-74%), and marked (>75%)
    - High GTC (moderate or marked) carries increased risk for breast cancer
- Mass (space-occupying lesion in two or more imaging planes):
  - ○ Size
  - ○ Shape (oval, round, lobulated, irregular)
  - ○ Orientation (parallel vs. non-parallel)
  - ○ Margins (circumscribed, not circumscribed (indistinct, microlobulated, angularl, spiculated)

Supplementary Information The online version contains supplementary material available at https://doi.org/10.1007/978-3-031-66274-4_6.

L. Schafer · B. Jakomin · P. J. Slanetz (✉)
Division of Breast Imaging, Department of Radiology, Boston University Medical Center, Boston, MA, USA
e-mail: Bernadette.jakomin@bmc.org; priscilla.slanetz@bmc.org

V. Dialani
Division of Breast Imaging, Department of Radiology, Beth Israel Deaconess Medical Center, Boston, MA, USA
e-mail: vdialani@bidmc.harvard.edu

- Lesion boundary (abrupt interface, echogenic rind, echogenic pseudocapsule)
  ○ Echogenic rind—band of echogenic tissue of variable thickness surrounding all or part of mass of any shape; reflects desmoplastic reaction and/or peritumoral edema; associated with malignancy and fat necrosis (Fig. 6.1); when seen, include rind in measurement of mass size
  ○ Echogenic pseudocapsule—uniformly thin echogenic line surrounding an oval circumscribed mass, such as a fibroadenoma (Fig. 6.2)
- Echo pattern (anechoic, hyperechoic, heterogeneous, isoechoic, hypoechoic, mixed solid and cystic)
- Posterior features (none, enhancement, shadowing)
- Vascularity (avascular, internal, peripheral)
- Calcifications (within mass, outside mass, intraductal)
- Associated findings (skin thickening/retraction, duct changes, edema, architectural distortion, lymphadenopathy, echogenic rind, echogenic pseudocapsule)
- Elasticity assessment (soft, intermediate, hard)

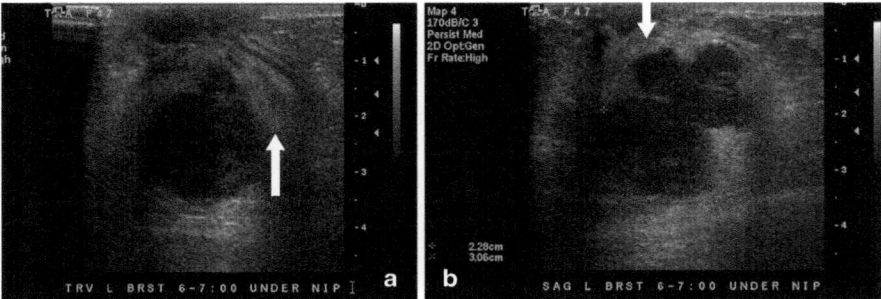

Fig. 6.1 75-year-old women with a palpable mass. Ultrasound (**a**) transverse and (**b**) sagittal images show an hypoechoic; antiparallel; mass with irregular margins, heterogeneous internal echotexture; echogenic rind (white arrows). This is highly suspicious for malignancy—biopsy showed triple negative invasive ductal cancer

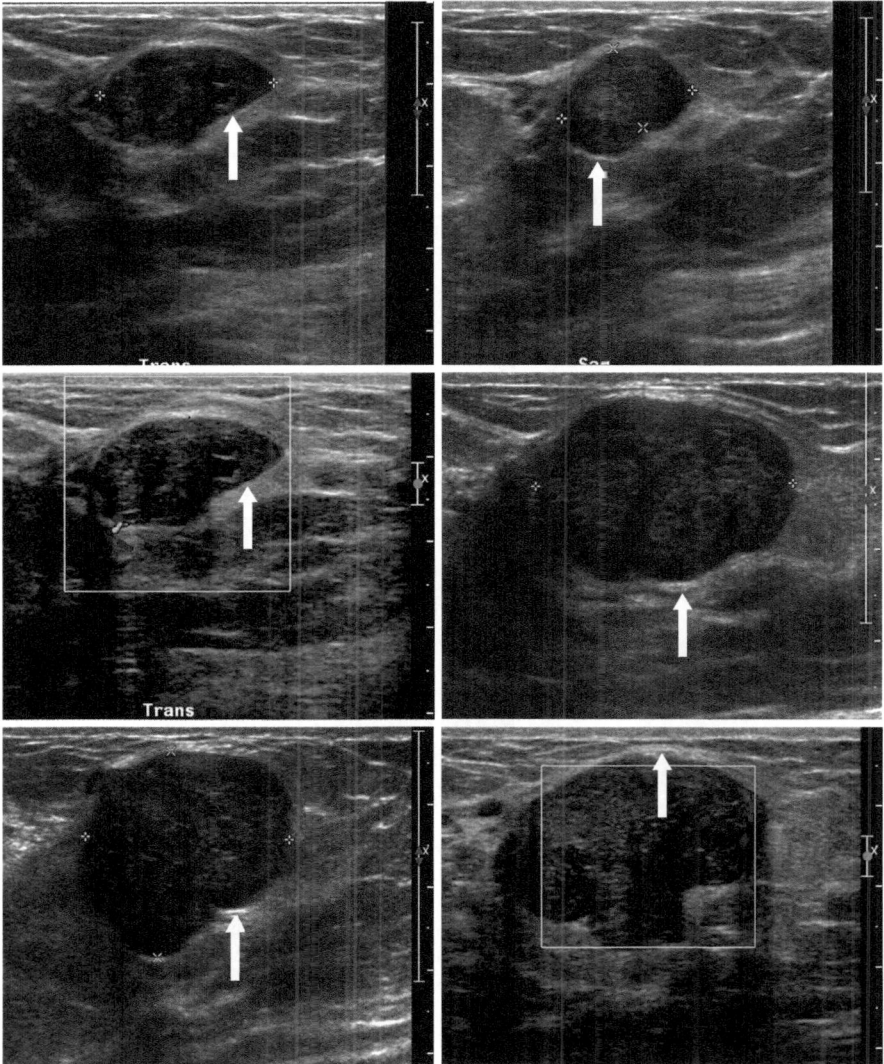

Fig. 6.2 Round to oval well-circumscribed hypoechoic masses with gentle bi- or tri-lobulations; homogeneous internal echotexture; parallel; posterior acoustic enhancement, and thin echogenic pseudocapsule (white arrows), suggestive of benign fibroadenomas

Non-mass finding (lesion)—sonographic finding that does not fulfill criteria of mass (Fig. 6.3); reproducible entity seen in two planes that correlates with finding on mammography, MRI or CEM; 10-54% chance of malignancy; invasive lobular carcinoma (ILC) and DCIS being more common than invasive ductal carcinoma (IDC)

- Size—may be difficult to measure
- Shape/Margin —No shape or margin descriptors
- Echogenicity—hypoechoic, isoechoic, hyperechoic, mixed
- Distribution—regional, focal, linear, segmental; segmental is most predictive feature of malignancy
- Orientation—parallel, not parallel
- Associated findings predictive of malignancy —echogenic rind, hypervascularity on Doppler, architectural distortion, posterior acoustic shadowing, duct extension, calcifications
- Associated clinical variable (nipple discharge, palpable)—increased probability of malignancy

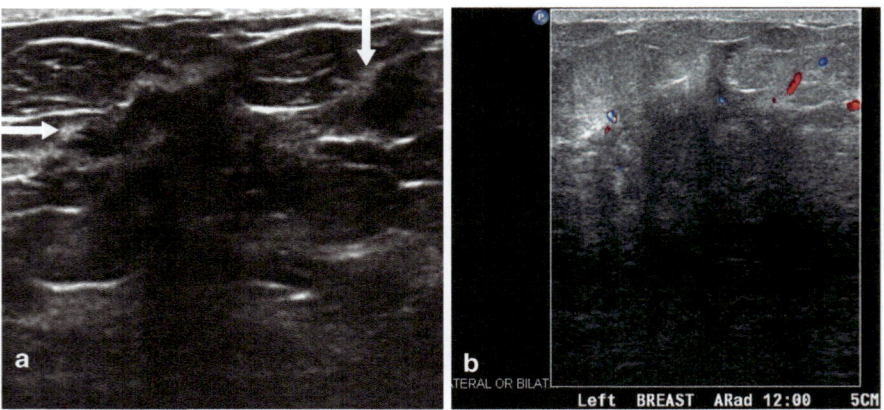

Fig. 6.3 48-year-old woman with left-sided bloody nipple discharge. (a) Transverse ultrasound image shows a non-mass hypoechoic, antiparallel lesion with posterior acoustic shadowing, ductal extension (arrows), and an echogenic rind and (b) increased peripheral vascularity on Doppler image. This lesion is highly suspicious for malignancy. Biopsy yielded invasive lobular carcinoma

Lymph nodes:

- Location—intramammary, axillary level I, II, III; internal mammary; supraclavicular
- Morphology
  - Normal—fatty hilum with smooth uniform cortex less than 3 mm (Fig. 6.4a); intramammary nodes may be up to 1 cm in size while axillary nodes may be up to 2–2.5 cm in size
  - Abnormal—cortical to hilar relationship; > 3 mm cortex, asymmetric cortical thickening, rounding, and absence of fatty hilum concerning for malignancy (Fig. 6.4b); echogenic foci may represent calcifications; may be enlarged but normal size with thickened cortex or loss of fatty hilum often warrant biopsy

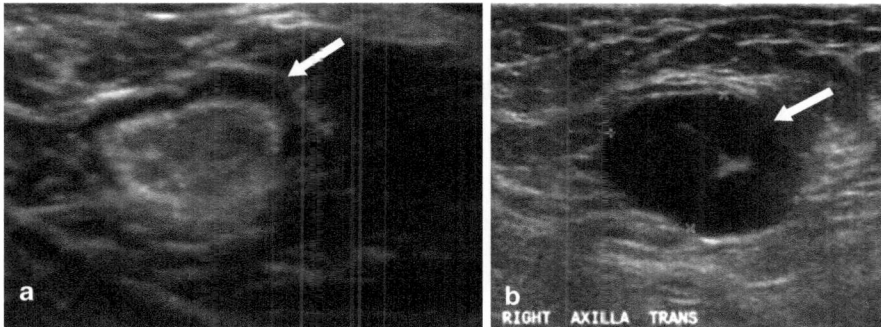

Fig. 6.4 **Lymph nodes.** (a) Normal—fatty hilum and cortical thickness of < 3 mm (arrow). (b) Abnormal—loss of fatty hilum and cortical thickness of > 3 mm (arrow)

BENIGN VS. MALIGNANT IMAGING FEATURES

- Likely benign—round or oval shape; circumscribed margins; gentle bi- or tri-lobulations; thin capsule; anechoic or intensely hyperechoic; homogeneous internal echotexture; parallel; posterior acoustic enhancement (Figs. 6.5, 6.6, and e6.1)
- Likely malignant—irregular, ill-defined or spiculated shape; microlobulated or angular margins; markedly hypoechoic; antiparallel; heterogeneous internal echotexture; posterior acoustic shadowing; calcifications; echogenic rind; ductal extension; internal hypervascularity (Figs. 6.7, 6.8, 6.9, e6.2, and e6.3)

  Any malignant feature should prompt biopsy!

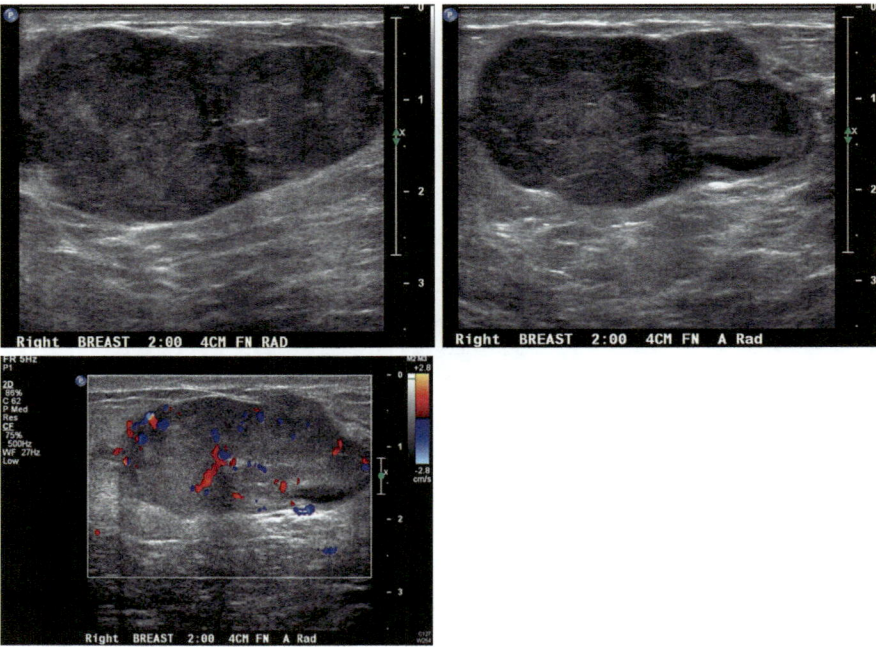

Fig. 6.5 22-year-old pregnant woman with a palpable lump in her right breast at 37 weeks. Note the circumscribed hypoechoic mass with gentle lobulations, posterior acoustic enhancement typical of a lactating adenoma

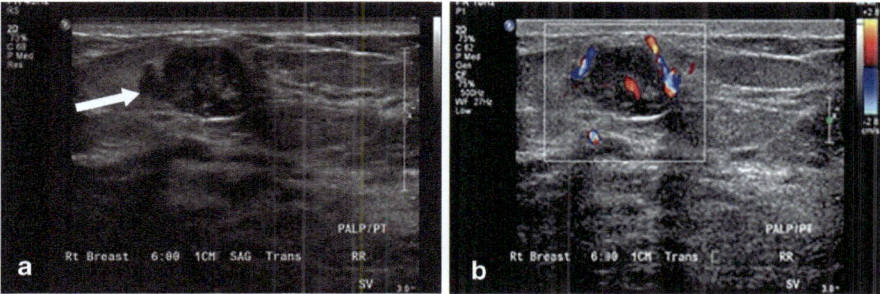

Fig 6.6 32-year-old patient with lump in the right breast. (a) Hypoechoic, well-defined lobulated mass with angular margins (arrow) and (b) increased central and peripheral vascularity on power Doppler. Biopsy revealed a fibroadenoma

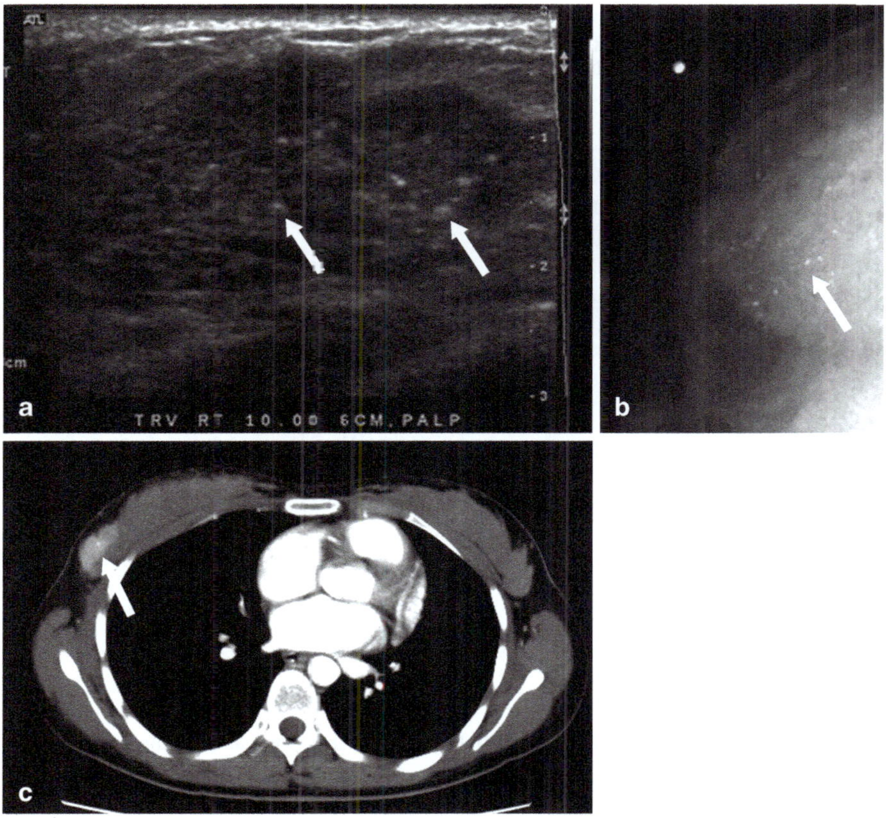

Fig. 6.7 25-year-old 38 weeks pregnant woman with a palpable lump in the right breast. (a) Initial ultrasound showed a loculated heterogeneous mass with punctate echogenic foci (arrows) suggesting calcifications. (b) Magnified CC view confirms suspicious micro-calcifications. Biopsy revealed grade 3 invasive ductal carcinoma. The patient delivered. (c) Staging CT shows the enhancing cancer in the outer right breast (arrow). Patient underwent surgery followed by radiation treatment and chemotherapy

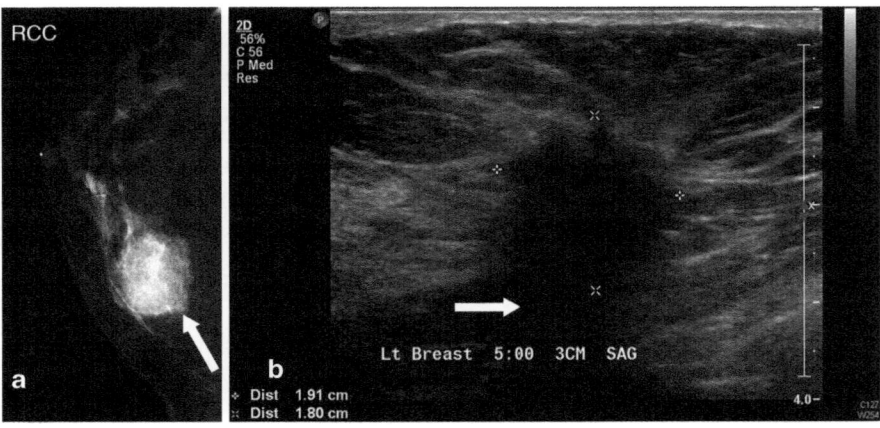

Fig. 6.8 68-year-old woman with a palpable lump in the right breast. (a) CC view shows a round ill-defined mass (arrow). (b) Ultrasound shows a hypoechoic, spiculated mass with posterior acoustic shadowing (arrow). This is highly suspicious for malignancy—biopsy showed invasive ductal cancer—Grade 2

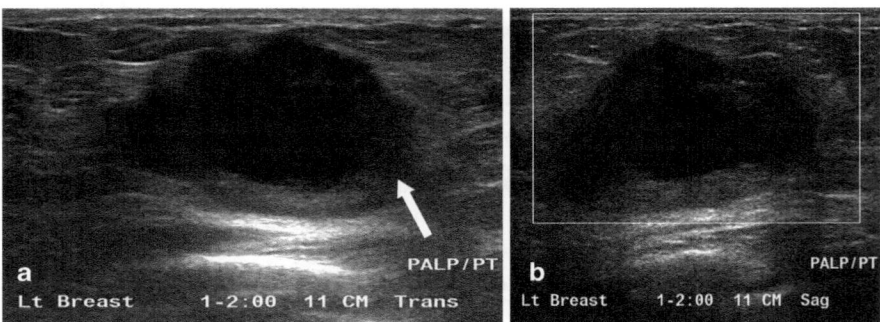

Fig. 6.9 38-year-old woman with a palpable lump. (a) Ultrasound showed an irregular mixed solid and cystic mass (arrows) with (b) no significant increased vascularity on power Doppler image. Biopsy showed grade 2 infiltrating ductal carcinoma. The patient underwent neoadjuvant chemotherapy

Further Readings

1. American College of Radiology BIRADS atlas. https://www.acr.org/Clinical-Resources/Reporting-and-Data-Systems/Bi-Rads.
2. Stavros AT, Thickman D, Rapp CL, Dennis MA, Parker SH, Sisney GA. Solid breast nodules: use of sonography to distinguish between benign and malignant lesions. Radiology. 1995;196:123–34.

Breast Magnetic Resonance Imaging (MRI)

Priscilla J. Slanetz, Patrick Tivnan,
and Vandana Dialani

INDICATIONS

- Assessment of silicone implant integrity (non-contrast)
- High-risk screening (Figs. 7.1, 7.2, 7.3, and 7.4)
- Determination of disease extent (Figs. 7.5, e7.1, and e7.2)
- Identification of breast primary with known positive axillary node (Fig. 7.6)
- Problem-solving (Fig. 7.7)
- Monitoring response to neoadjuvant chemotherapy (Figs. 7.8 and e7.3)
- Post-surgical margin assessment (Fig. 7.9)

Supplementary Information The online version contains supplementary material available at https://doi.org/10.1007/978-3-031-66274-4_7.

P. J. Slanetz (✉) · P. Tivnan
Division of Breast Imaging, Department of Radiology, Boston University Medical Center, Boston, MA, USA
e-mail: priscilla.slanetz@bmc.org

V. Dialani
Division of Breast Imaging, Department of Radiology, Beth Israel Deaconess Medical Center, Boston, MA, USA
e-mail: vdialani@bidmc.harvard.edu

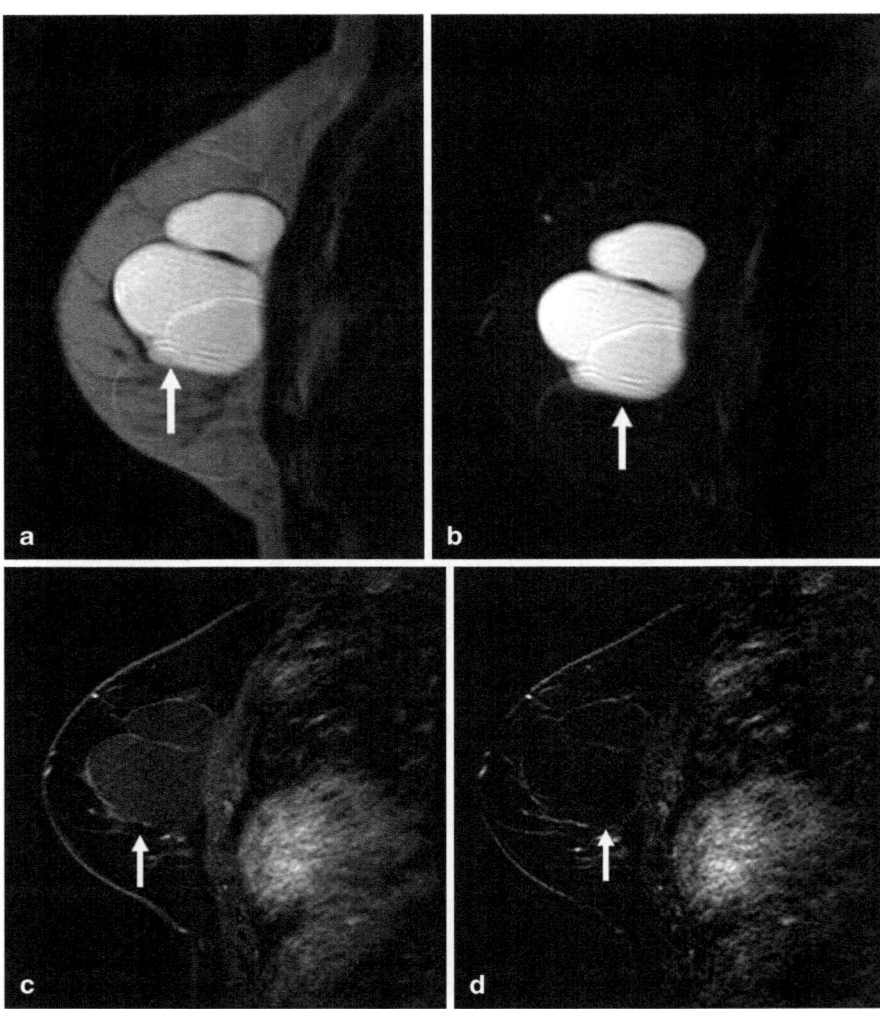

Fig. 7.1 High-risk screening—Benign cysts. (a) T2-weighted nonfat saturated, (b) fat-saturated, (c) postcontrast fat saturated T1, and (d) subtraction postcontrast sagittal images. Note the well-circumscribed T2 bright non-enhancing masses (arrow) consistent with cysts

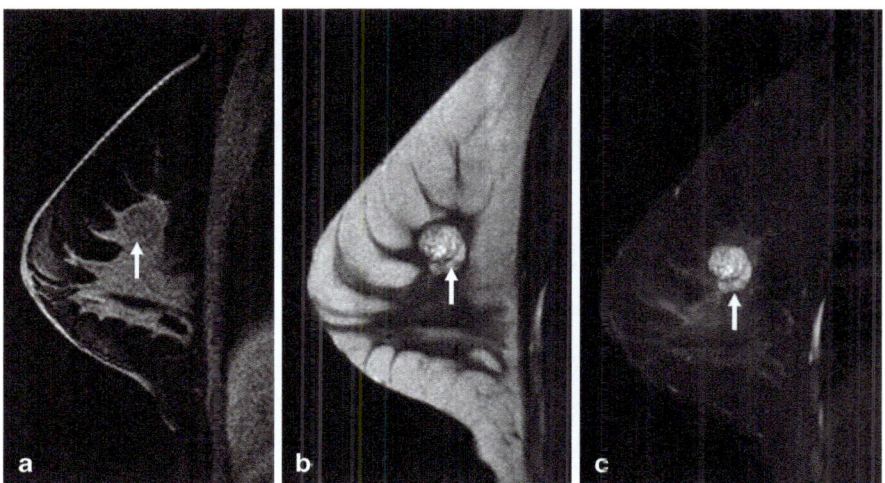

Fig. 7.2 High-risk screening—fibroadenoma. (**a**) T1-weighted, (**b**) T2-weighted, and (**c**) post-contrast fat saturated T1 sagittal images. Note the well-circumscribed T2 bright enhancing mass with typical non-enhancing internal septations (arrow) typical of a fibroadenoma

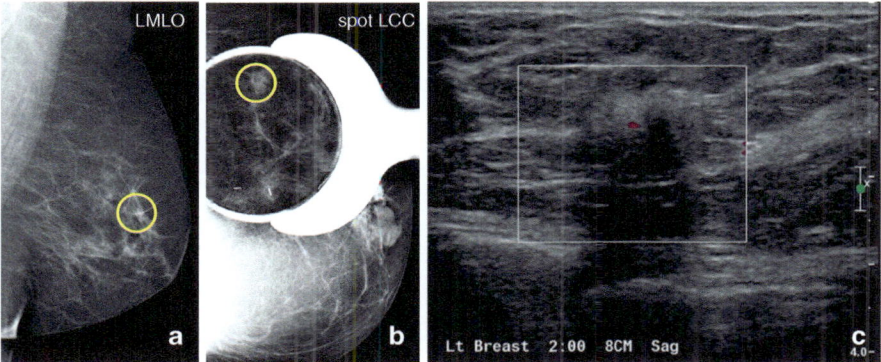

Fig. 7.3 High-risk screening. (**a**) MLO view shows a subtle spiculated mass (circle). (**b**) Additional imaging with spot CC view shows an irregular mass (circle), and (**c**) ultrasound shows an irregular hypoechoic mass with echogenic rind, central vascularity and posterior shadowing, highly suspicious for cancer. Biopsy showed invasive ductal cancer—grade 1

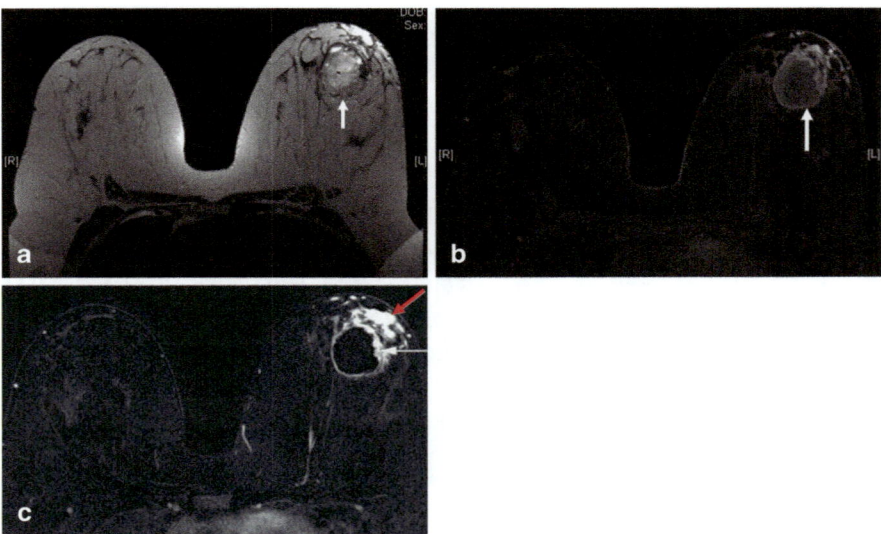

Fig. 7.4 High-risk screening—cancer. (**a**) T2-weighted nonfat-saturated, (**b**) T1-weighted pre-contrast, and (**c**) postcontrast fat-saturated T1 axial images. Note the T2 bright heterogeneous enhancing mass with irregular rim of enhancement (arrow), typical of necrotic cancer and adjacent non-mass enhancement (red arrow-additional close finding, extent less than 2 cm in total)

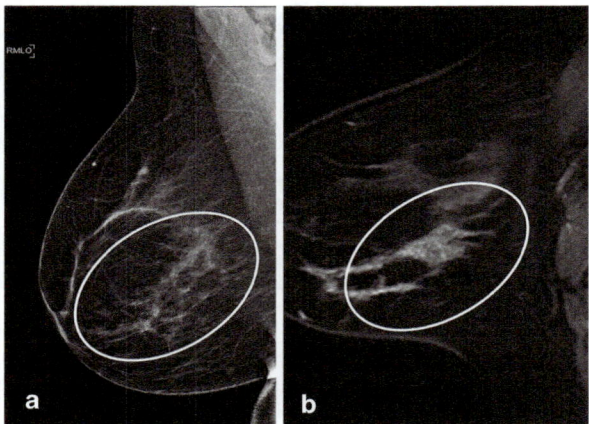

Fig. 7.5 Extent of disease— (**a**) MLO view shows extensive pleomorphic calcifications (circle), extending from nipple to chest wall. Biopsy showed DCIS. (**b**) Sagittal postcontrast fat-saturated T1-weighted MRI shows enhancement corresponding to the calcifications on mammography. No other suspicious enhancement is seen in either breast other than that corresponding to the segmental calcifications

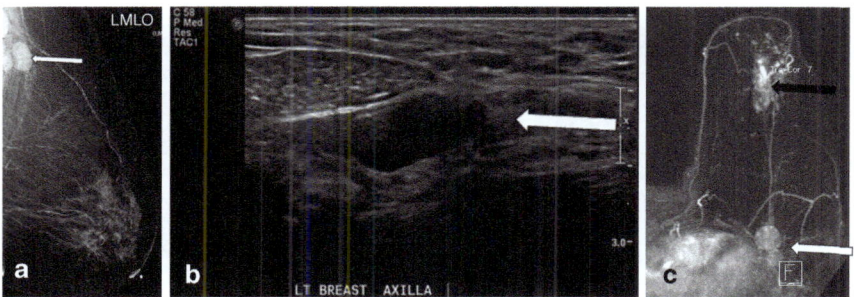

Fig. 7.6   **68-year-old woman with a palpable left axillary mass (arrow).** (a)Left MLO mammogram shows left axillary mass (white arrow) with no definite breast mass. (**b**) Ultrasound shows a hypoechoic lymph node with replacement of the fatty hilum. No primary breast malignancy was seen on whole breast US. (**c**) Axial T1-weighted postcontrast MR image of the left breast and axilla shows clumped non-mass enhancement (black arrow) and a rounded axillary lymph node (white arrow). Biopsy confirmed invasive ductal carcinoma with metastasis to the ipsilateral axillary lymph node

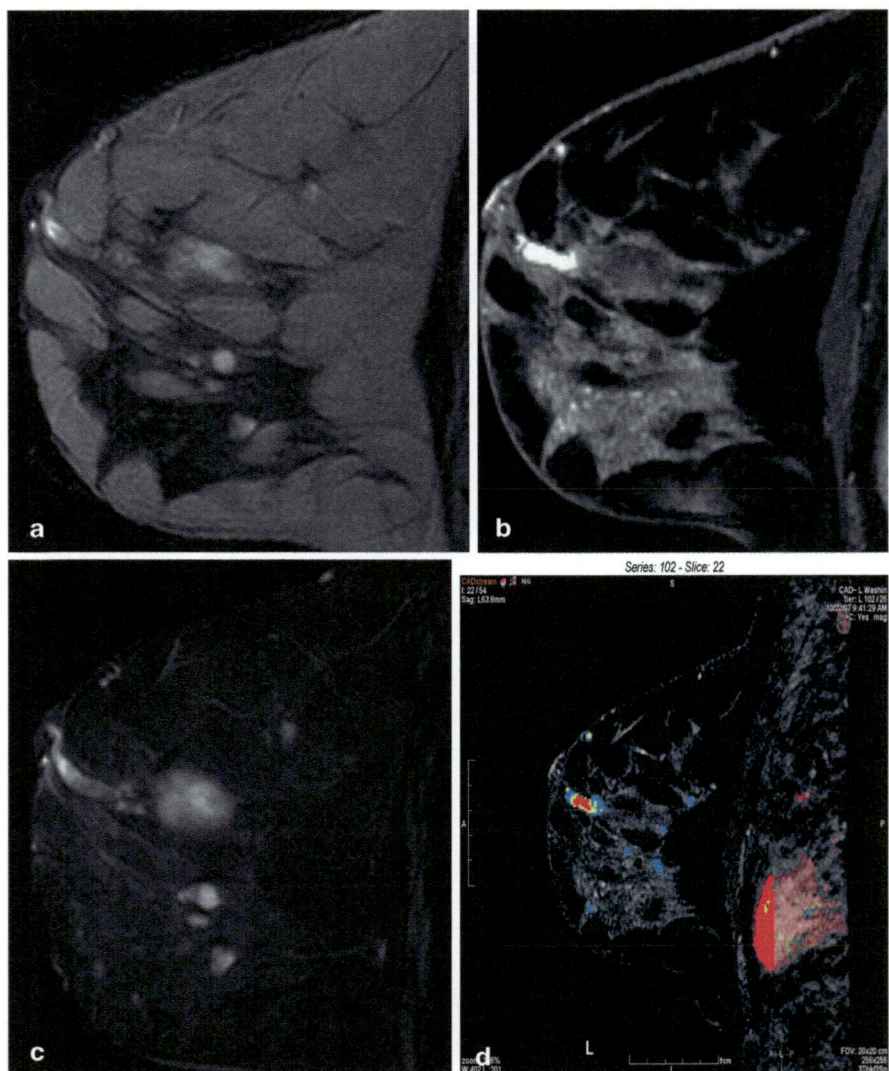

Fig. 7.7 **Problem solving-62-year-old with nipple discharge-negative mammogram and ultrasound**. (**a**) Sagittal nonfat-saturated T2-weighted image shows fluid within the duct and a filling defect which shows enhancement on the (**b**) T1 fat-saturated sagittal image, (**c**) subtraction image and (**d**) washout kinetics on the kinetic map. Biopsy revealed an intraductal papilloma without atypia

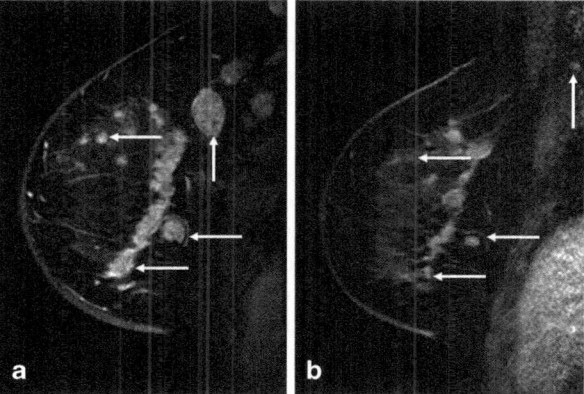

Fig. 7.8 Neoadjuvant—partial response—49-year-old female patient presented with inverted right nipple, bloody nipple discharge, and increasing right breast firmness over 1.5 years with a diagnosis of Grade 3 invasive ductal carcinoma (ER/PR positive, Her2 negative). Partial response is appreciated on the post treatment MRI after 10 weeks of neoadjuvant chemotherapy (**b**) compared to the pretreatment MRI (**a**) with decrease in tumor load and reduction in size of the involved lymph nodes (arrows). Patient subsequently was diagnosed with distant metastatic disease to liver, spine, and brain

Fig. 7.9 Surgical margin assessment—72-year-old woman with invasive ductal cancer status post breast conservation with posterior and lateral positive margins. Sagittal T2-weighted nonfat-saturated image shows a surgical seroma (black arrow) and hypodense enhancing non-mass enhancement and enhancing masses posterior and lateral to the seroma cavity consistent with residual disease (white arrows)

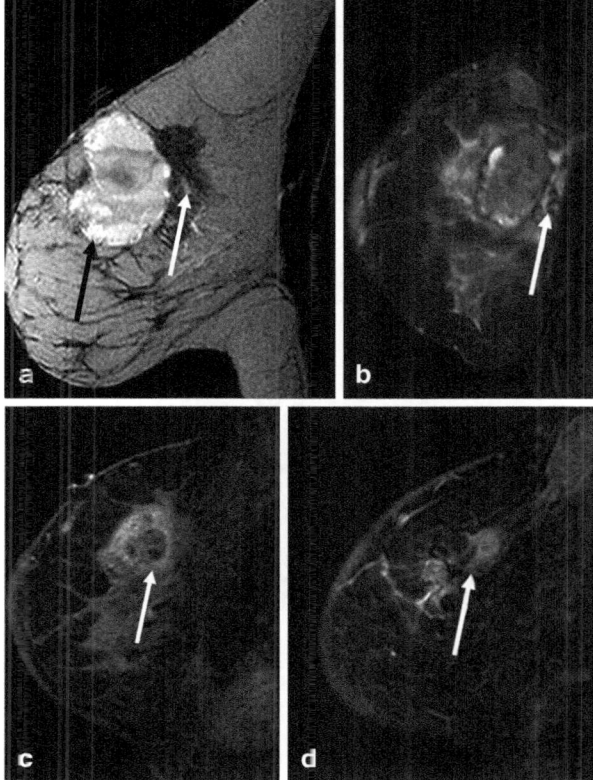

LOGISTICS

Performed on 1.5–3 T magnet using dedicated breast coil and intravenous contrast (except when evaluating silicone implant integrity) (Fig. 7.10)

- Logistics[1]—Breasts pendant and centered in dedicated breast coil to maximize spatial resolution. Sequences- Full protocol includes ocalizer, axial T1-weighted non-fat saturated, axial T2-weighted with or without fat saturation, dynamic 3D fat-suppressed axial or sagittal T1-weighted gradient-echo (at least 2 post), ± diffusion-weighted imaging (DWI)
    - ○ Administer IV gadolinium 0.1 mmol/kg at 3 cc/s; first postcontrast at 60–120 seconds (90 sec peak)
    - ○ Image day 5–15 of menstrual cycle in premenopausal patients to minimize hormonal effect on gadolinium uptake in breast tissue for screening, if possible; imaging not delayed for diagnostic cases due to menstrual cycle

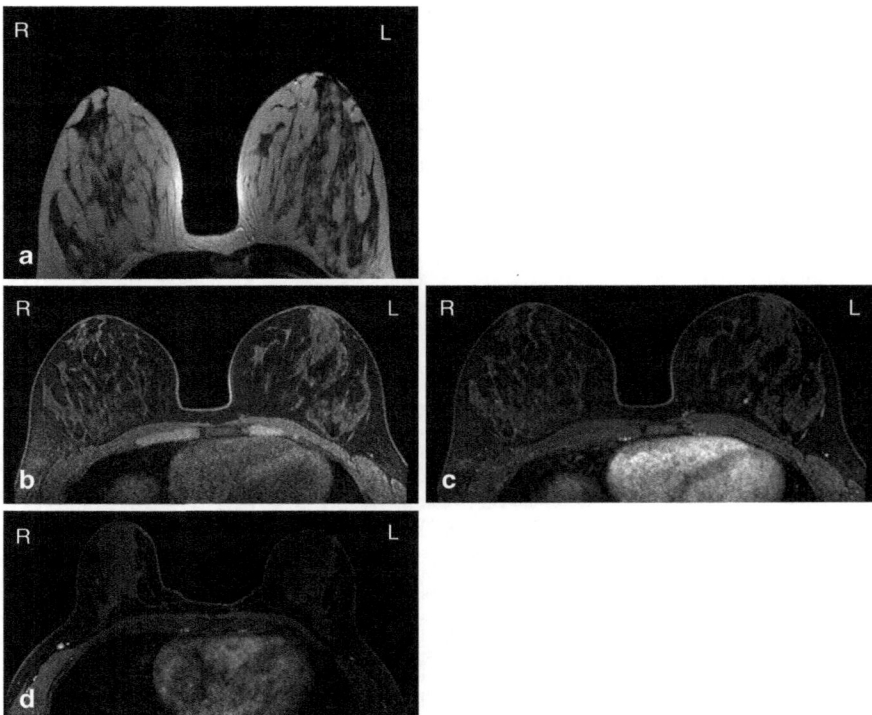

Fig. 7.10 (**A**) **Axial T1-weighted: (a) nonfat-suppressed, (b) fat-suppressed precontrast image, and (c) postcontrast-enhanced images from breast MRI performed on a 1.5 T magnet.** (**B**) (**d**)Axial contrast-enhanced T1-weighted fat-suppressed image from breast MRI performed on a 3 T magnet

- Post-processing—sagittal reformat, subtraction of pre- and postcontrast sequences, maximum intensity projection (MIP), kinetic map
- Clinical history—obtain clinical indication, risk factors, prior surgery, prior radiation or chemotherapy, and current use of chemoprevention (e.g., tamoxifen/aromatase inhibitors decrease background uptake)
- Interpretation combines lesion morphology and enhancement kinetics to determine management
  - Correlate with prior and recent breast imaging
  - Amount of fibroglandular tissue—almost entirely fatty, scattered fibroglandular tissue, heterogeneous fibroglandular tissue, extreme fibroglandular tissue
  - Background parenchymal enhancement—minimal (<25%), mild (26–50%), moderate (51–75%), marked (≥76%) (Fig. 7.11); symmetric vs. asymmetric
  - Morphology
    - Small mass—< 0.5 cm size mass or focal non-mass enhancement not felt to be background
    - Mass—space occupying with defined shape and convex outward contour
      - Size
      - Shape (oval, lobulated, round, irregular)
      - Margins (circumscribed, non-circumscribed- indistinct or spiculated)
      - Enhancement pattern (homogeneous, dark internal septations, heterogeneous, thick rim enhancement)
      - T2 features—hyperintense, not hyperintense (isointense or hypointense, as compared to normal lymph node)

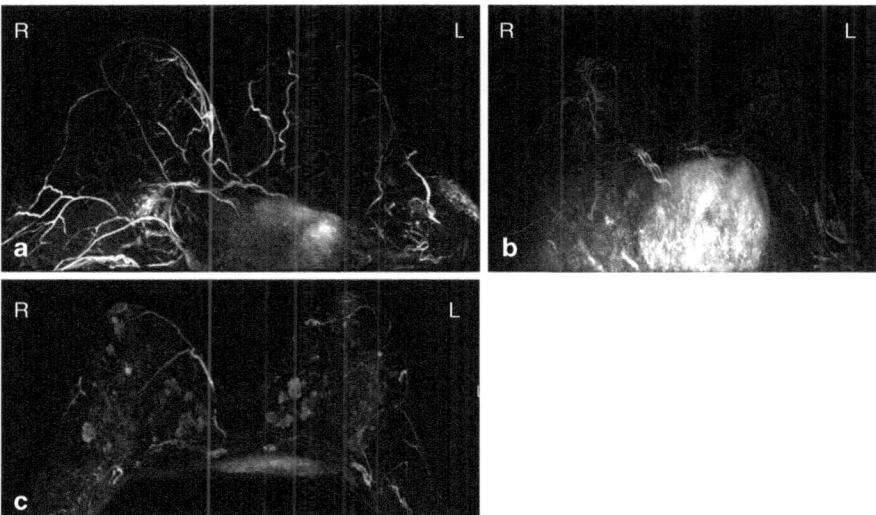

Fig. 7.11 Maximum intensity projection images from breast MRI. (**a**) Mild background parenchymal enhancement. (**b**) Asymmetric moderate background parenchymal enhancement. (**c**) Marked background parenchymal enhancement

- Irregular shape, non-circumscribed margins, heterogeneous internal enhancement, lack of T2 hyperintensity worrisome for malignancy; warrants biopsy
  - Oval or lobulated, circumscribed, homogeneous internal enhancement, dark internal septations, T2 hyperintensity, not new or increasing favors benign; follow-up imaging reasonable
- Non-mass enhancement—area of enhancement distinct from background without features of a mass; describe distribution (focal, linear, segmental (triangular enhancement with apex pointing toward nipple), regional (more than one quadrant but not following segmental or linear distribution), diffuse (2 or more quadrants)) and internal enhancement pattern (homogeneous, heterogeneous, clumped, clustered ring))
  - For NME, as only seen 30% on US, MR guided biopsy best management; For masses, up to 82% are reliably seen by US so can try US or manage with MR biopsy
  - Additional close findings (ACF)—≤ 2 cm away from known malignancy with total extent under 2 cm and no change in management; describe along with relationship to known malignancy (Fig. 7.4)
  - Additional ipsilateral findings—> 2 cm from known malignancy and/or increase total extent to > 2 cm; leads to management change (Fig. e7.1)
  - Kinetics—early phase and delayed phase (persistent/progressive (6–17% malignant), plateau (30–50% malignant), washout (57–80% malignant)) (Fig. 7.12)
- Diffusion-weighted imaging (DWI)—measures disruption of water movement across cell membrane; restricted diffusion in cancers (low signal on ADC map) (Fig. 7.13)
- Assess lymph nodes - no criteria for size or cortical thickness on MRI but suspicious features include increase in size, non-circumscribed margin, or absence of fatty hilum; asymmetric from contralateral side; describe location and approximate number
- Assess for other findings such as signal voids, high T1 signal within ducts, pectoralis and chest wall involvement (i.e. loss of fat plane, extension into muscle or chest wall with enhancement), nipple retraction, skin involvement, peritumoral edema (increased T2 signal around tumor)
- Look for incidental non-breast findings—sternum, internal mammary nodal chain, lung, mediastinum, chest wall, spine, and abdomen (Fig. e7.4); occur in 16–34% cases, of which 20% malignant

Abbreviated protocol—5–8 min imaging; localizer, single precontrast and postcontrast T1-weighted fat-saturated acquisition ± T2-weighted sequence; similar cancer detection to full protocol in retrospective studies

Ultrafast imaging—acquire dynamic data every 5 seconds for 30–60 seconds after administration of intravenous gadolinium

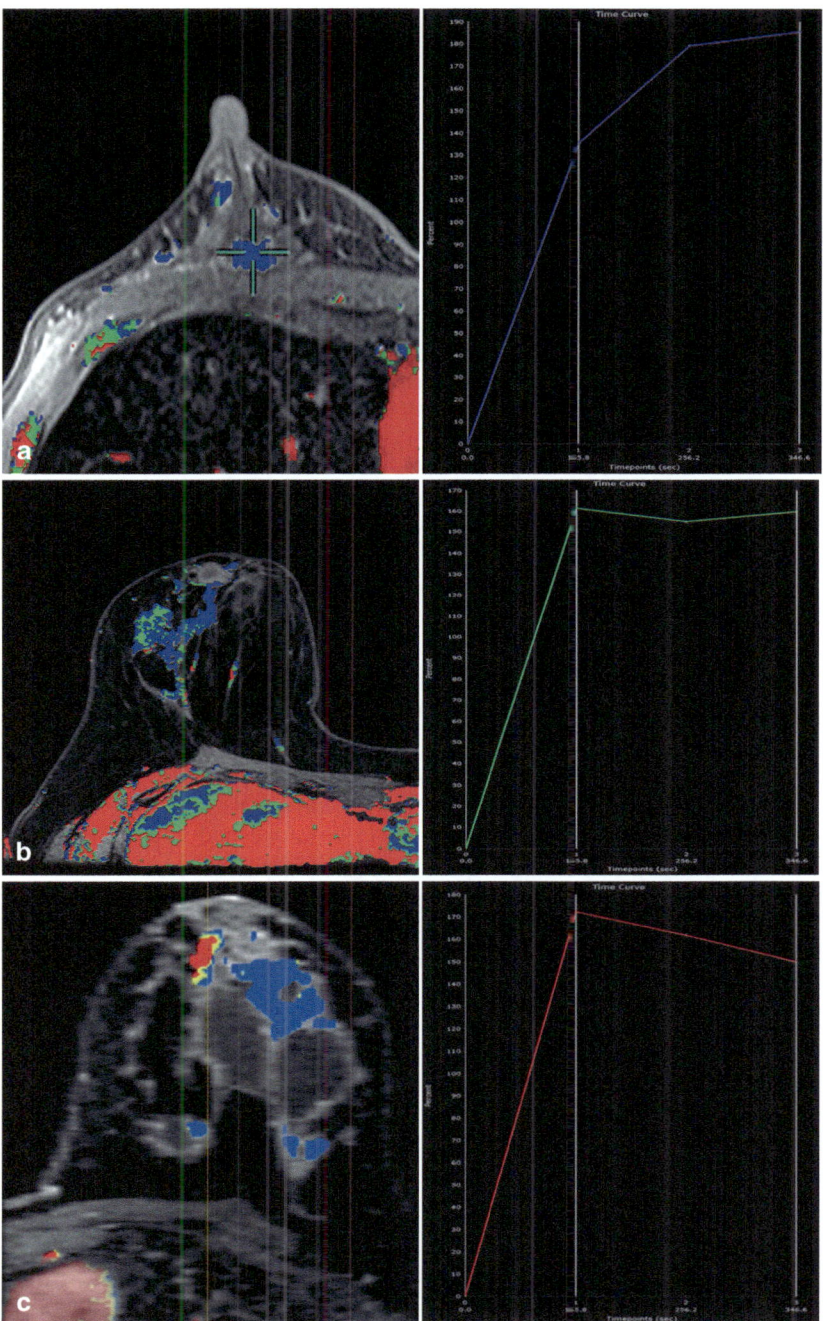

Fig. 7.12 **Typical kinetic curves encountered on breast MRI—persistent (a),** plateau (b), and washout (**c**). Although there is overlap, malignancies more often demonstrate mixed kinetics being proedominantly plateau and washout. However, lower grade malignancies (such as DCIS and invasive lobular cancer) may show persistent kinetics, and sometimes even can be below threshold on the kinetic map

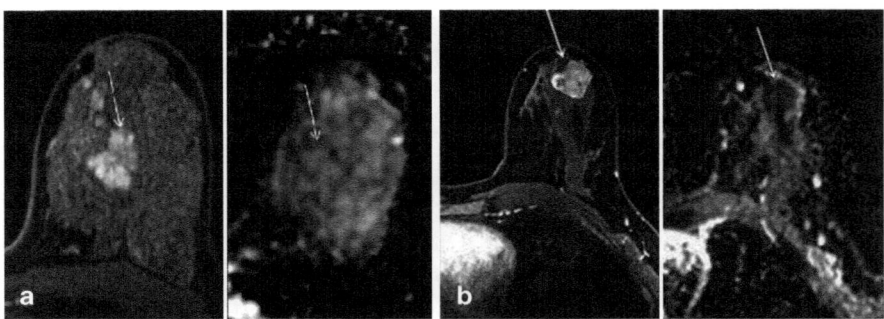

Fig. 7.13 (a) **Diffusion-weighted imaging of a fibroadenoma.** Postcontrast image (left) and diffusion *b* value-1000 image (right) show no restricted diffusion (arrows). (**b**) Diffusion-weighted imaging of an invasive ductal carcinoma. Postcontrast image (left) and diffusion *b* value-1000 image (right) show restricted diffusion (arrows)

Non-contrast Study

For assessing integrity of silicone implants; acquire axial T2-weighted, axial and sagittal STIR-silicone selective and silicone-suppressed sequences

- Interpretation - no BIRADS assessment for implant exam
  - ○ Normal—location (prepectoral or retro/subpectoral (Fig. 7.14); radial folds (infolding of implant envelope); intact envelope and capsule; small peri-implant fluid collection non-specific (Fig. e7.5)
  - ○ Intracapsular rupture—linguine sign (collapsed envelope floating in silicone contained by capsule) (Fig. 7.15)
  - ○ Extracapsular rupture—disrupted capsule with silicone extending into breast tissue ± linguine sign (Fig. 7.16); silicone in axillary and internal mammary lymph nodes

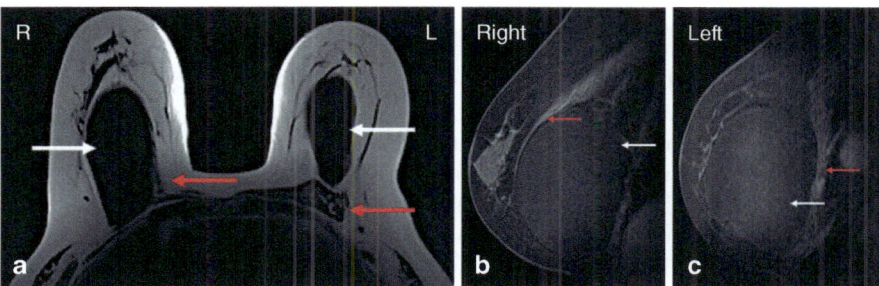

Fig. 7.14 Normal silicone implants. (**a**) Axial image-right subpectoral silicone implant and left prepectoral silicone implant. (**b**, **c**) Sagittal image. Note: relation of the implant (white arrows) under the muscle on the right and in front of the pectoralis muscle (red arrow) on the left

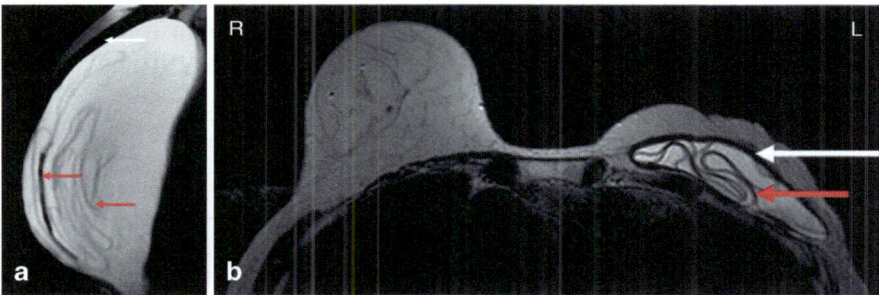

Fig. 7.15 Implant with intracapsular rupture. (**a**) Sagittal and (**b**) axial image shows the collapsed elastomere shell (red arrows); however, the capsule is intact (white arrow) and the rupture remains contained within the capsule

Fig. 7.16 Implant with extracapsular rupture. Note the extracapsular herniation of the implant (red arrows) and intracapsular rupture (white arrows)

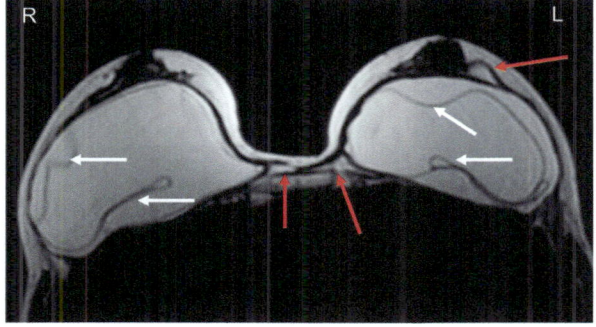

ARTIFACTS

- Suboptimal positioning—breast not centered in coil and tissue adjacent to coil resulting in high signal (Fig. 7.17)
- Motion—movement between or during acquisition leading to misregistration on subtraction and limiting utility of kinetic map (Fig. 7.18)
- Metallic susceptibility—loss of signal due to presence of ferromagnetic metal (e.g., biopsy or surgical clips, sternotomy wires) (Fig. 7.19)
- Wrap around (aliasing or phase wrap)—FOV too small leading to signal from tissue outside FOV superimposing on structures within FOV due to misregistration, occurs in phase-encoding direction (Fig. e7.6)
- Suboptimal fat suppression—due to field inhomogenity (corrected with shimming) or selecting incorrect peak (fat suppresses at frequency 3.5 ppm below water peak); more commonly seen when entirely fatty or presence of silicone or saline implants (Fig. e7.7)
- Zebra (moiré)—phase interference due to signal from tissue outside FOV wrapping into FOV and poor magnet shimming causes phase shift between tissue within and outside of FOV such that rapid phase shifting causes in/out of phase (white and black lines) (Fig. e7.8)
- Radiofrequency interference—RF signal penetrates shield due to leak resulting in noisier image or zipper artifact (high signal foci in center of image)
- Chemical shift—at fat-fluid interface due to difference in resonance frequency of hydrogen in fat vs. water with spatial misregistration in frequency-encoding direction; appears as black line at water-fat interface due to shift in opposite direction (Fig. e7.9)

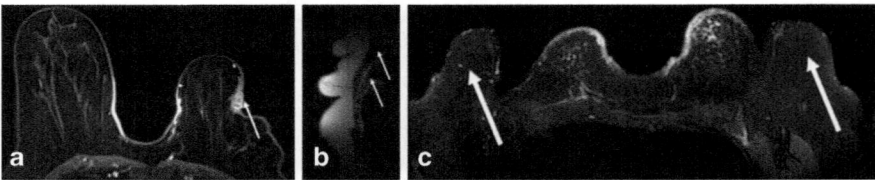

Fig. 7.17 Suboptimal position. (**a**) Nipple touching the coil and breast tissue outside of the coil (**b**, **c**; white arrows)

Fig. 7.18 Motion artifact—movement between or during acquisition leading to misregistration (white arrows)

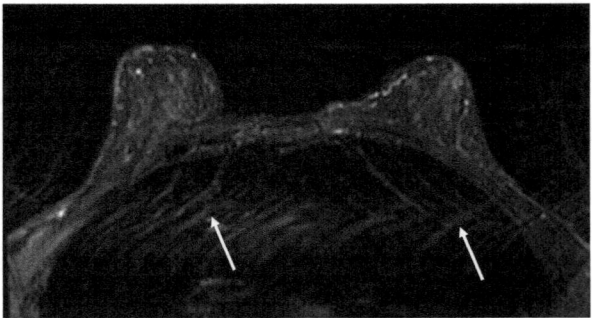

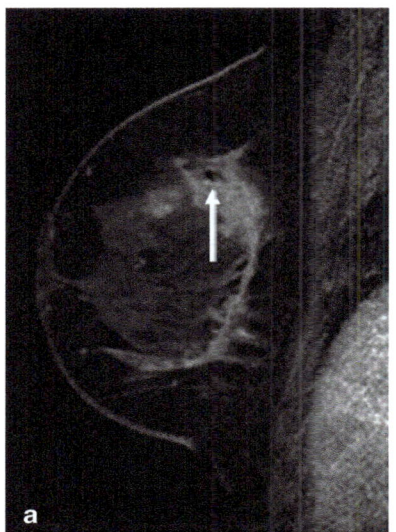

Fig. 7.19 Signal voids. (a) Signal void from percutaneous titanium biopsy clip (white arrow). (b) Metallic artifact from wire localization performed with a non-compatible stainless steel needle: (b) T1-weighted fat-saturated gradient echo image post needle insertion (white arrow) (c) with corresponding susceptibility sequence (white arrow)

BENCHMARKS

Screening and diagnostic (see Refs. [3, 4] for further details)

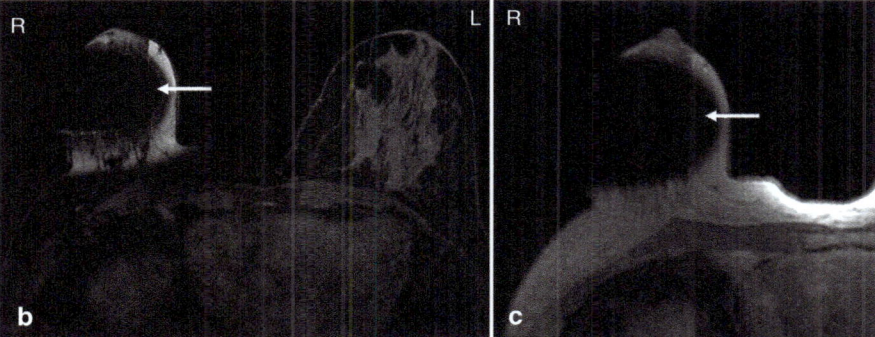

Performance measure	BIRADS benchmark
Cancer detection rate (CDR)	20–30/1000
PPV$_2$	15%
PPV$_3$	20–50%
Sensitivity	>80%
Specificity	85–90%
% Minimal cancer	>50%
% Node negative invasive cancer	>80%

Further Readings

1. Mann RM, Cho N, Moy L. Breast MRI—state of the art. Radiology. 2019;292:520–36.
2. Harvey JA, Hendrick E, Coll JM, Nicholson BT, Burkholder BT, Cohen MA. Breast MR imaging artifacts: how to recognize and fix them. Radiographics. 2007;27:S131–45.
3. Lee JM, Ichikawa L, Valencia E, et al. Performance benchmarks for screening breast MR imaging in community practice. Radiology. 2017;285:44–52.
4. Neill BL, Gavenonis SC, Motazedi T, et al. Auditing a breast MRI practice—performance measures for screening and diagnostic breast MRI. J Am Coll Radiol. 2014;11:883–9.

Image-Guided Breast Interventions

8

Donna Lee Selland, Patrick Tivnan, and Priscilla J. Slanetz

Minimally invasive method to biopsy suspicious findings seen on imaging can be performed using any modality (mammography, US, or MR; rarely, CT or nuclear imaging).

BIRADS 4 and 5 lesions warrant biopsy; BIRADS 3 may be biopsied depending on patient or physician concern, patient history, or patient inability to comply with follow-up.

Radiologic-pathologic correlation key to ensure adequate sampling and to guide management.

Biopsy Logistics

- Patient preparation—check allergies (latex, local anesthesia); some hold anticoagulation but no increased risk of major complications if performed on these medications
- Choice of modality—biopsy using modality that "sees" the target the best
- Informed consent—includes discussion of potential risks: bleeding and infection; milk fistula if lactating; non-diagnostic sample; potential allergic reaction to local anesthesia or percutaneous biopsy clip (extremely rare); implant rupture (if have implants)

Supplementary Information The online version contains supplementary material available at https://doi.org/10.1007/978-3-031-66274-4_8.

D. L. Selland · P. Tivnan · P. J. Slanetz (✉)
Division of Breast Imaging, Department of Radiology, Boston University Medical Center, Boston, MA, USA
e-mail: donna-lee.selland@bmc.org; priscilla.slanetz@bmc.org

- Anesthesia—local with 1–2% lidocaine ± epinephrine; rarely, conscious sedation
- Sterile field
- Number of samples—obtain on average 4–12 tissue samples (most often 4–5 cores)
- Place percutaneous biopsy clip at site of biopsy
  - Most clips are made of titanium but some are stainless steel or contain nickel
  - Some clips embedded in other materials can cause foreign body reaction/allergic reaction
- Apply compression to achieve hemostasis
- Cover needle entry with steri-strips ± sterile bandage
- Provide instructions for care at home (ice, Tylenol, no heavy lifting/exercising for 24 h, shower next day)
- Post-procedure mammogram obtained (typically CC and lateral), unless < 30 years old

Biopsy Options

- Fine needle aspiration:
  - Primarily for axillary lymph nodes (Fig. e8.1); rarely, vascular breast mass in anticoagulated patient
  - 3–5 passes with 22–25 gauge needle
  - Aspirates sent routinely to cytology; also sent for flow cytometry in RPMI fluid if lymphoma is of concern

- Cyst aspiration
  - ○ Performed if cyst is symptomatic or if appears complicated
  - ○ 18–20 gauge needle placed into cyst for drainage (Fig. 8.1)
  - ○ Fluid only sent to cytology if bloody, lesion does not completely resolve, or patient requests
  - ○ If atypia on cytology, follow-up imaging in 3 months; if cyst recurs, surgical excision to exclude malignancy

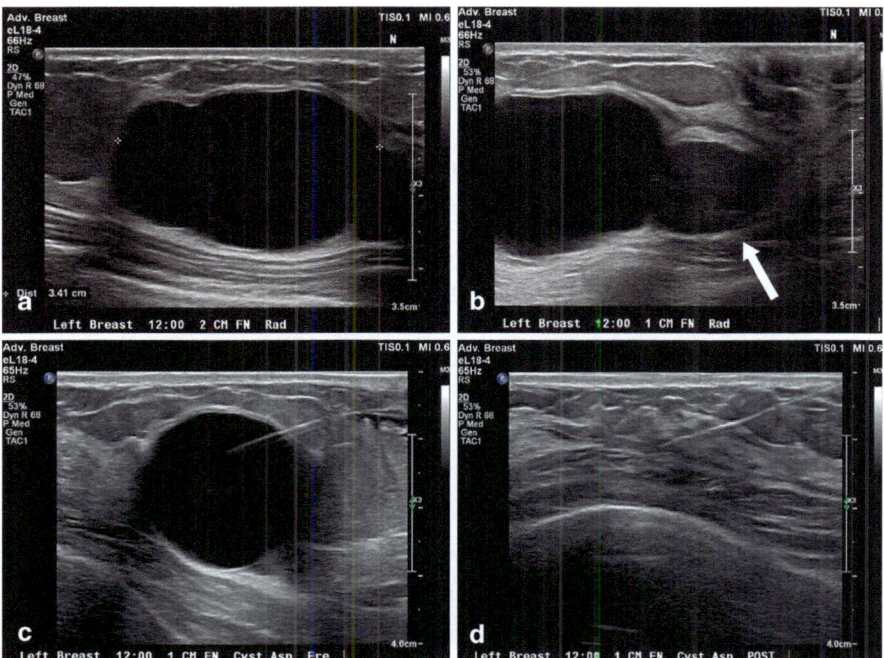

Fig. 8.1 Ultrasound-guided cyst aspiration. 39-year-old female with focal left breast pain. Ultrasound shows 3.5 cm simple cyst (**a**) with an adjacent circumscribed homogeneously hypoechoic mass suggestive of a complicated cyst (**b**; arrow). Aspiration was recommended to exclude a solid lesion. Under ultrasound guidance using an 18 g spinal needle (**c**), the cyst was drained with no residual lesion after aspiration (**d**). The aspirated fluid was discarded as it was straw colored

- Aspiration: to drain abscess (aspirate sent for microbiology) (Fig. 8.2) and symptomatic seroma, hematoma, or lymphocele
- Core needle biopsy
  - ○ Advantages—avoids surgical biopsy ≥ 70–80%; false negative rate of 1–2% comparable to surgery; can differentiate in situ from invasive cancer; can reliably determine cancer receptor status; faster, less painful, and less costly than surgery; minimal recovery time; permits definitive surgical planning minimizing chance of additional surgery if cancer diagnosis
    - Ultrasound guided—primarily for masses and axillary nodes, sometimes for segmental calcifications
      - ▪ 14–16 gauge spring-loaded needle (Fig. 8.3) or 8–12 gauge vacuum-assisted device (Fig. 8.4); use no-throw technique if close to chest wall
      - ▪ For axilla, use 14-16-gauge no-throw device
      - ▪ Vacuum device gives larger tissue sample and hence lower upgrade rates from high risk lesion to malignancy; however, more expensive
        - Ideal for mixed solid and cystic mass, intraductal mass, small vascular lesion, and calcifications
      - ▪ Perform specimen radiograph if biopsy calcifications

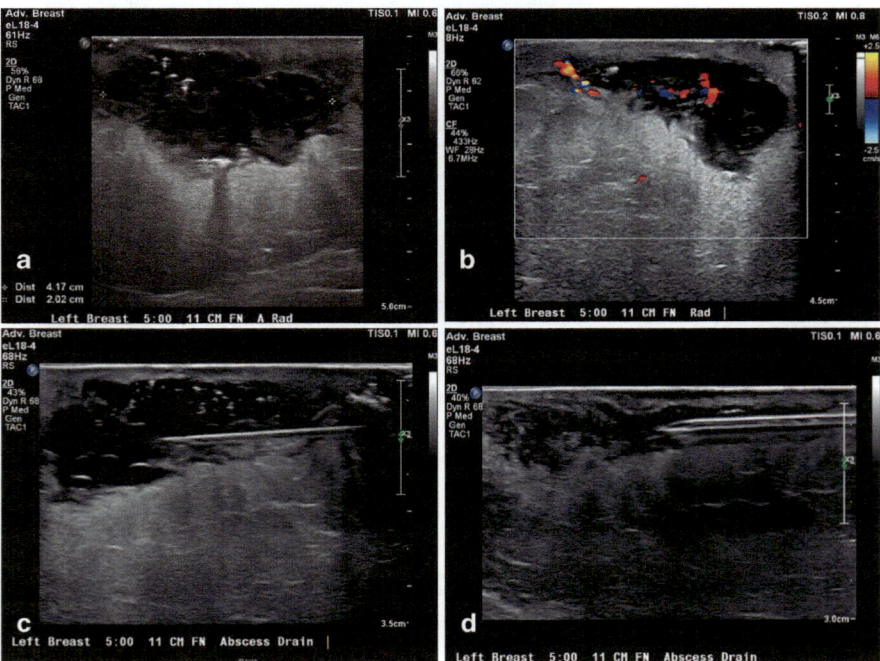

Fig. 8.2 Ultrasound-guided abscess drainage. 47-year-old female with left breast erythema and pain. Ultrasound at 5:00 11 cm from the nipple demonstrates a heterogeneous fluid collection measuring up to 4.2 cm (**a**) with surrounding hyperemia (**b**) consistent with a breast abscess. Ultrasound-guided aspiration (**c**) was performed with an 18 g needle yielding 6 cc of purulent fluid with a small residual collection (**d**) at the end of the procedure. The fluid was sent for Gram stain and culture revealing a polymicrobial infection

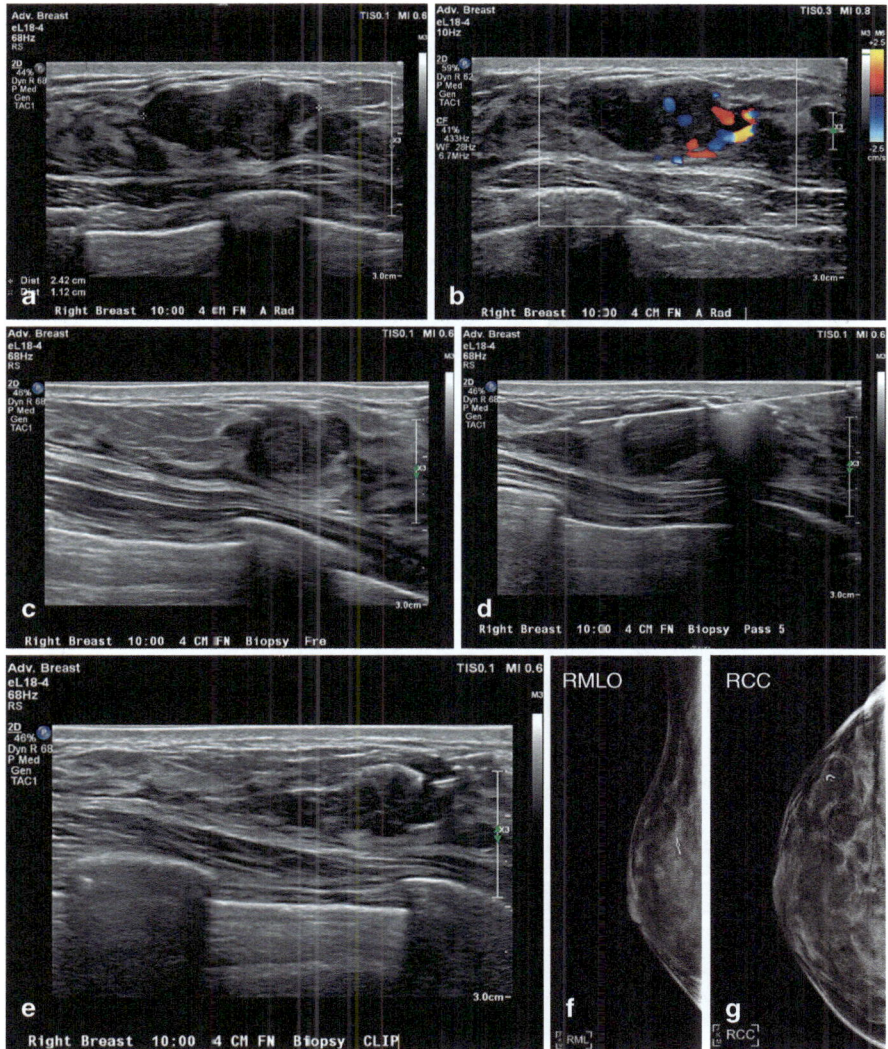

Fig. 8.3 **Ultrasound-guided right breast biopsy**. 43-year-old with palpable right breast mass. Ultrasound revealed an oval macrolobulated hypoechoic parallel mass at 10:00 4 cm from the nipple (**a**) with internal flow (**b**) and for which biopsy was recommended (BIRADS 4a). On a subsequent day, the same mass (**c**) was biopsied using a 14 gauge spring-loaded device (**d**). An eye-shaped clip was placed after the biopsy (**e**). Post-biopsy mammogram demonstrates the clip within the right upper outer breast (**f, g**; mass was mammographically occult). Pathology revealed fibroadenoma

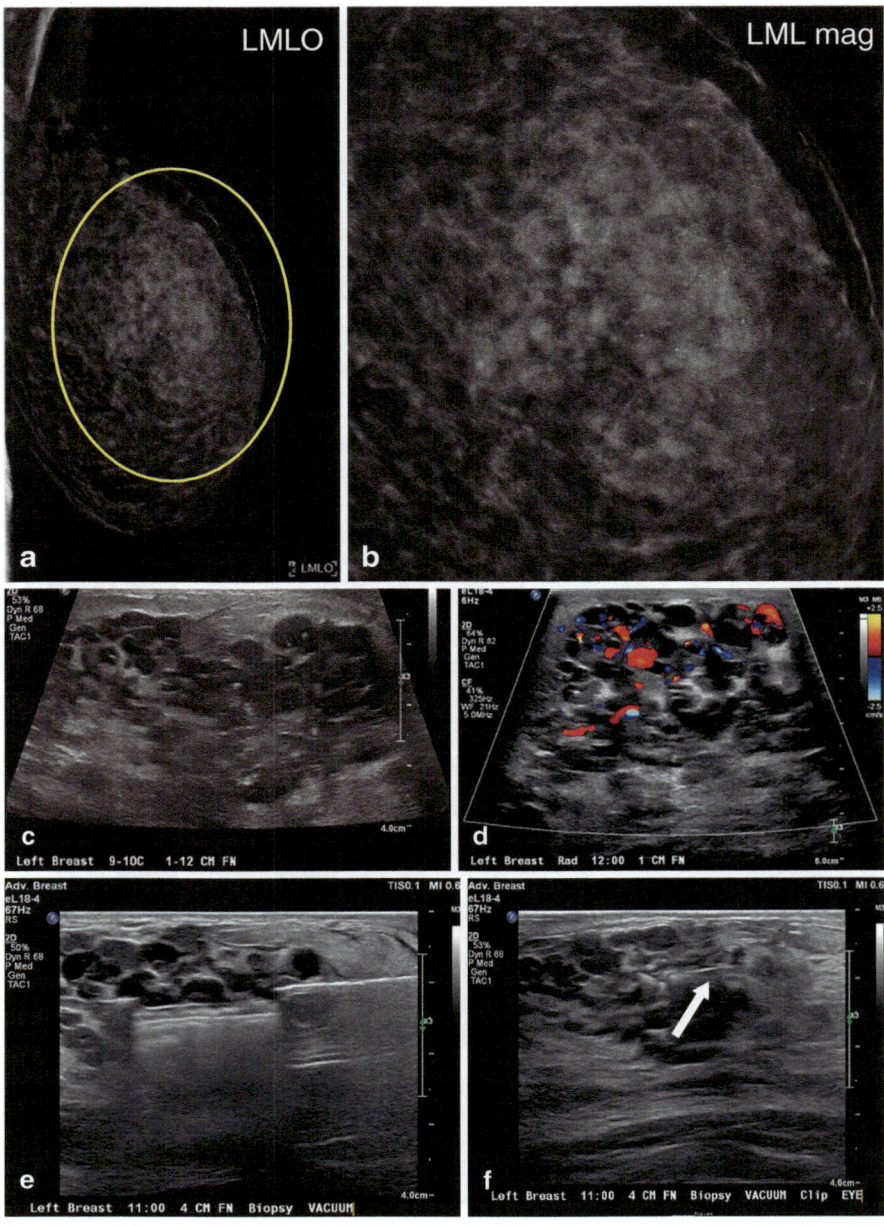

Fig. 8.4 **Ultrasound-guided vacuum-assisted core biopsy**. 39-year-old female with palpable left breast mass for 3 months. MLO (**a**) and lateral magnified (**b**) views show global asymmetry (circle) with associated calcifications in the upper left breast in the area of concern. Ultrasound shows multiple dilated ducts with microcalcifications (**c**) and hypervascularity in the surrounding breast tissue (**d**). Biopsy with a spring-loaded device gave discordant results, and therefore, vacuum-assisted biopsy was performed (**e**) using a 9-gauge needle. An eye-shaped clip was placed (**f**; arrow). Radiography of the excised tissue shows numerous calcifications (**g**; circles) within the excised tissue. Post-procedure ML (**h**) and CC (**i**) views show the eye-shaped clip (arrow) adjacent to the clip placed during the spring-loaded procedure. Pathology confirmed papillary ductal carcinoma in situ

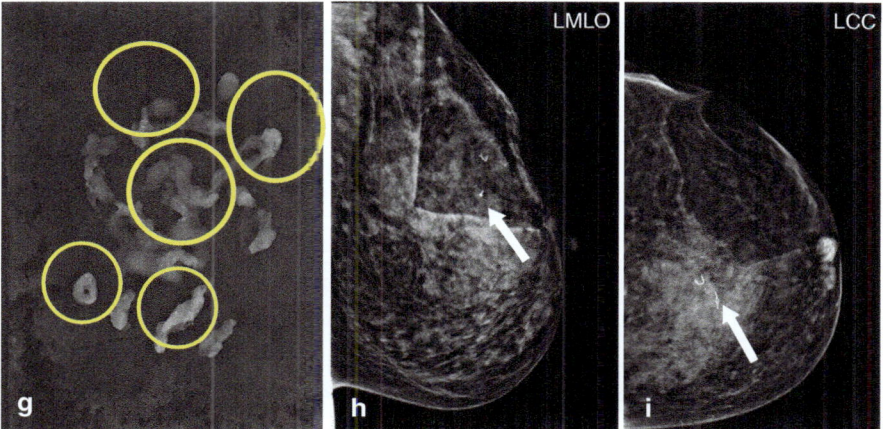

Fig. 8.4 (continued)

- Documentation—image of lesion in orthogonal planes with and without calipers; image of needle prior to biopsy; image of needle passing through lesion and in orthogonal plane for first pass; image of needle passing through lesion for each subsequent pass
- Stereotactic/tomosynthesis guided—primarily for calcifications, distortion, and masses not seen on US
  - Breast compression thickness of at least 2.3 cm, if using vacuum device; can biopsy thinner breast if use lateral arm (needle enters parallel to detector rather than orthogonal to detector)
  - Either acquire scout and stereo pair for targeting (2D stereotactic biopsy) (Fig. 8.5) or single tomosynthesis scout (tomosynthesis-directed) (Fig. 8.6)
  - If lesion superficial, inject additional local anesthesia in skin to increase thickness or advance needle deeper into tissue so lesion in proximal part of bowl
  - If lesion far posterior, either use lateral arm (Fig. e8.2) or put arm through hole (if table)
  - Prone table
    - Patient lies prone with breast pendant through hole in table
    - 300 lb weight limit for hydraulic lift; 450 lb weight limit for table
    - Difficult to biopsy lesions close to chest wall and in axilla
- Upright/add-on
  - Patient seated upright with breast compressed
  - No weight limit but patient may experience vasovagal reaction
  - Improved access to lesions near chest wall and in axillary region
- MR guided (Fig. 8.7)
  - Used to biopsy MR-detected lesions
  - Patient lies prone with breast pendant and mildly compressed in biopsy grid
  - Intravenous gadolinium administered to identify target for biopsy
  - Sterile technique and 1–2% lidocaine for local anesthesia

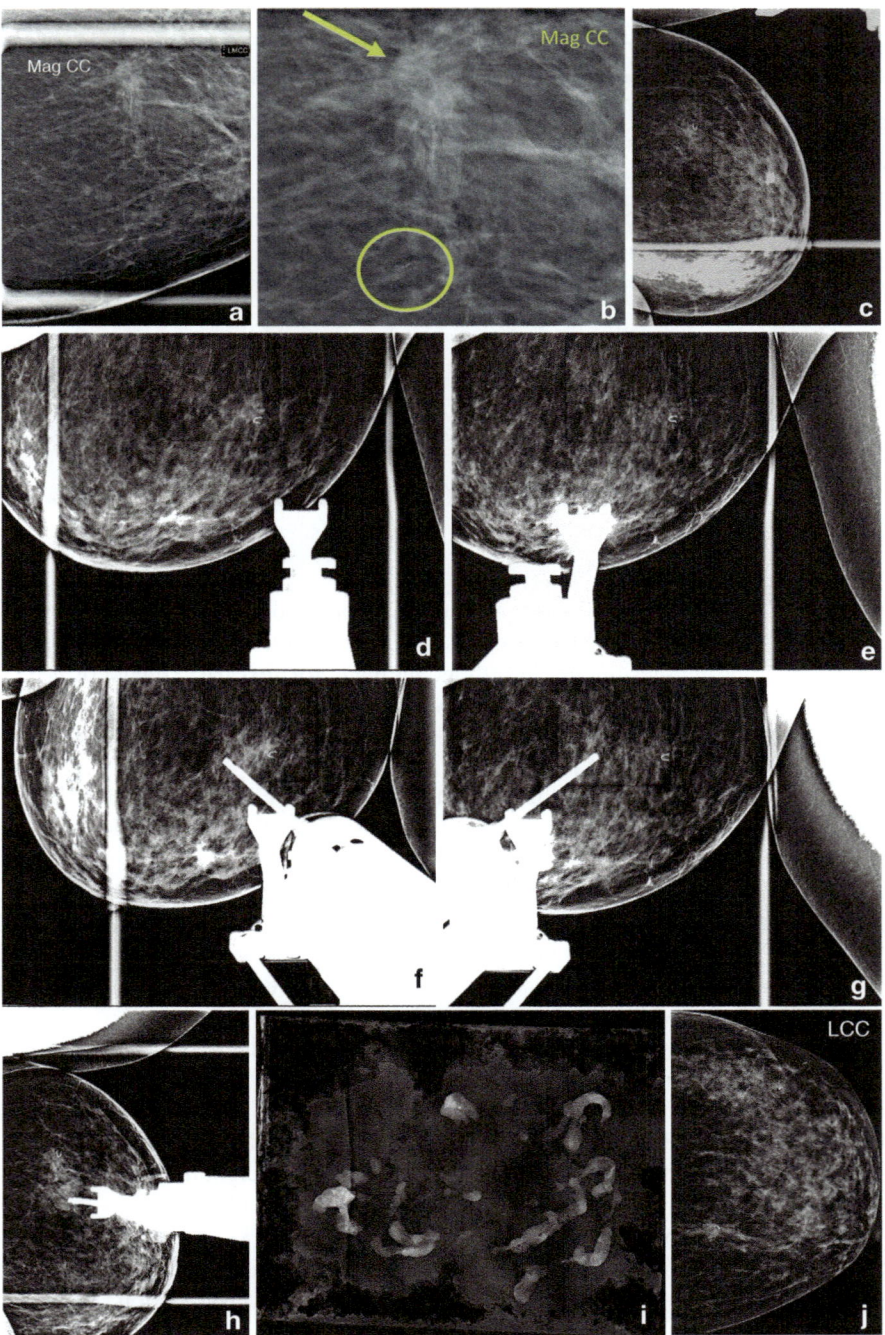

Fig. 8.5 Stereotactic core biopsy. 51-year-old with a spiculated right breast outer mass (**a**; arrow) and linear heterogeneous calcifications 4 cm inferior and 2 cm medial to the mass (**b**; circle). The spiculated mass was biopsied under ultrasound. The calcifications were biopsied under stereotactic guidance. Scout CC view (**c**), initial stereo pair (**d, e**), and post-needle placement stereo pair (**f, g**) were acquired. Vacuum-assisted biopsy was performed with post-biopsy imaging demonstrating post-biopsy changes (**h**). Radiography of the excised tissue shows several calcifications (**i**). Post-biopsy post-clip placement CC view (**j**) Post biopsy post clip placement CC views confirmed a rod-shaped marker in the lateral right breast at the site of biopsy. Pathology revealed high-grade DCIS

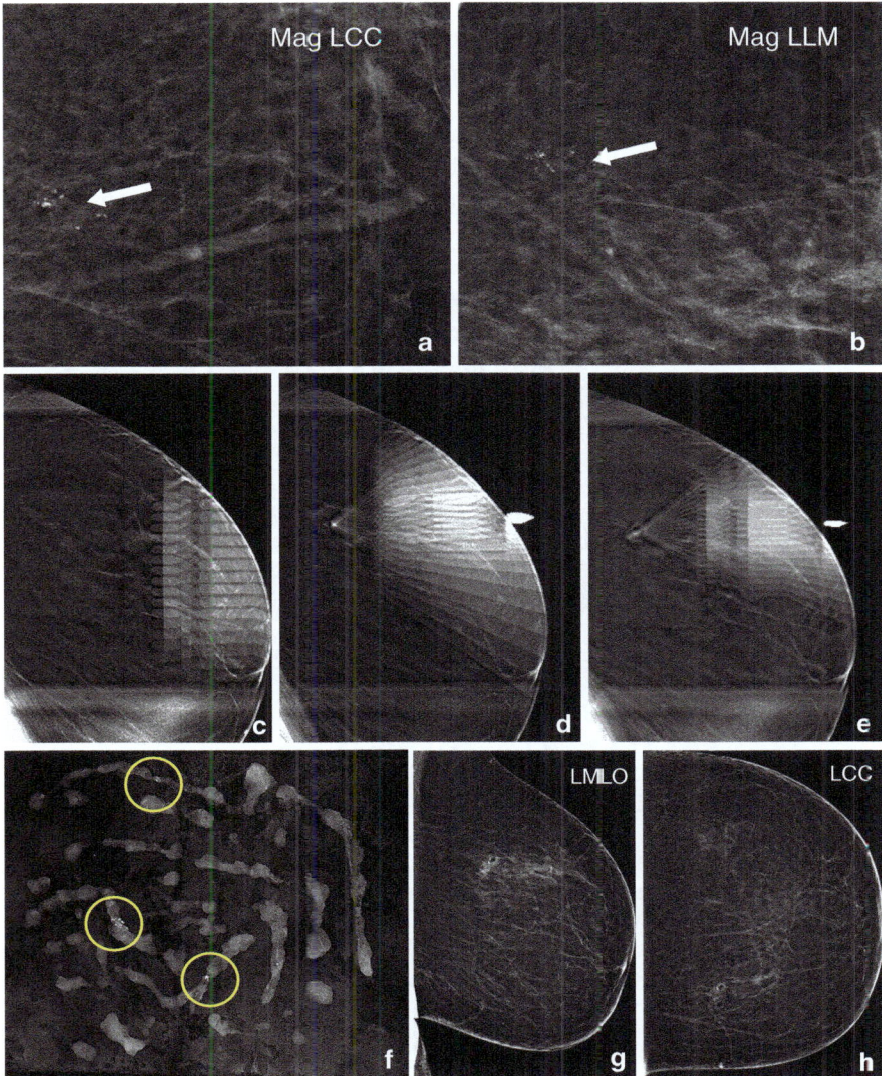

Fig. 8.6 Tomosynthesis-directed core biopsy. 58-year-old female with grouped left upper inner coarse heterogeneous calcifications (arrows) seen on CC (**a**) and ML (**b**) magnification views. Tomosynthesis biopsy was recommended (BIRADS 4b). From a medial approach, tomosynthesis biopsy was undertaken with scout image (**c**), prebiopsy (**d**), and post-biopsy post-clip placement (**e**). Radiography of the excised tissue confirms calcifications (**f**. circles). Post-biopsy post-clip placement ML (**g**) and CC (**h**) views demonstrate appropriate post-biopsy changes in the upper inner left breast with appropriately placed biopsy clip. Biopsy results showed calcified fibroadenoma

- Images acquired to ensure accurate needle placement and adequate sampling
- 10–12 cores obtained using MR-compatible 9-gauge vacuum-assisted device
- MR-compatible biopsy clip placed
- Post-procedure mammogram obtained
- Note: risk of hematoma/bleeding higher with MR biopsy as biopsy targets vascular lesions

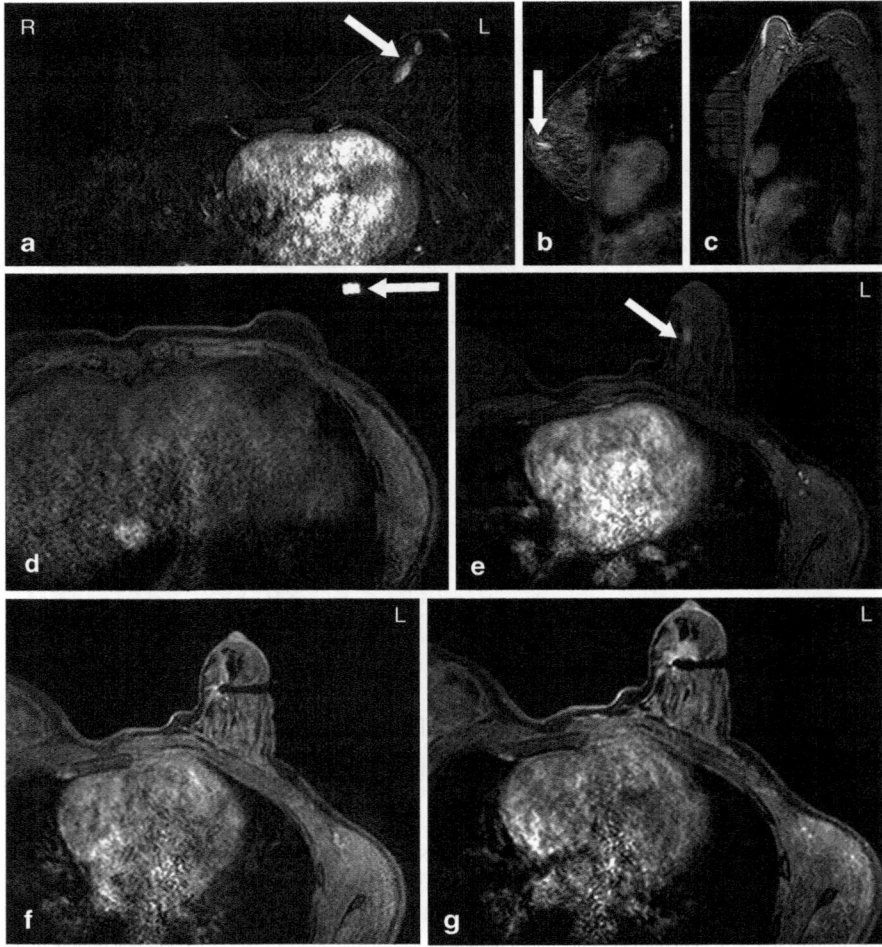

Fig. 8.7 MRI-guided core biopsy. 21-year-old female with focal left breast pain and diagnostic breast MR demonstrating an indeterminate tubular enhancing mass (arrows) in the central left breast on axial subtracted (**a**) and sagittal post-contrast (**b**) sequences. MR-guided biopsy was performed using a 9-gauge vacuum-assisted device. The patient's left breast was placed in the biopsy grid with mild compression (**c**) and the fiducial was visualized (**d**; arrow). After administration of IV gadolinium, the mass was re-identified (**e**; arrow). A 9-gauge needle was advanced into the lesion (**f**) and after biopsy, post-biopsy changes were confirmed (**g**). Pathology showed fibroadenoma and pseudoangiomatous stromal hyperplasia (PASH) which was felt to be concordant

- Preoperative localization
  - Performed using mammography, US, or MRI, rarely CT
    - Needle
      - 20-gauge needle/hook wire combination
      - Using mammography (Fig. 8.8)
        - ◆ Breast placed in compression grid with approach being the shortest distance to target
        - ◆ Needle placed and depth confirmed in orthogonal projection (tip 1.5–2 cm past lesion)
        - ◆ Hook wire deployed
      - Using ultrasound (Fig. e8.3)
        - ◆ Lesion identified
        - ◆ Needle placed through the lesion with tip 1.5 cm past lesion
        - ◆ Hook wire deployed under direct visualization
        - ◆ Post-procedure one-view mammogram obtained with wire parallel to detector
    - Seed/reflector/tag
      - Can be placed using mammography (Fig. e8.4) or US (Fig. e8.5); MRI (if device compatible)
      - Similar to performing needle localization with benefit of seed/reflector/tag placement days before surgery
      - Confirm signal from seed/reflector/tag once placed (depending on device) prior to discharging patient
- Percutaneous therapy
  - Most commonly used to manage benign breast lesions such as fibroadenomas, but not widely available; may have role for managing < 2 cm invasive cancers in non-operative patients but not routinely offered
    - Excision (Fig. e8.6)—use 8-9-gauge vacuum device; 92–99% effective
    - Cryoablation (Fig. e8.7)—freeze lesions; 93% effective
    - Radiofrequency ablation—ablate with RF pulse; 73% reduction in size

Management

- Radiologic-pathologic correlation guides management
- Lesions on FNA/core biopsy that necessitate surgical excision include:
  - Malignancy
  - Atypia, such as atypical ductal hyperplasia, florid and pleomorphic lobular neoplasia, atypical papillary lesions, flat epithelial atypia (unless incidental)
  - Complex sclerosing lesion/radial scar (unless incidental)
  - Fibroepithelial lesions (cellular fibroadenomas and phyllodes)
  - Papillary lesions with atypia
- Issue addendum to report with follow-up and management recommendations and communicate results to referring provider ± patient

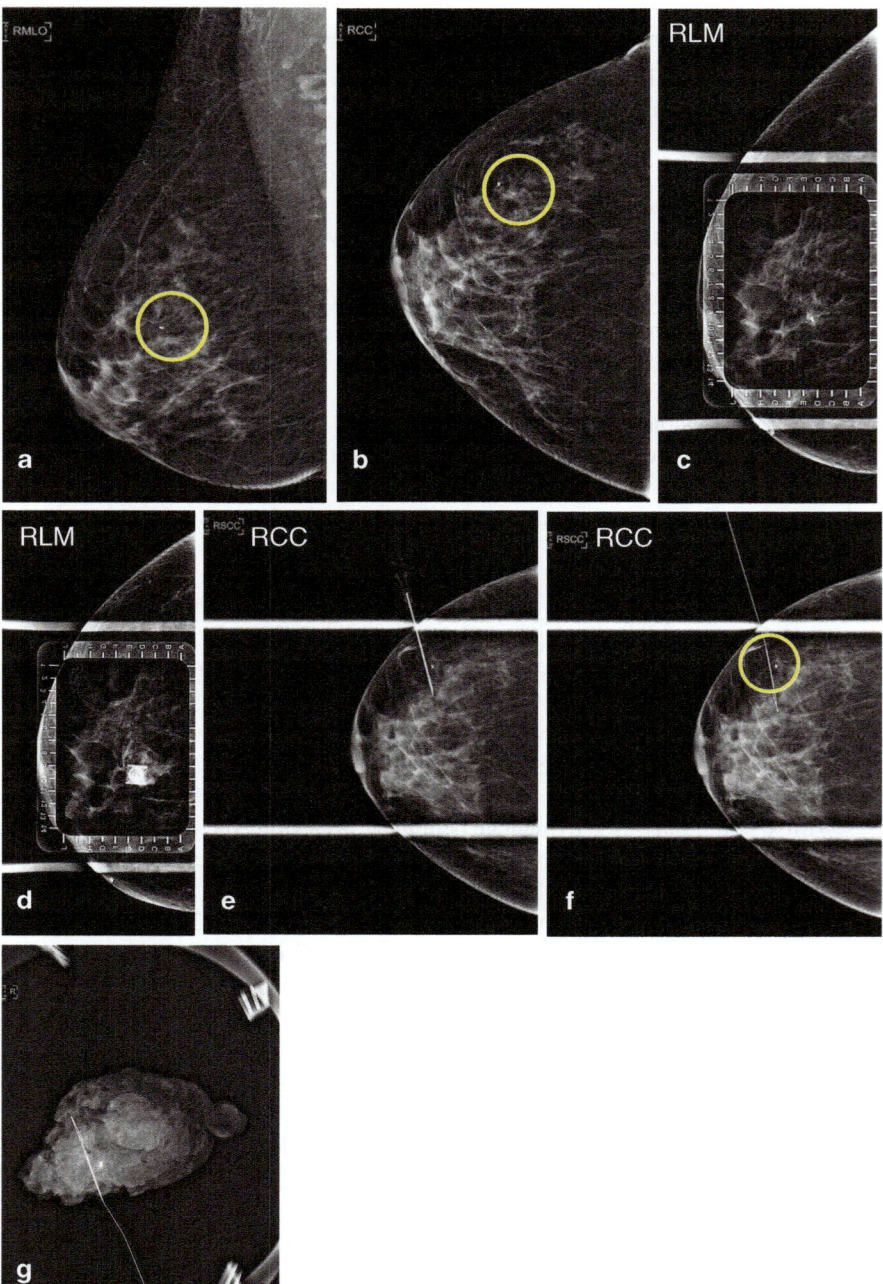

Fig. 8.8 Mammographically guided wire localization. 64-year-old presenting for localization of right upper outer calcifications revealing radial scar and atypical ductal hyperplasia on core biopsy. Right MLO (**a**) and CC (**b**) views demonstrate the biopsy clip in the upper outer right breast with adjacent residual calcifications (circles). The breast was placed in the alpha-numeric grid using a lateral approach (**c**). A 5 cm Kopans needle was advanced into the breast (**d**) with the depth confirmed in the orthogonal plane (CC; **e**) prior to deployment of the hook wire adjacent to the clip and residual calcifications (**f**; circle). Radiography of the excised tissue showed the clip, residual calcifications, and wire (**g**). These results were immediately conveyed to the surgeon in the operating room

Outcomes Analysis

In order to evaluate and improve performance, practices monitor the following parameters:
- Total number of procedures
- Total number of cancers found
- Total number of benign lesions found
- Total number of biopsies requiring repeat biopsy (open or repeat needle biopsy)
  - Insufficient sample, discordance, atypia/radial scar, other
- Total number of complications
  - Hematomas requiring surgical intervention
  - Infections requiring treatment
  - Other

Optimal performance measures include:

- PPV3: 25–40%
- Stage 0 or 1 cancers: >50%
- Minimal cancers: >30%
- Node positivity: <25%

References

1. BIRADS atlas. 5th ed. American College of Radiology; 2013. https://www.acr.org/Clinical-Resources/Reporting-and-Data-Systems/Bi-Rads.
2. Yeh ED, Frost EP, Raza S, Birdwell RL, Geiss CS. Avoiding pitfalls, maximizing success at image-guided breast interventions: a pictorial review. Curr Prob Diagn Radiol. 2017;46:161–9.

Benign Breast Disease

Priscilla J. Slanetz, Bernadette Jakomin,
and Patrick Tivnan

Benign breast disease affects over one million women in the USA annually who typically present with palpable lump, focal pain, nipple discharge, or incidental finding on routine mammography

Some benign diagnoses, such as atypical ductal hyperplasia, atypical lobular hyperplasia, and lobular carcinoma in situ, increase a woman's subsequent lifetime risk for developing breast cancer up to 4–5×

Supplementary Information The online version contains supplementary material available at https://doi.org/10.1007/978-3-031-66274-4_9.

P. J. Slanetz (✉) · B. Jakomin · P. Tivnan
Division of Breast Imaging, Department of Radiology, Boston University Medical Center, Boston, MA, USA
e-mail: Priscilla.slanetz@bmc.org; Bernadette.jakomin@bmc.org

SEBACEOUS AND EPIDERMOID INCLUSION CYST

- Benign cystic mass located in dermis or subcutaneous tissues differentiated on pathology
  - Sebaceous cysts—arise in sebaceous gland (Fig. 9.1a–e)
  - Epidermoid inclusion cysts—proliferation of squamous epithelium in dermis (Fig. 9.1f–j)
- Typically present with inflamed palpable superficial mass
- Imaging appearance of sebaceous and epidermoid inclusions cysts identical
  - Mammography—non-calcified circumscribed superficial mass
  - Ultrasound—cystic to hypoechoic mass with peripheral vascularity, overlying skin thickening, and visible tract to skin surface
  - MRI—enhancing superficial mass often with associated focal skin thickening
- Core biopsy contraindicated due to leaked contents inciting local inflammatory response
- Require surgical excision if recurrent symptoms

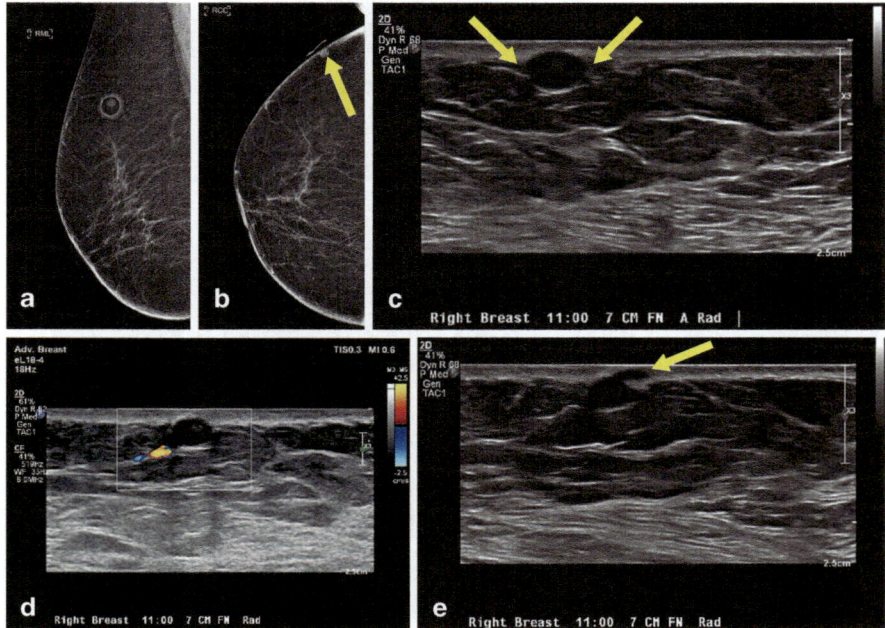

Fig. 9.1 (a–e) **Sebaceous and epidermoid inclusion cyst**. 62-year-old female presenting for screening. RML (**a**) and CC (**b**) views demonstrate round radio-opaque skin marker corresponding to skin lesion. Oval circumscribed dense mass resides in the skin in the upper outer right breast (arrow). Ultrasound demonstrates oval circumscribed anechoic cyst with "claw sign", thus dermal, (**c**, arrows) without internal vascularity (**d**) and a tract extending to the skin surface (**e**, arrow) at 11:00 8 cm from the nipple.

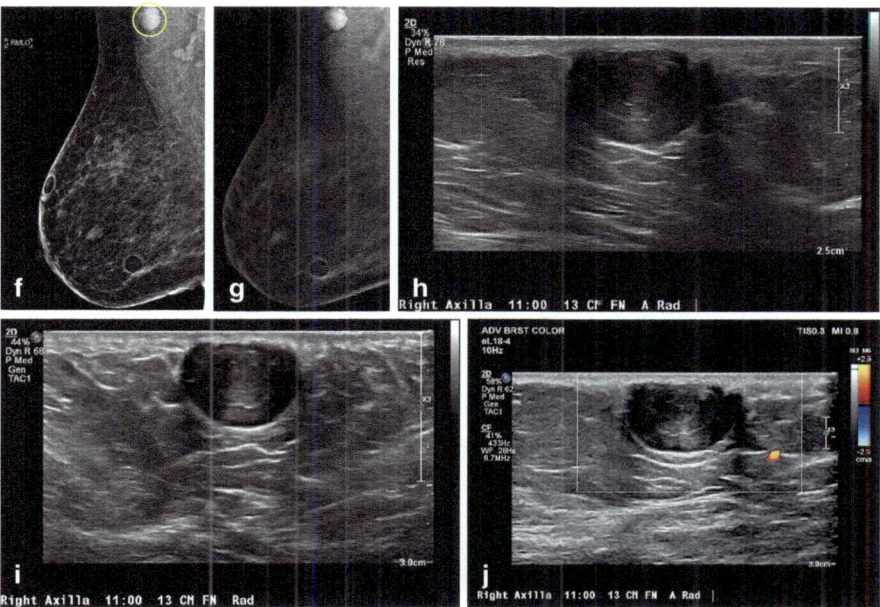

Fig. 9.1 (continued) (**f–j**) 45-year-old female with palpable lump. RMLO view (**f**) demonstrates dense oval circumscribed mass in the right axilla (circle) that localizes superficially on tomosynthesis image (**g**). Ultrasound at 11:00 demonstrates oval circumscribed hypoechoic subcutaneous mass with characteristic internal lamellar or "onion skin" appearance (**h, i**) without internal vascularity (**j**) representing an epidermoid inclusion cyst. Internal lamellated keratin accounts for this appearance

BREAST INFECTION

- **Cellulitis**—infection localized to skin related to insect bite, pimple, or inflamed dermal cyst
- **Mastitis**—inflammation of the breast tissue, most commonly related to breast-feeding (Fig. 9.2)
- Most common risk factors include lactation, diabetes, smoking, and obesity
- **Abscess**—collection of pus in breast tissue in patients with mastitis (Figs. 9.3 and e9.1)
  - Zuska-Atkins disease—recurrent periareolar abscesses with fistulas to skin (Fig. e9.2); associated with smoking

Fig. 9.2 (a–e) **Mastitis.** 47-year-old female presenting with left breast swelling and erythema. MLO (**a, b**) and CC (**c, d**) views demonstrate global asymmetry in lower outer left breast with trabecular thickening and skin thickening (yellow circles) which contrasts to the normal right breast (**a, c**). Ultrasound demonstrates large region of subcutaneous edema and skin thickening without focal fluid collection (**e**). The patient received antibiotics and her left mastitis resolved

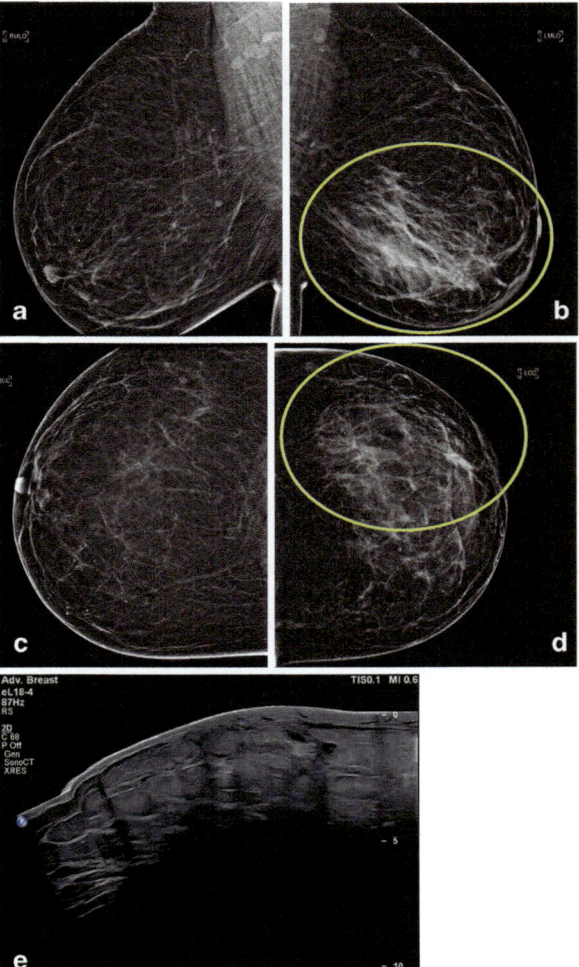

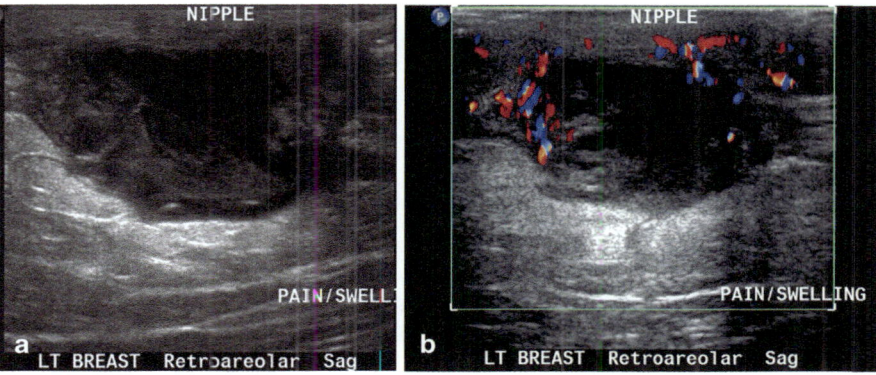

Fig. 9.3 (**a, b**) **Breast abscess**. 27-year-old female lactating patient with subareolar lump and erythema. US reveals complex fluid collection (**a**) with marked peripheral vascularity (**b**) consistent with abscess. The patient underwent aspiration of the abscess and was placed on antibiotics

- ○ Granulomatous mastitis—rare inflammatory presumed autoimmune process in women of childbearing age characterized by microabscesses and granuloma formation, sometimes associated with *Corynebacterium diphtheriae* colonization; may develop fistulas to skin (Fig. 9.4)
    - • Treatment with steroids ± antibiotics ± methotrexate
- • Imaging
    - ○ Mammography—skin thickening and trabecular thickening with focal mass if abscess present
    - ○ Ultrasound—skin thickening, dilated lymphatics, loss of soft tissue planes, and focal complex fluid collection (abscess)
- • Treated with warm compresses, antibiotics and percutaneous drainage of abscess
- • Fluid from abscess typically sent for microbiology (gram stain, aerobic and anaerobic culture, and sensitivity)

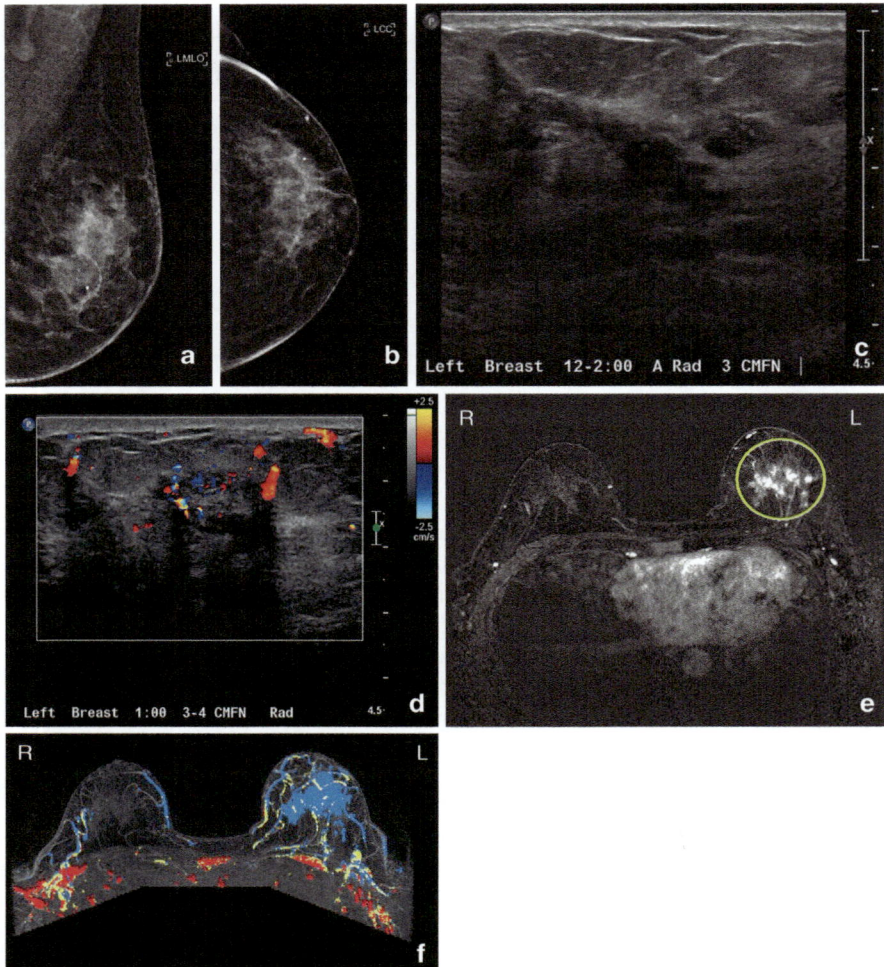

Fig. 9.4 (a–f) **Granulomatous mastitis**. 38-year-old female with 4 cm palpable lump in left upper outer breast. LMLO (**a**) and LCC (**b**) views demonstrate global asymmetry in the left upper outer breast corresponding to the palpable lump (metallic BB on skin). US demonstrates ill-defined heterogeneity involving 12:00–2:00 (**c**) with color demonstrating increased vascularity (**d**). MRI (axial T1-weighted post contrast) demonstrates extensive heterogeneous non-mass enhancement involving the left upper outer and upper inner quadrants (**e**; circle) with predominantly persistent enhancement kinetics (**f**). Biopsy confirmed granulomatous mastitis

BREAST TRAUMA

- **Contusion/hematoma**
  - Focal bleeding within breast tissue resulting in fat stranding and/or mass
  - Commonly presents as a palpable lump after trauma (Fig. 9.5)
  - Resolves spontaneously

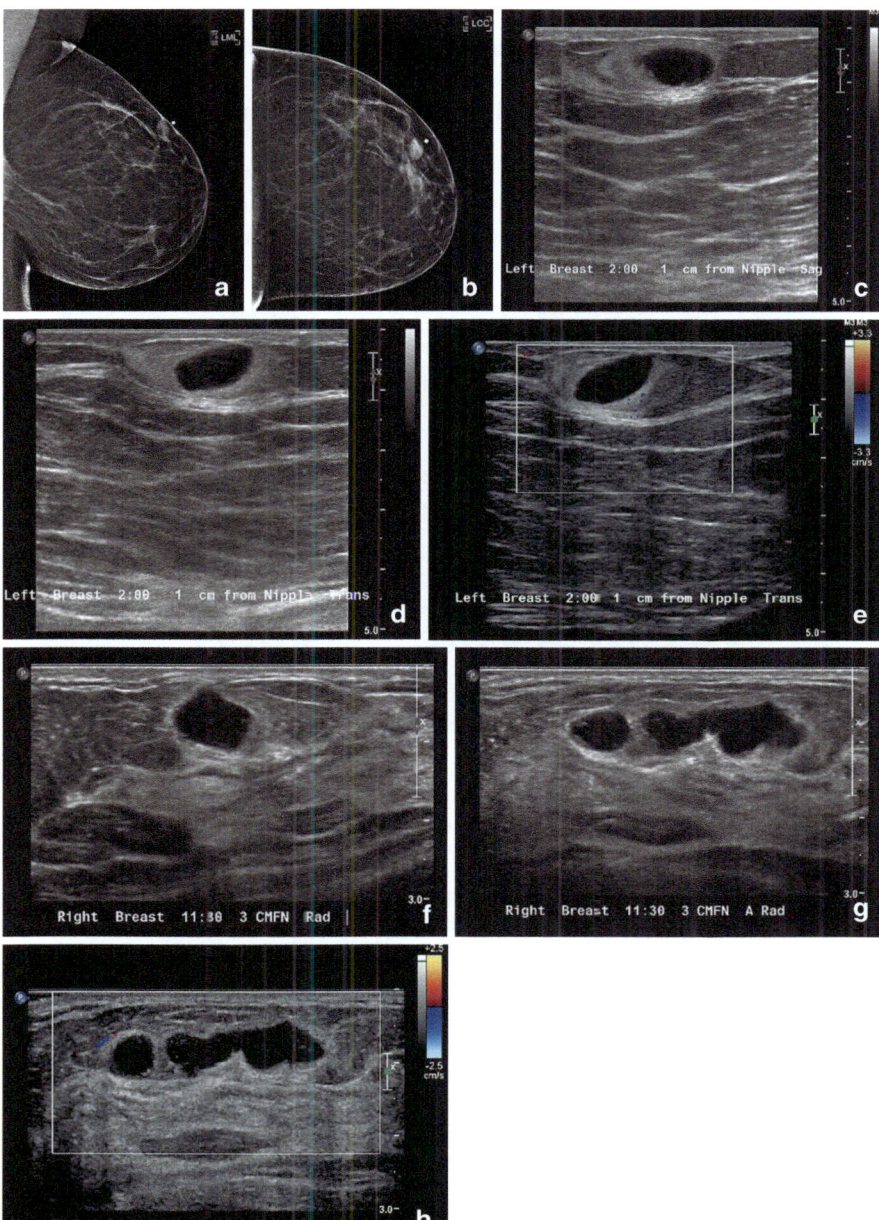

Fig. 9.5 (a–e) **Hematoma**. 33-year-old female with palpable mass in left breast with visible bruise on skin. LML (**a**) and LCC (**b**) views demonstrate oval circumscribed mass deep to skin at site of palpable lump (metallic BB). US demonstrates superficial oval circumscribed avascular mass with anechoic center and echogenic periphery (**c–e**). (**f–h**) 85-year-old female with palpable mass in the upper outer right breast with bruising at site after right breast trauma. US demonstrates oval avascular mass with central fluid component with low level internal echoes and subtle peripheral echogenicity (**f–h**)

- **Fat necrosis**
  - ○ Injury to breast fat from trauma, surgery, biopsy, or radiation therapy so correlation with clinical history essential in order to avoid intervention
  - ○ Typically presents as a painful palpable lump but often asymptomatic
  - ○ Imaging
    - • Mammography—oil cysts (Figs. 9.6, e9.3, e9.4, and e9.5); lucent-centered and coarse dystrophic calcifications (Fig. 9.7); developing asymmetry (Fig. e9.6); rarely spiculated mass (Fig. 9.8) or distortion

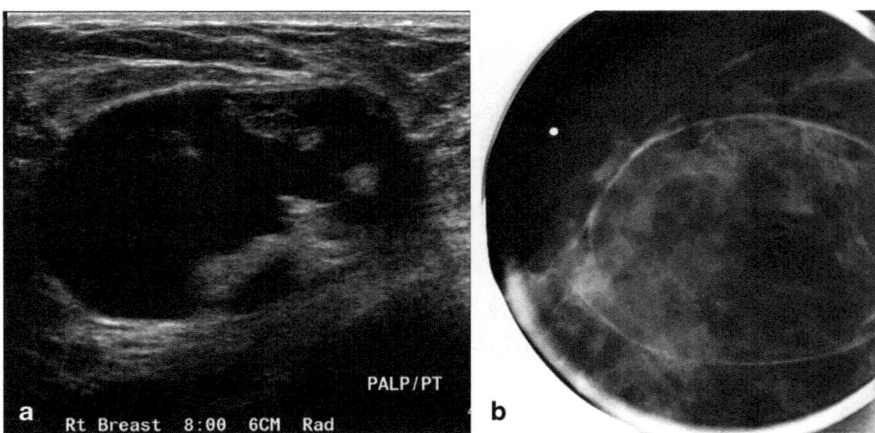

Fig. 9.6 (**a**, **b**) **Oil cyst**. 33-year-old female with a palpable right breast lump 1 month after a motor vehicle accident. US (**a**) showed mixed solid and cystic mass with internal nodular components. Tangential CC spot compression view (**b**) confirmed a radiolucent mass consistent with an oil cyst

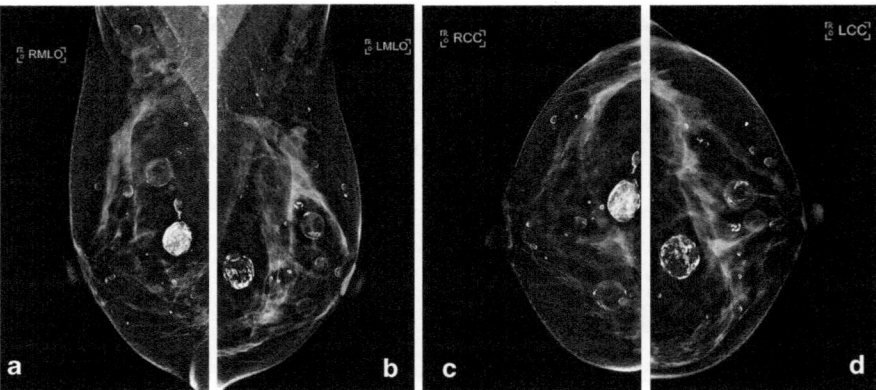

Fig. 9.7 (**a–d**) **Fat necrosis**. 45-year-old female status post bilateral breast reduction. MLO (**a**, **b**) and CC (**c**, **d**) views demonstrate scattered areas of fat necrosis/oil cysts with and without rim and dystrophic calcifications secondary to breast reduction

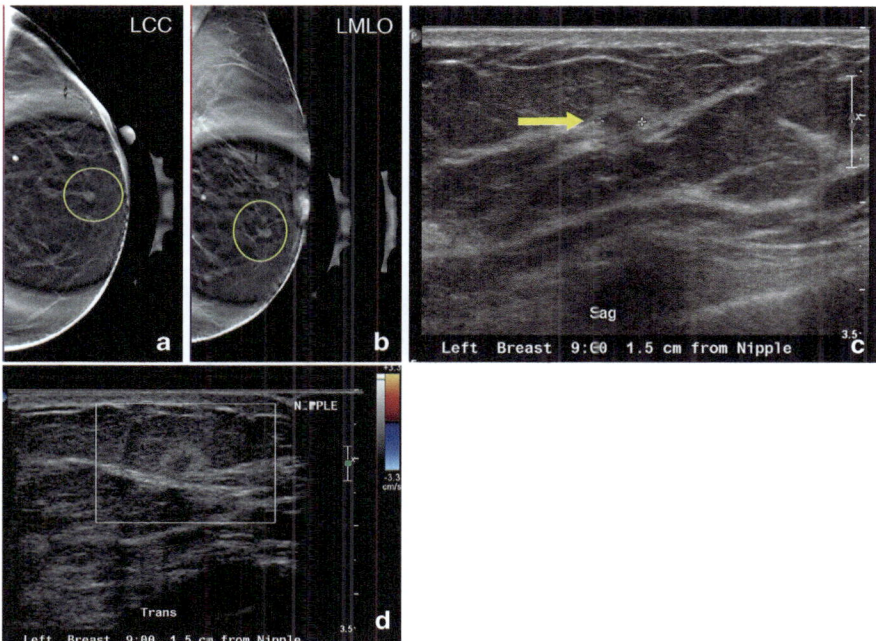

Fig. 9.8 (**a–d**) Fat necrosis. 76-year-old female with history of left breast grade 3 invasive ductal cancer status post lumpectomy, radiation and 5 years of anastrozole. Spot compression LCC (**a**) and LMLO (**b**) views with tomosynthesis demonstrate a 5 mm spiculated mass at 9 o'clock at anterior depth. US demonstrates a 5 mm round irregular hypoechoic mass with an echogenic rind (**c**; arrow) and no internal vascularity (**d**). Biopsy confirmed fat necrosis

- Ultrasound—oil cysts range from anechoic to mixed solid and cystic; coarse calcifications may cause posterior acoustic shadowing; heterogeneous mass with scattered cystic and echogenic areas, rarely irregular shadowing mass
- MRI—area or mass with internal fat that follows T1 and T2 signal characteristics of fat (Fig. e9.7)
  ○ Manage conservatively as symptoms usually improve with time

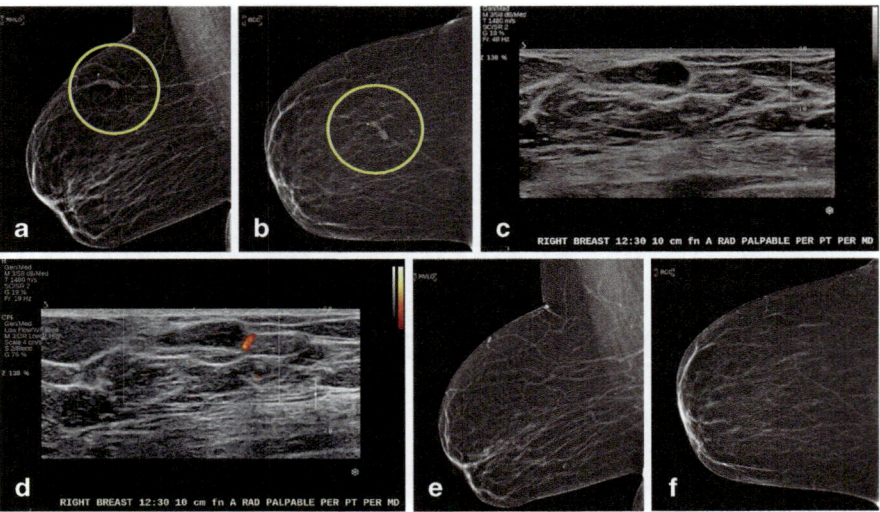

Fig. 9.9 (a–f) **Mondor's disease (thrombophlebitis).** 66-year-old female presenting with painful palpable mass in the upper outer right breast, designated by BB. RMLO (**a**) and RCC (**b**) views demonstrate a dilated tubular structure contiguous with a vein in the upper central right breast (yellow circles). Ultrasound of the palpable abnormality demonstrates superficial tubular noncompressible hypoechoic structure without internal vascularity (**c, d**) corresponding to a thrombosed vein. Patient was conservatively treated for pain with anti-inflammatory and analgesics for superficial thrombophlebitis. Follow-up right mammogram in 6 months demonstrates resolution of the thrombosed vein (**e, f**)

Mondor's Disease

- Superficial thrombophlebitis of breast vein typically due to trauma or recent surgery which presents as superficial tender palpable cord or string of tissue; may also see skin dimpling on clinical exam when acute
- Imaging (Fig. 9.9)
    - Mammography—tubular beaded opacity corresponding to thrombosed vein
- Ultrasound—distended or dilated non-compressible superficial vein with no vascular flow on Doppler
- Treat with warm compresses, NSAIDs, and sometimes antibiotics, if infection is of concern
- Will resolve spontaneously

FIBROCYSTIC CHANGES

- Fluid collection contained by breast lobule, most commonly seen in premenopausal women during latter half of menstrual cycle and in perimenopausal women
- Simple cyst—entirely anechoic mass with or without thin septations (Fig. 9.10)
- Clustered microcysts—grouped cysts (Fig. 9.11)

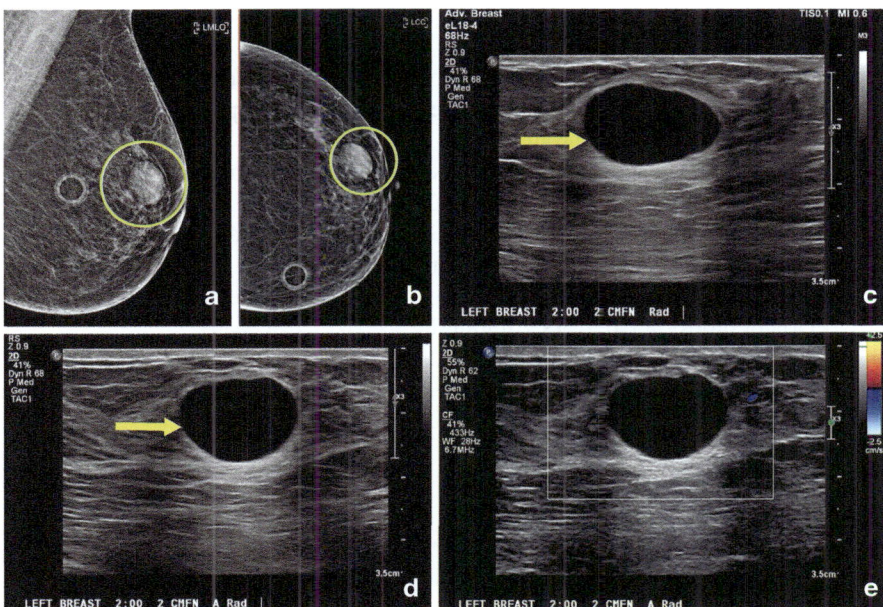

Fig. 9.10 **Simple cyst** (**a–e**). 65-year-old female with palpable mass in left breast. LMLO (**a**) and LCC (**b**) views demonstrate an oval circumscribed mass in the upper outer left breast corresponding to the palpable mass (yellow circles). Ultrasound demonstrates an oval parallel anechoic mass with posterior enhancement and without internal vascularity representing a simple cyst (**c–e**; yellow arrows)

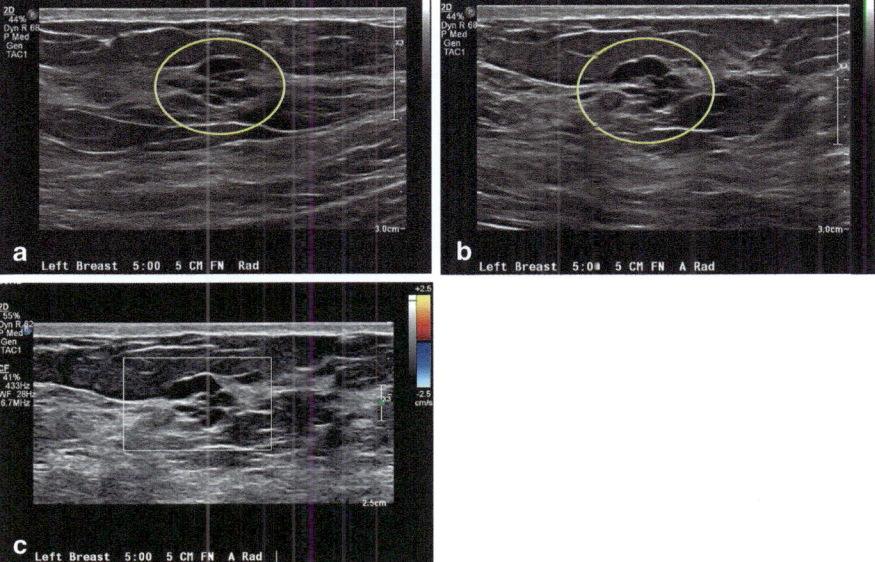

Fig. 9.11 (**a–c**) **Clustered microcysts**. 27-year-old female with palpable lump left lower outer breast. Ultrasound demonstrates a collection of small anechoic cysts without internal vascularity (**a–c**; yellow circles)

- Complicated cyst—homogeneous internal echoes with <2% chance of malignancy (Fig. 9.12)
  - ○ Either aspirate to rule out solid lesion or follow-up imaging in 3–6 months
  - ○ Fluid sent to cytology if bloody or lesion does not completely resolve; patient may also request to send fluid
- Complex cyst—cystic mass with thickened or nodular internal septations with ≅ 30% chance of malignancy (Fig. e9.3)
  - ○ Percutaneous core biopsy indicated, most often with vacuum-assisted device
- Milk of calcium—calcium precipitating out within cyst resulting in "teacup" appearance or layering on the 90° projection (Figs. 9.13, e9.8, and 9.14)
  - ○ Do not biopsy—BIRADS 2 finding!

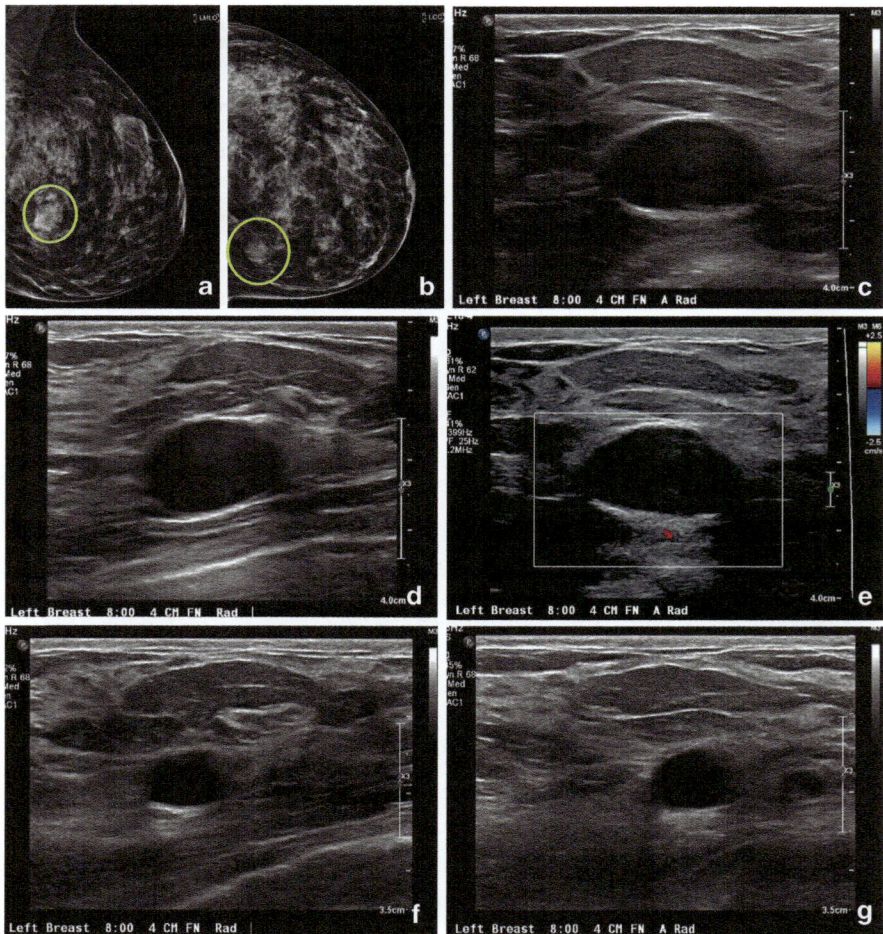

Fig. 9.12 (**a–g**) **Complicated cyst**. 44-year-old female with oval mass in medial central left breast at posterior depth (yellow circles) on screening mammogram (**a, b**). Ultrasound demonstrates oval circumscribed hypoechoic mass with low level internal echoes and posterior enhancement (**c, d**). Color Doppler image shows no internal vascularity (**e**). On follow-up imaging, the complicated cyst significantly decreased in size (**f, g**)

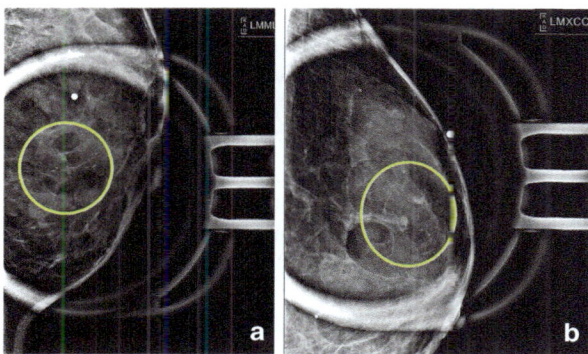

Fig. 9.13 (a, b) **Milk of Calcium/Layering Calcifications**: 50-year-old female with screen detected group of calcifications. LML magnification view (**a**) demonstrates group of layering calcifications centrally and anteriorly (yellow circle). LXCCL magnification view (**b**) demonstrates the group of calcifications to be less distinct/amorphous representing milk of calcium (yellow circle)

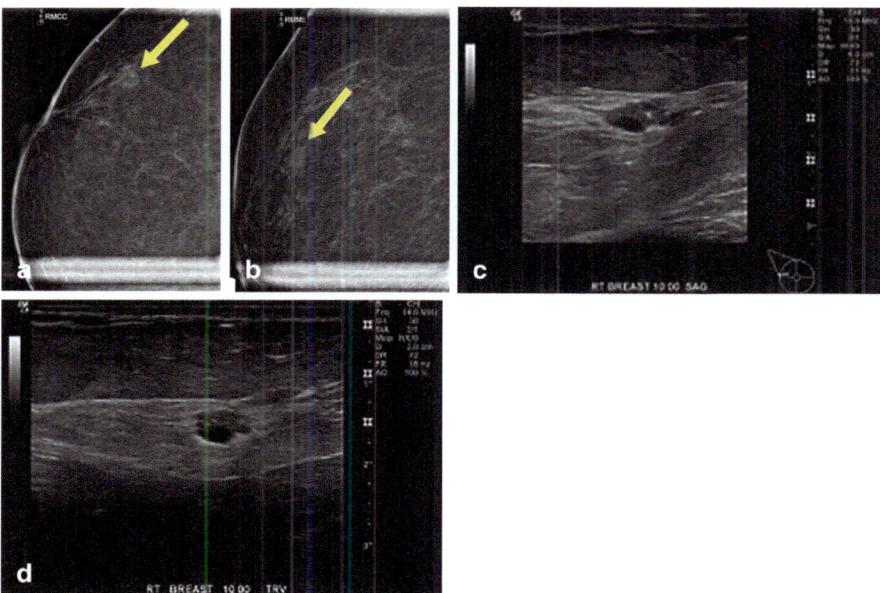

Fig. 9.14 **Apocrine cysts with calcium oxalate**. 49-year-old female with low attenuation mass containing calcifications (arrows; **a**, **b**). Ultrasound (**c**, **d**) showed cystic appearing mass with echogenic foci. Biopsy confirmed apocrine cysts with calcium oxalate

- Apocrine metaplasia—variant of fibrocystic change presenting as solid-appearing mass containing multiple microcystic areas (Fig. e9.9)
  - ○ Recommend follow-up imaging in 6 months to assess for fluctuation—BIRADS 3

- Imaging
  - Mammography—circumscribed iso-dense mass and/or focally grouped to diffusely scattered calcifications which layer ("teacup") on the lateral projection
  - Ultrasound—anechoic mass with thin barely perceptible wall and posterior acoustic enhancement
  - MRI—(Fig. e9.10)
    - T2 bright, T1 isointense non-enhancing or rim-enhancing mass
    - T2 dark, T1 bright non-enhancing mass consistent with proteinaceous cyst

PSEUDOANGIOMATOUS STROMAL HYPERPLASIA (PASH)

- Hormonally sensitive benign stromal proliferation with slit-like spaces lined by spindle shaped fibroblasts and myofibroblasts resembling endothelial cells
- Primarily seen in premenopausal and perimenopausal women
- Most often found incidentally on breast biopsy performed for another lesion (non-tumoral) but may also present as a mass or developing asymmetry on imaging (tumoral)
- Imaging (tumoral form)
  - Mammography—circumscribed mass or developing asymmetry (Fig. 9.15)
  - Ultrasound—circumscribed isoechoic to hypoechoic mass often with posterior acoustic enhancement and sometimes micro- to macro-cystic spaces (Fig. e9.11)
  - MRI—focal enhancing mass or clumped non-mass enhancement with persistent or plateau kinetics and variable T1-weighted and T2-weighted signal characteristics
- Management—routine screening, but if enlarges, repeat biopsy

⟶

Fig. 9.15 Pseudoangiomatous stromal hyperplasia (PASH) (a–k). 44-year-old female with palpable mass fluctuating with menstrual cycle in upper outer quadrant right breast. RMLO view 5 years prior (**a**), current RMLO (**b**) and current RXCCL (**c**) views demonstrate new asymmetry in upper outer right breast at posterior depth corresponding to palpable mass (yellow circles). Ultrasound at 10:00, 10 cm from the nipple demonstrates oval hyperechoic area (**d, e**; oval) with internal vascularity (**f**). Ultrasound-guided biopsy was performed with post clip placement RML view showing accurate position of clip (**g**; yellow circle). Pathology demonstrated PASH. 43-year-old female recalled from screening mammogram with spot compression tomosynthesis RMLO (**h**) and RCC (**i**) images of right breast showing oval mass in central outer right breast at posterior depth (circle). Ultrasound demonstrates heterogeneous oval mass at 9:00 6 cm from the nipple (**j, k**; yellow arrows). Pathology following ultrasound-guided core biopsy confirmed PASH

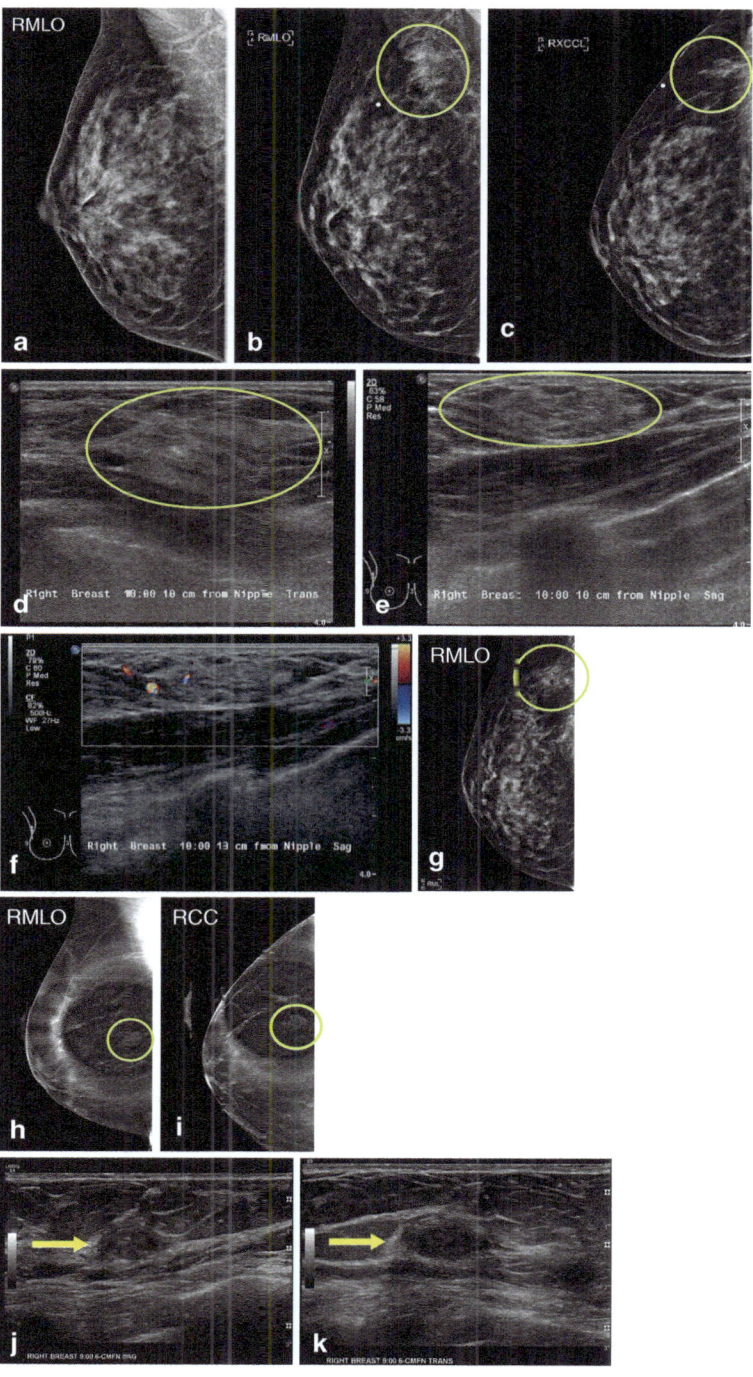

FIBROADENOMA

- Most common benign neoplasm in women in their 20s and 30s
- Typically < 3 cm palpable lump that can fluctuate with menstrual cycle or enlarge during pregnancy; may be found incidentally on mammography (Fig. 9.16)
- Most often solitary but up to 20% multiple
- Juvenile variant—in girls 10–18 years; rapidly enlarging breast lump up to 10 cm in size
- Imaging
  - Mammography—circumscribed mass which can develop coarse (popcorn-like) calcifications (Fig. 9.17)
  - Ultrasound—circumscribed homogeneously hypoechoic mass sometimes with posterior acoustic enhancement and variable peripheral and internal vascularity
    - Presence of marked internal vascularity, heterogeneous internal echotexture, or cystic spaces warrant biopsy to exclude circumscribed malignancy or phyllodes
  - MRI—classic appearance is T2 hyperintense, T1 isointense circumscribed homogeneously enhancing mass with dark internal septations and Type 1 or 2 kinetics, less often has Type 3 kinetics, and heterogeneous internal enhancement (Fig. e9.12)
- Management—follow-up imaging or biopsy depending on patient preference or imaging features; excise if symptomatic or if biopsy-proven fibroadenoma enlarges given concern for phyllodes

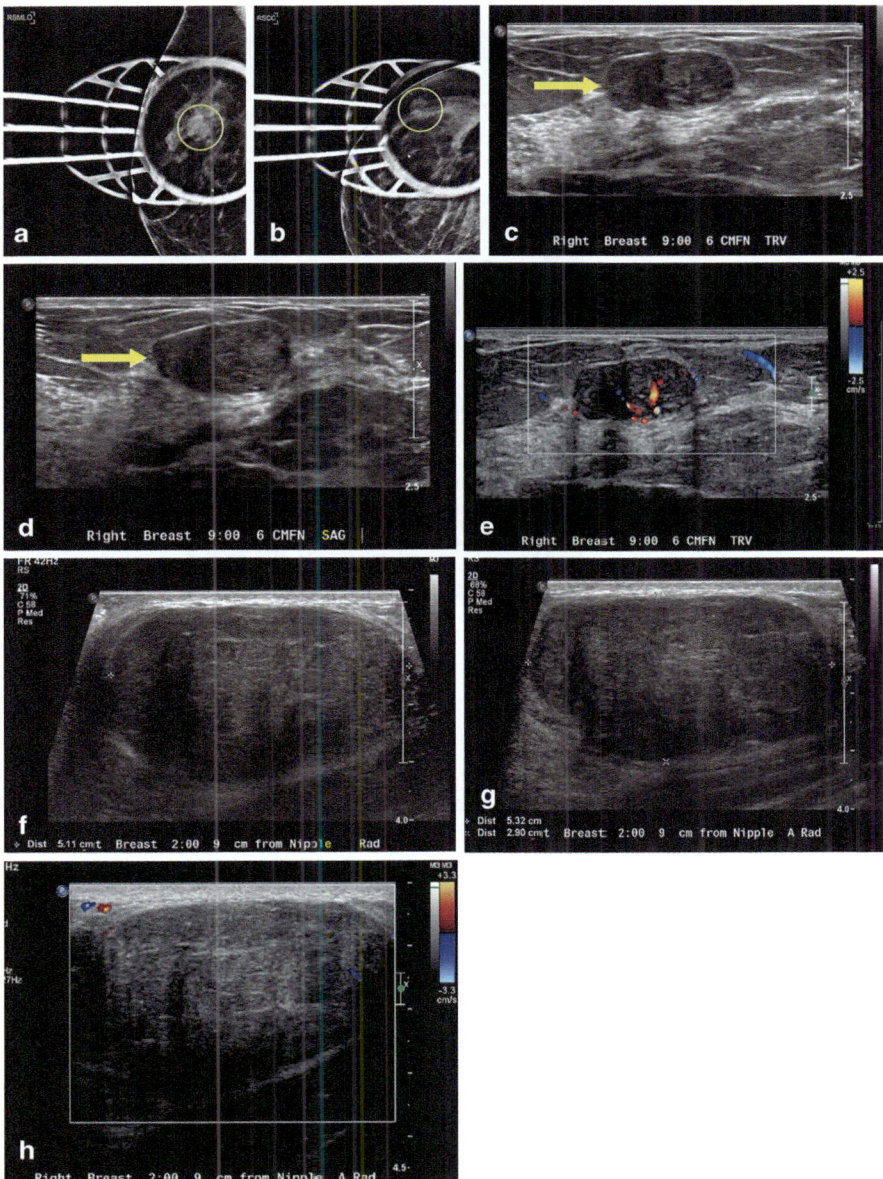

Fig. 9.16 Fibroadenoma. (**a–h**) 46-year-old female with palpable mass in right breast. Spot compression RMLO (**a**) and RCC (**b**) views demonstrate oval mass in upper outer quadrant of right breast (yellow circles). Targeted ultrasound at 9:00, 6 cm from the nipple demonstrates oval circumscribed hypoechoic mass (**c, d**, yellow arrows) with internal vascularity (**e**). Pathology following ultrasound-guided core biopsy demonstrated fibroadenoma. 17-year-old female with targeted ultrasound of a palpable mass at 2:00 in the right breast demonstrates 5 cm oval circumscribed hypoechoic mass (**f, g**) without internal vascularity (**h**). The mass was surgically excised and shown to represent a juvenile fibroadenoma

Fig. 9.17 Fibroadenoma. 55-year-old female with coarse (popcorn-like) calcifications in the central upper posterior breast (**a**, **b**; arrows) consistent with an involuted fibroadenoma

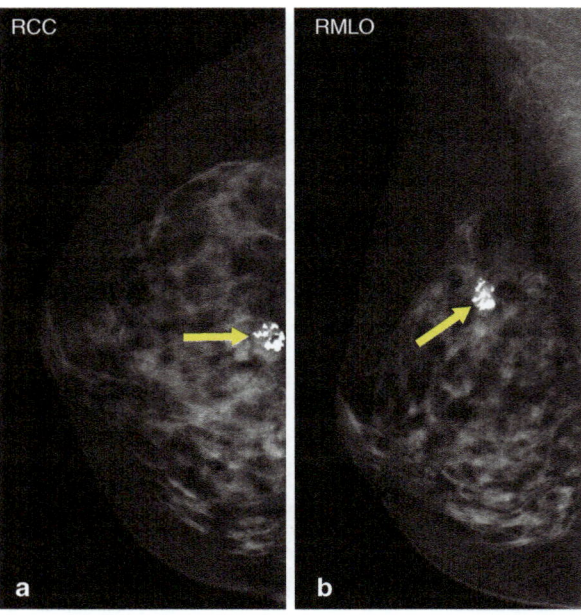

TUBULAR ADENOMA

- Rare epithelial benign tumor indistinguishable from fibroadenoma on presentation and imaging (Fig. e9.13)
- Typically seen in premenopausal women but have also been reported in postmenopausal women
- Managed conservatively when diagnosed on core biopsy

PHYLLODES

- Locally aggressive rare nearly always benign fibroepithelial neoplasm most often seen in women in third and fourth decades characterized by "leaf-like" proliferation of connective tissue
- Up to 10% may be malignant
- Classic history—rapidly enlarging palpable mass over few weeks but can be found incidentally on imaging (Fig. 9.18)
- Difficult to distinguish from cellular fibroadenoma on core biopsy histopathology

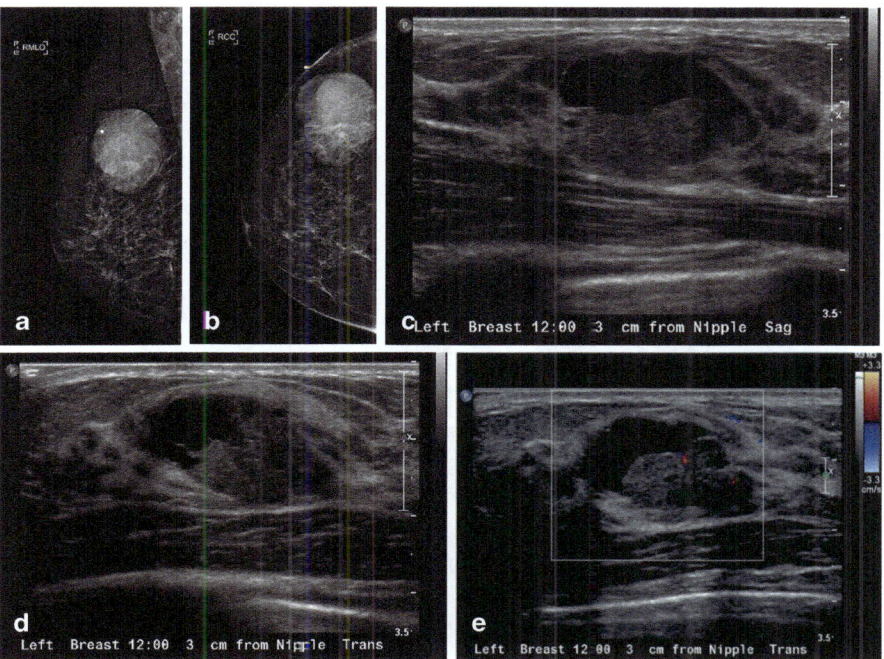

Fig. 9.18 Phyllodes tumor. (**a–e**) 58-year-old female with palpable mass in the upper outer quadrant of the right breast with RMLO (**a**) and RCC (**b**) views demonstrating large circumscribed mass. Patient underwent right mastectomy for malignant phyllodes. 29-year-old female with palpable lump at 12:00 in the left breast. Targeted left breast ultrasound demonstrates an oval circumscribed mixed cystic and solid mass at 12:00 3 cm from the nipple (**c, d**) with internal vascularity in the solid component (**e**). Pathology demonstrated benign phyllodes tumor

- Imaging
  - ○ Mammography—circumscribed mass typically without associated calcifications
  - ○ Ultrasound—circumscribed hypoechoic mass with heterogeneous internal echotexture and microcystic spaces
- Managed with wide surgical excision to achieve clear margins as has high local recurrence rate

FIBROEPITHELIAL LESION

- Comprised of cellular fibroadenomas and phyllodes tumors
- When found on core biopsy, surgical excision indicated (Figs. 9.19 and e9.14)

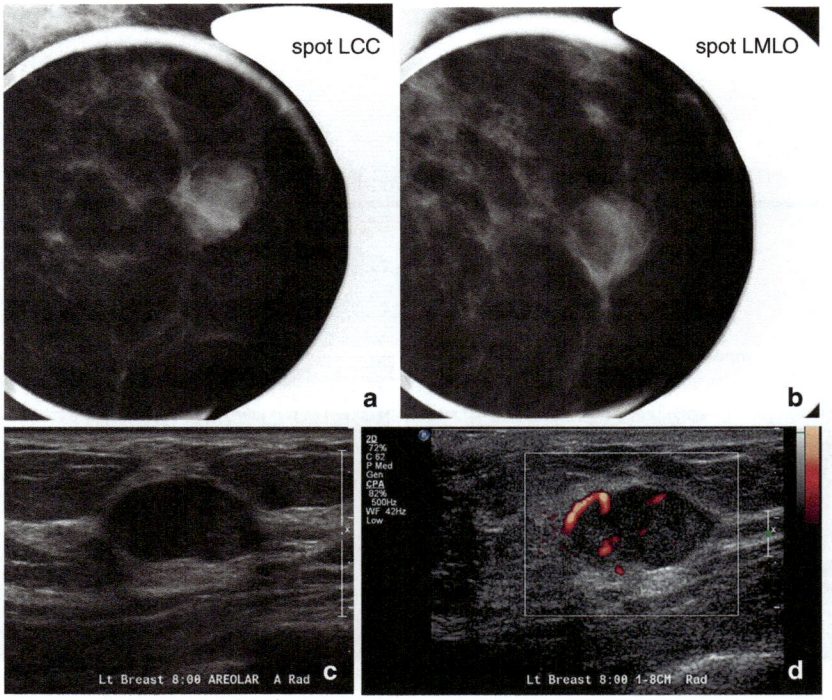

Fig. 9.19 **Fibroepithelial lesion**. 46-year-old female recalled from screening for left breast mass. Spot compression CC (**a**) and MLO (**b**) views confirm circumscribed mass in the inner central left breast. US (**c**, **d**) showed a hypoechoic oval mass with internal vascularity at 8:00. Biopsy revealed fibroepithelial lesion. Subsequent excision confirmed fibroadenoma

SCLEROSING ADENOSIS

- Benign lobulocentric proliferation of glands, tubules, and stroma
- Most often found incidentally on biopsy for other causes (Fig. 9.20)
- "Nodular" variant presents as palpable and mimics fibroadenoma on imaging (Fig. e9.15)
- Managed conservatively when diagnosed on core biopsy

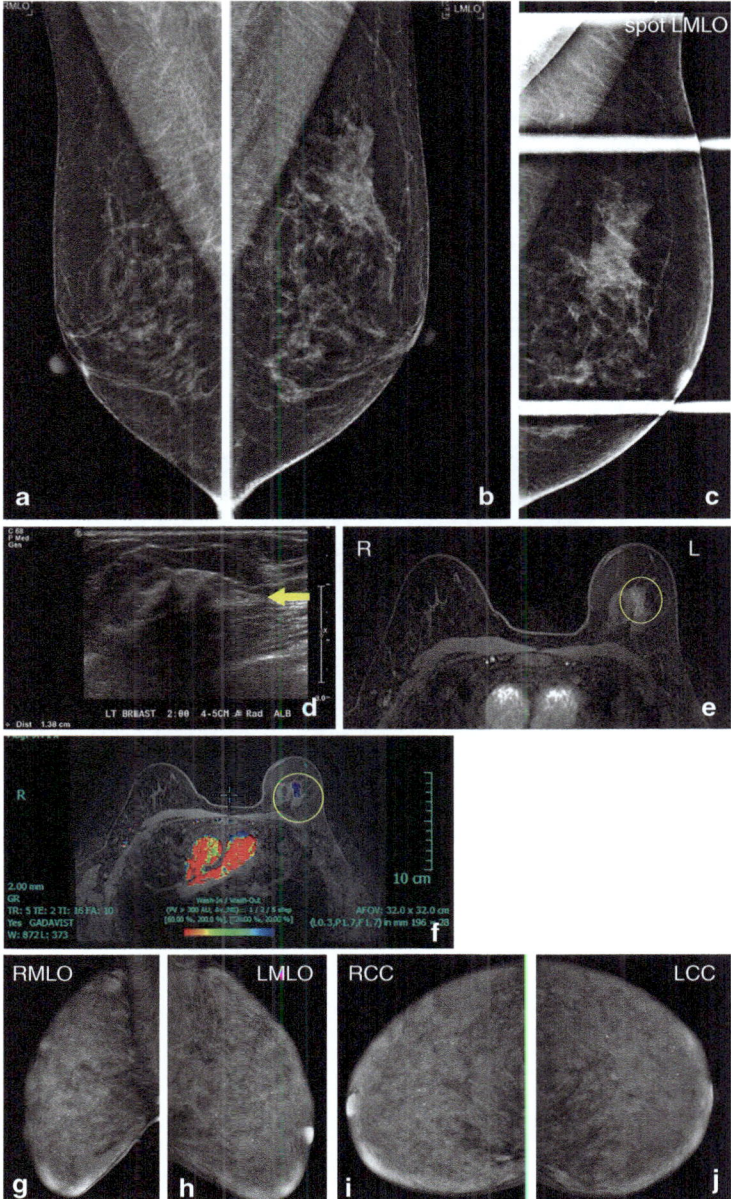

Fig. 9.20 **Sclerosing adenosis**. (**a**–**j**) 40-year-old female screening mammogram with asymmetry in the left upper breast (**a**, **b**) persisting on spot compression MLO view (**c**). Ultrasound demonstrates heterogeneous mass with indistinct margins and posterior acoustic shadowing at 2:00 (**d**). MRI was performed for further evaluation, demonstrating non-mass enhancement (**e**) with persistent enhancement kinetics corresponding to the finding on mammography and ultrasound (**f**). Biopsy confirmed sclerosing adenosis. 53-year-old female with MLO (**g**, **h**) and CC (**i**, **j**) views demonstrating extremely dense breasts with bilateral diffuse scattered calcifications consistent with sclerosing adenosis

HAMARTOMA

- Also referred to as fibroadenolipoma or "breast within a breast" as lesion is comprised of fat, connective tissue and glandular tissue
- May be palpable and enlarge over time
- Does not require biopsy for diagnosis as pathognomic on imaging
- Imaging
  - Mammography—encapsulated circumscribed oval mass containing fat and soft tissue densities; rarely, calcifications (Figs. 9.21 and e9.16)
  - Ultrasound—encapsulated circumscribed mass of mixed echotexture
- Managed conservatively

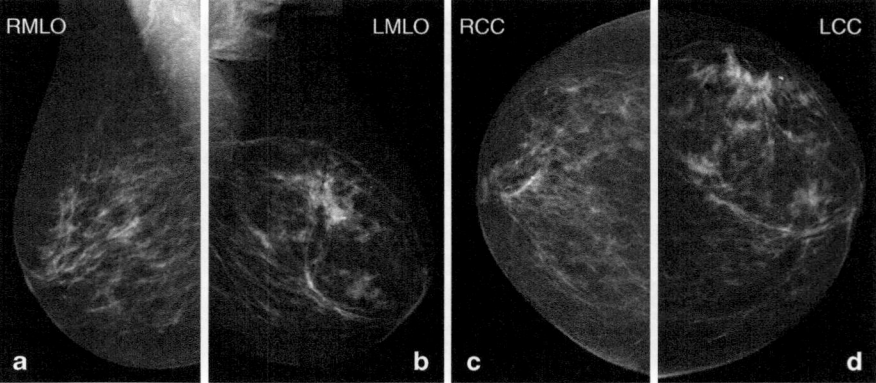

Fig. 9.21 **Hamartoma**. 53-year-old female for screening. MLO (**a, b**) and CC (**c, d**) views show a large encapsulated mass comprised of fat and soft tissue density in the entire upper outer left breast consistent with a hamartoma or fibroadenolipoma

LIPOMA

- Fatty encapsulated mass that typically presents as palpable mass on exam
- Can enlarge over time and may be multiple
- Imaging
  - Mammography—Thin-rimmed fat-containing mass (Figs. 9.22 and e9.17)
  - Ultrasound—most often homogeneously echogenic mass, but may be isoechoic; often can appreciate rim of encapsulation
- Managed conservatively but may be excised if enlarge or become cosmetic issue

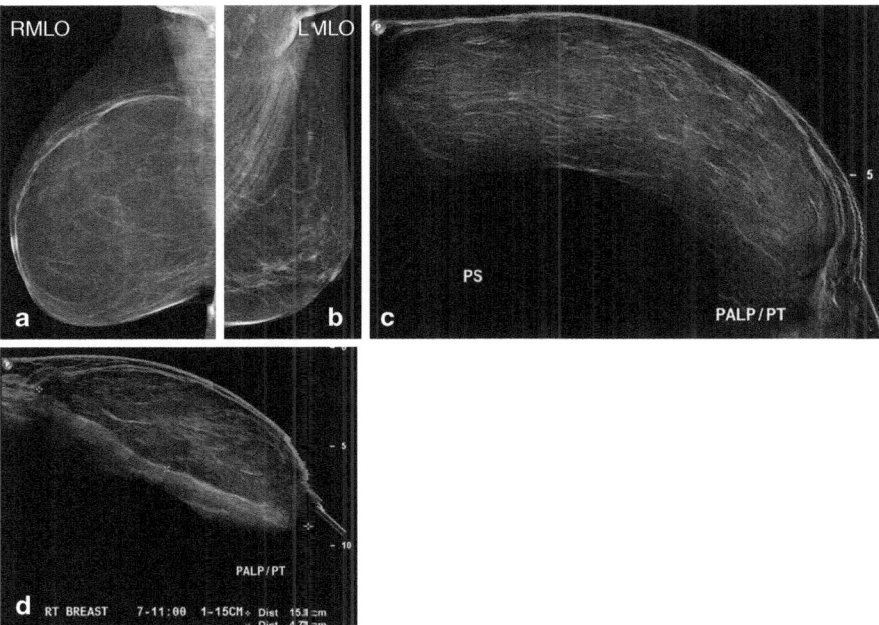

Fig. 9.22 Lipoma. 67-year-old with asymmetrically enlarged right breast. MLO views (**a, b**) show large radiolucent encapsulated mass in the right breast consistent with lipoma. Notice how the right breast is much larger than the left breast due to the lipoma US (**c, d**) shows corresponding 15 cm isoechoic encapsulated mass. The patient opted for surgical excision given asymmetric breast size

INTRAMAMMARY LYMPH NODE

- Benign < 1 cm reniform circumscribed mass with fatty hilum nearly always found in the upper outer breast; other locations warrant further characterization with imaging (Fig. 9.23)
- May enlarge or become denser due to reactive hyperplasia or due to other inflammatory or malignant diseases (Fig. 9.24)
- Imaging
  - ○ Mammography—reniform low attenuation mass with a fatty notch in upper outer breast
  - ○ Ultrasound—hypoechoic cortical rim less than 0.3 cm in diameter with central echogenicity; occasional trilaminar appearance with alternating echogenic, hypoechoic, and then echogenic fat centrally
- Manage conservatively unless enlarging, abnormal morphology, or cortical thickness exceeds 0.3 cm prompting biopsy

Fig. 9.23 Intramammary lymph node. (a, b) 69-year-old female for routine screening mammogram. RMLO and RCC tomosynthesis images demonstrate oval circumscribed mass with a fatty hilum in the upper outer right breast at mid depth representing an intramammary lymph node (yellow circles)

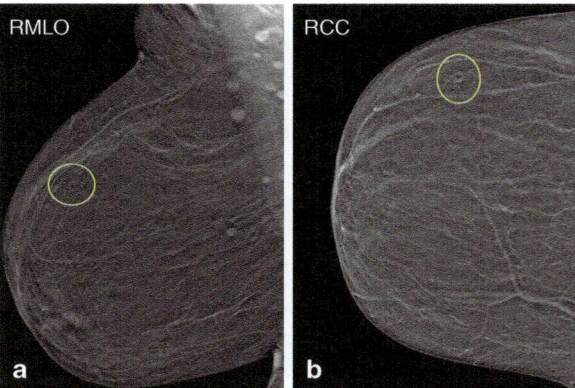

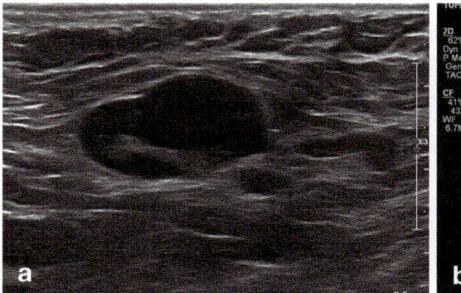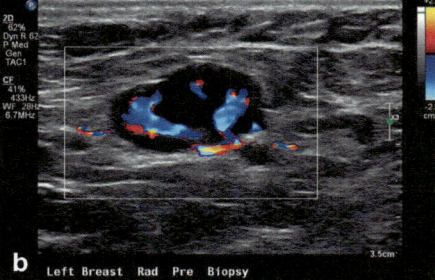

Fig. 9.24 COVID lymphadenopathy. 54-year-old with strong family history. Screening MRI (not shown) showed enlarged nodes in the superior left axilla. Ultrasound (**a, b**) confirmed a 2 cm lymph node with a 0.8 cm thickened cortex. Given recent COVID vaccination, the finding was consistent with reactive lymphadenopathy. The patient opted for biopsy given her family history, which confirmed reactive lymphadenopathy

DUCT ECTASIA

- Benign dilatation with fluid within one or more milk ducts
- Common cause of clear nipple discharge
- Most often asymptomatic, but when marked, may be etiology for nipple discharge
- Can develop periductal mastitis due to inflammatory reaction to ductal fluid
- Nodular appearance within the duct may represent chronic inflammatory infiltrates or solid intraductal mass often leading to biopsy
- Imaging
  - Mammography—retroareolar tubular low attenuation branching structures tapering into breast periphery (Fig. 9.25)
    - Internal nodular appearance if chronic inflammatory infiltrates (Fig. 9.26)
  - Ultrasound—dilated ducts filled with fluid or proteinaceous debris
  - MRI—T2 hyperintense fluid within dilated ducts; ductal enhancement if periductal mastitis (Fig. 9.27)
- Managed conservatively with no need for follow-up imaging

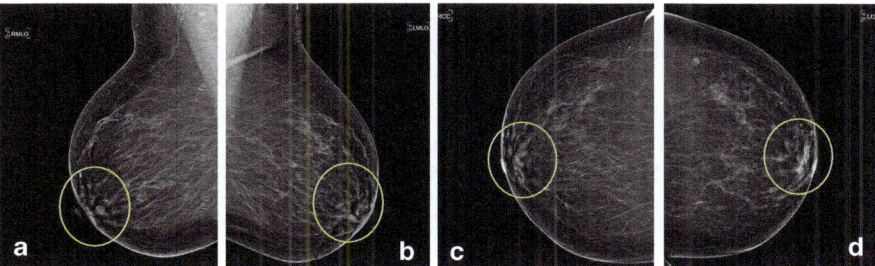

Fig. 9.25 Ductal ectasia (a–d) 72-year-old female presenting for routine screening mammogram. Bilateral subareolar tubular structures radiating from the nipple (a–d; yellow circles) represent ductal ectasia and demonstrated stability for over 7 years

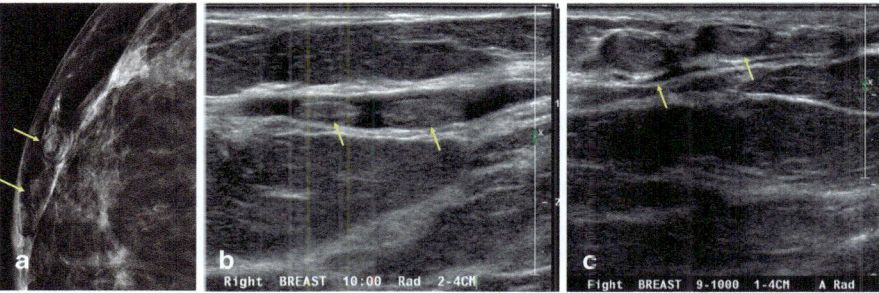

Fig. 9.26 Chronic inflammatory infiltrates. 54-year-old asymptomatic female for screening. Magnified CC view shows dilated retroareolar tubular structure with internal fatty and soft tissue density (a; arrows). US (b, c) show dilated duct with multiple avascular intraductal masses (arrows) at 9–10:00 in the right breast consistent with chronic inflammatory infiltrates

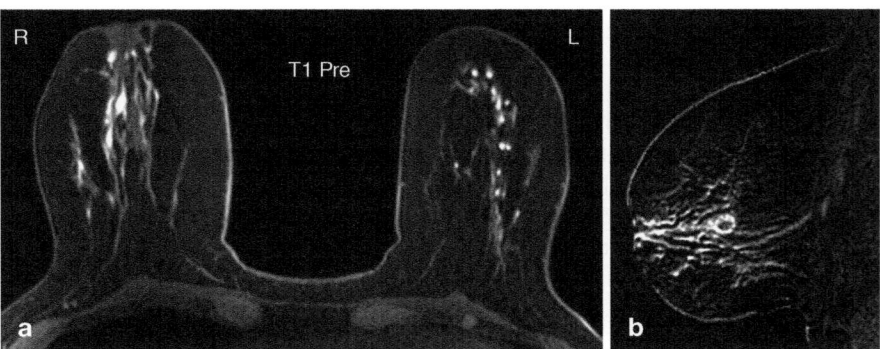

Fig. 9.27 Periductal mastitis. 59-year-old female with elevated prolactin found to have T1-hyperintense material within dilated ducts on axial MR pre-contrast image (**a**) and enhancement surrounding the ducts on post-contrast sagittal subtraction image (**b**). Findings consistent with periductal mastitis

PAPILLOMA/PAPILLOMATOSIS

- **Intraductal papilloma**
  - Benign neoplasm central lactiferous duct consisting of arborizing fronds with well-developed fibrovascular cores
  - Most common cause of spontaneous nipple discharge (most often bloody) typically found in women ages 30–50 years; rarely palpable
  - No increased risk for malignancy
  - Imaging
    - Mammography—< 1 cm circumscribed to slightly irregular mass which may have associated coarse calcifications, solitary dilated duct, or grouped heterogeneous calcifications in subareolar location (Figs. 9.28, e9.18, and e9.19)
    - Ultrasound—< 1 cm iso- to hypoechoic intraductal vascular mass
    - MRI—< 1 cm enhancing intraductal mass with Type I–III kinetics
  - Do not need to be surgically excised unless associated atypia, symptomatic or enlarge
- **Papillomatosis**
  - Multiple peripheral papillomas in terminal duct lobular units
  - Most often occur in younger women who are asymptomatic; rarely present with nipple discharge or mass
  - Carry 1.5–2× increased lifetime risk for breast cancer
  - Imaging
    - Mammography—segmentally dilated ductal system with multiple small non-calcified masses (Fig. e9.20)
    - Ultrasound—segmental dilated ducts with multiple intraductal vascular masses
  - Management difficult due to multiplicity; most often followed on imaging with biopsy indicated if there is interval change

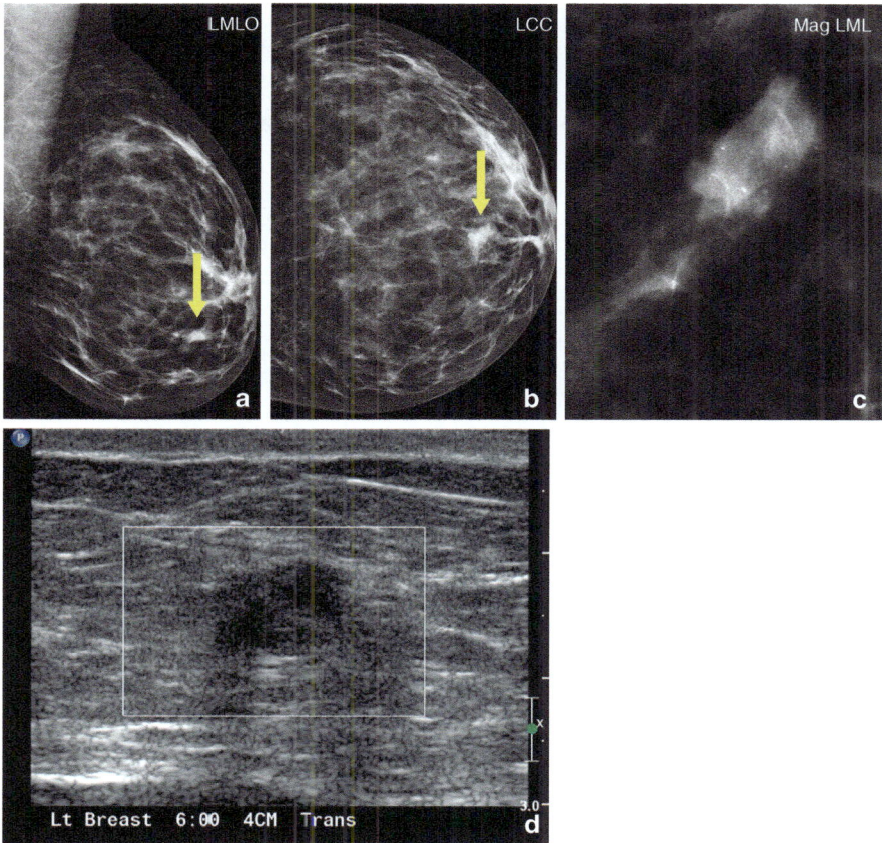

Fig. 9.28 **Intraductal papilloma**. 31-year-old female with left breast spontaneous yellowish nipple discharge. MLO (**a**) and CC (**b**) views show a solitary dilated retroareolar duct with an associated mass (arrow). Magnified lateral view (**c**) shows a mass with associated coarse round calcifications. US (**d**) identified a solid hypoechoic mass. Biopsy confirmed intraductal papilloma

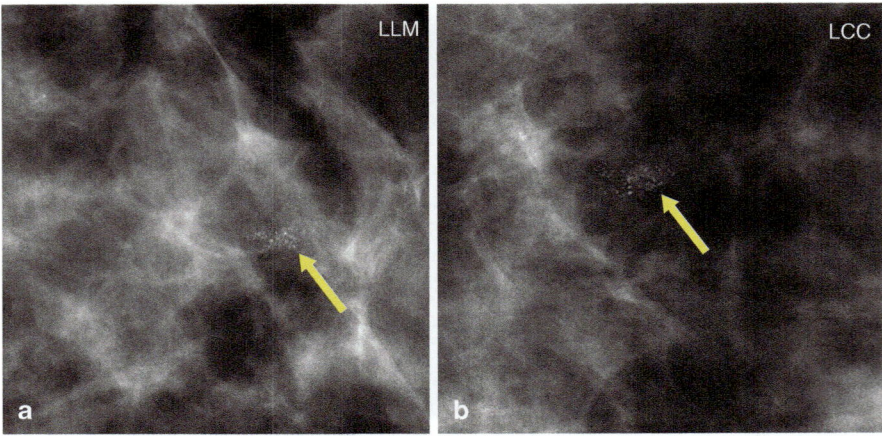

Fig. 9.29 **Atypical ductal hyperplasia (ADH).** 42-year-old female recalled from screening with left breast calcifications. Magnified lateral (**a**) and, CC (**b**) show grouped pleomorphic calcifications (yellow arrows). Biopsy confirmed ADH

HIGH RISK BENIGN LESIONS

- **HYPERPLASIA**
  - ○ Proliferative changes in terminal duct lobular unit that warrant surgical excision when atypia found on percutaneous core biopsy, unless determined to be incidental
  - ○ **USUAL DUCTAL HYPERPLASIA**
    - • Benign intraductal proliferation of epithelial cells
    - • Typically occult on imaging, although sometimes presents as grouped calcifications
    - • Most often found incidentally on biopsy for another lesion
  - ○ **ATYPICAL DUCTAL HYPERPLASIA**
    - • Epithelial proliferation in terminal duct lobular unit that borders on low grade ductal carcinoma in situ (DCIS)
    - • 4–5× increased lifetime risk for breast cancer when found on core biopsy
    - • Most commonly presents as grouped calcifications that can be round to pleomorphic; may be incidental
    - • Imaging
      - • Mammography—grouped round to pleomorphic calcifications (Fig. 9.29)
    - • Management—surgical removal when found on core biopsy as 10–40% may upgrade to DCIS upon excision

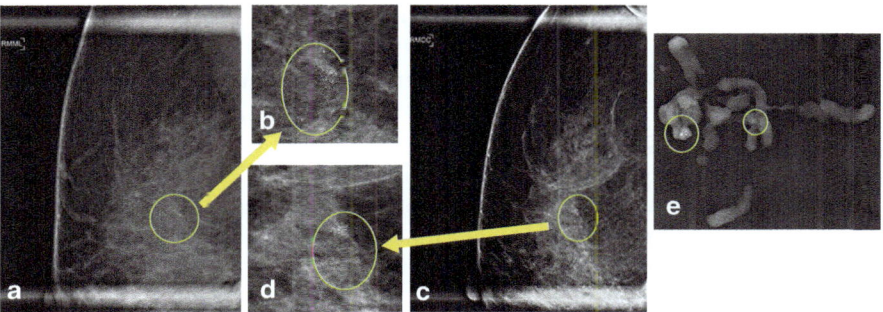

Fig. 9.30 (a–e) **53-year-old female recalled from screening mammogram for calcifications in the upper outer right breast**. Magnification RML (**a**, **b**) and RCC (**c**, **d**) views demonstrate a group of heterogeneous calcifications in the upper outer right breast with an additional smaller group of calcifications inferior and medial to the aforementioned calcifications (circles). Stereotactic guided core biopsy of the calcifications was performed with calcifications present in the specimen radiograph (**e**) and pathology demonstrated pleomorphic lobular carcinoma in situ. Surgical excision was subsequently performed

LOBULAR NEOPLASIA

- Proliferation of loosely cohesive epithelial cells in terminal duct lobular unit
- Consists of atypical lobular hyperplasia (ALH) and lobular carcinoma in situ (LCIS)
- **Atypical lobular hyperplasia**
  - Nearly always incidental as found on biopsy performed for other indications
  - Occult on imaging
  - 3–5× elevated lifetime risk for breast cancer
  - Usually surgically excised only if associated with other worrisome pathology
- **Lobular carcinoma in situ**
  - Typically found incidentally on biopsy of calcifications secondary to another etiology in predominantly premenopausal women
  - Most often multicentric and often bilateral if discovered in one breast
  - Considered to be risk factor for breast cancer as carries 7–10× elevation in lifetime risk
    - If develop cancer, most often invasive ductal cancer, although prevalence of invasive lobular cancers more than in average population
    - Not obligate precursor to invasive lobular cancer
  - Most often managed with surgical excision, especially if florid LCIS, as often associated with other concerning findings and then followed closely with imaging while on selective estrogen receptor modulators; can be followed on imaging if incidental and other findings are benign
- **Pleomorphic variant**
  - Presents with suspicious grouped or pleomorphic microcalcifications on mammography (Fig. 9.30)
  - Clinically behaves similar to DCIS so treated with surgical excision ± radiation therapy and treatment with selective estrogen receptor modulators

COMPLEX SCLEROSING LESION/RADIAL SCAR

- Sclerosing lesion with entrapment of benign glands and tubules by fibroelastotic stroma
  - Radial scar if ≤ 1 cm in size
  - Complex sclerosing lesion if > 1 cm size
- Most often present as architectural distortion or spiculated lesion with central lucency; may be incidental on biopsy for other reasons
- 2–10% associated with malignancy upon excision
- Imaging
  - Mammography—architectural distortion or spiculated mass with central lucency (Fig. 9.31)
  - Ultrasound—irregular hypoechoic mass with posterior acoustic shadowing
  - MRI—irregular T1 hypointense enhancing mass with Type I–III kinetics; can mimic malignancy (Fig. e9.21)
- Management—most often surgical excision if detected on core biopsy, unless incidental; follow up imaging reasonable if no atypia and biopsy performed with 8–9 gauge vacuum assisted device and at least 10–12 cores obtained

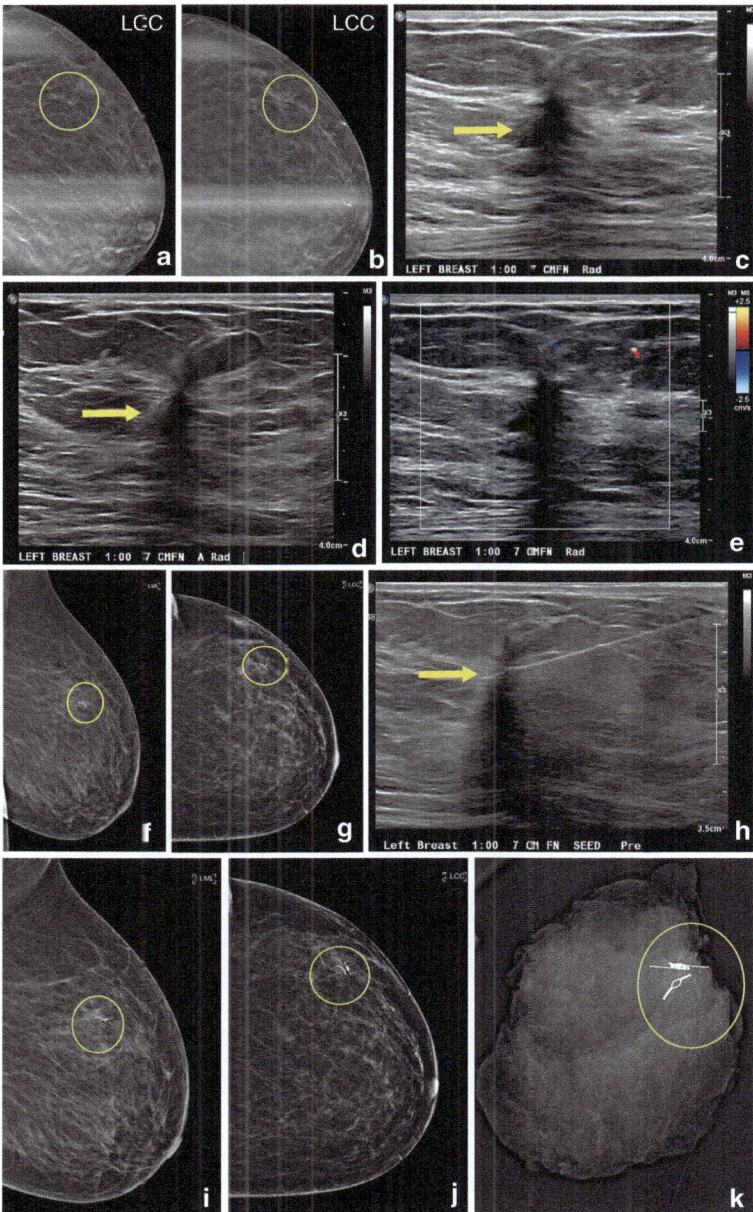

Fig. 9.31 Complex sclerosing lesion/radial scar (a–k). 48-year-old female screen detected architectural distortion in the upper outer left breast confirmed on LMLO and CC spot compression tomosynthesis views (**a**, **b**; yellow circles). Ultrasound at 1:00 demonstrates an irregular spiculated mass with posterior shadowing and no internal vascularity (**c–e**; yellow arrow). Ultrasound-guided biopsy was performed with LML and LCC post biopsy mammogram demonstrating accurate position of the eye shaped biopsy clip with respect to the architectural distortion (**f**, **g**; yellow circles). Pathology demonstrated radial scar. Ultrasound-guided Savi Scout reflector was placed for surgical excision (**h**) which was confirmed to be in appropriate position on LML and LCC views (**i**, **j**; yellow circles). Post lumpectomy specimen radiograph demonstrates excision of the architectural distortion, clip, and reflector (**k**; yellow circle) Final pathology revealed radial scar and post biopsy changes

RHEUMATOLOGIC DISEASES AFFECTING THE BREAST

- Comprised of systemic lupus erythematosus (SLE), dermatomyositis, rheumatoid arthritis, and sarcoidosis
- Often present with bilateral non-calcified axillary lymphadenopathy (Fig. 9.32); developing asymmetry or irregular mass may be seen (Fig. 9.33); if prior gold therapy for RA, can see high density material in nodes (Fig. 9.34); dystrophic calcifications may be seen in dermatomyositis (Fig. e9.22)
- Immunosuppressants ± steroids for management

Fig. 9.32 **Bilateral axillary nodes**. 50-year-old female for screening. MLO views (**a**, **b**) show bilateral dense prominent axillary nodes (arrows) consistent with systemic lupus erythematosus given clinical history

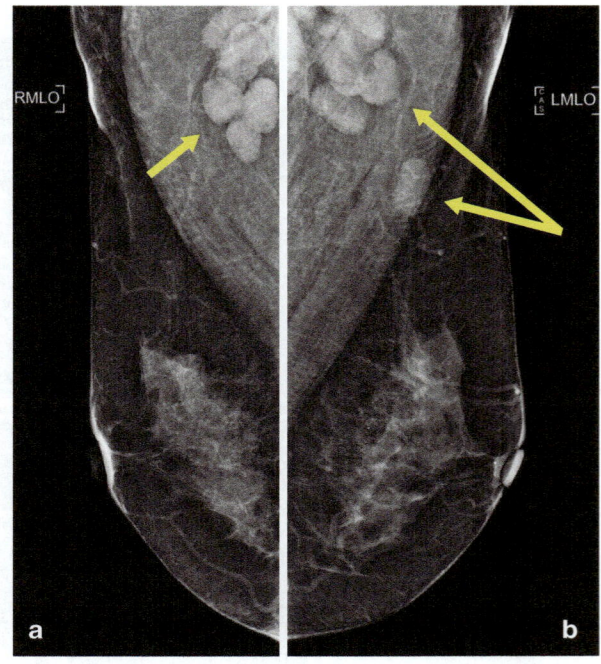

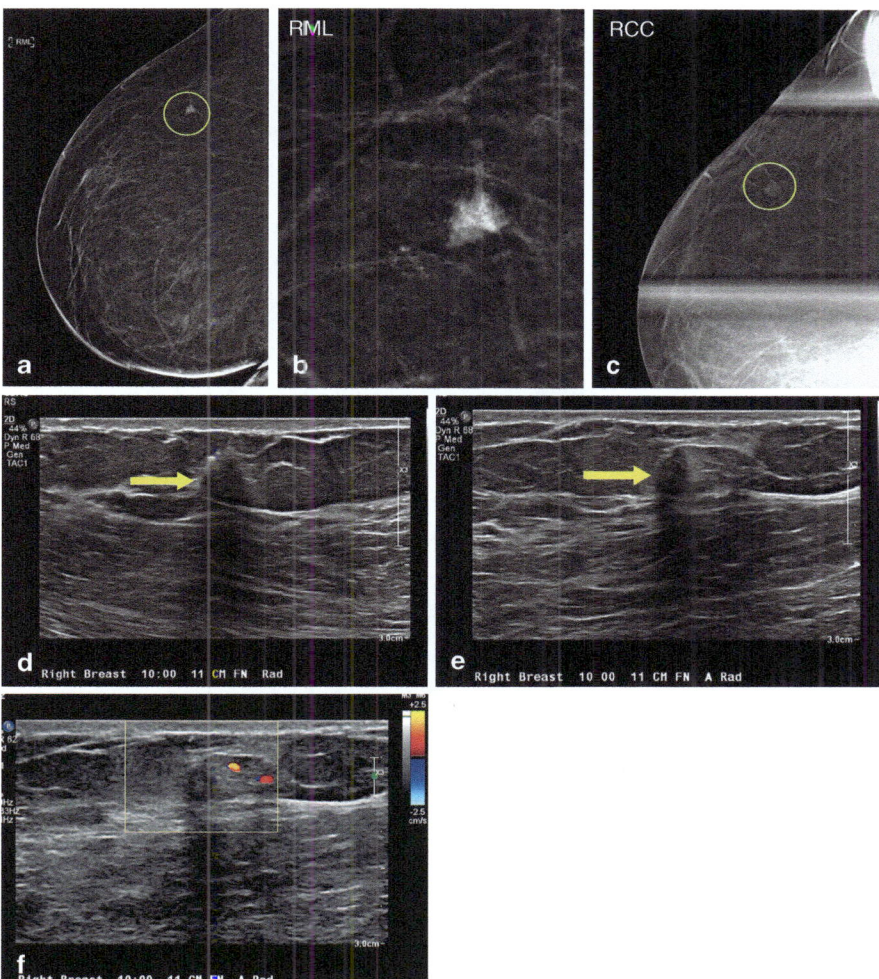

Fig. 9.33 **Sarcoidosis** (a–f). 42-year-old female with progressive lung sarcoidosis and recall from screening. RCC image (**a**), spot compression RML image (**b**) and tomosynthesis RCC slice (**c**) demonstrate a small irregular dense mass in upper outer right breast at mid depth (circle). Ultrasound demonstrates a taller than wide hypoechoic avascular irregular mass (arrow) with minimally angulated margins (**d–f**). Ultrasound core biopsy demonstrated non-necrotizing granulomatous inflammation with no ductal or lobular epithelium. AFB, PAS-GMS stains were negative for acid fast and fungal microorganisms. Findings were consistent with sarcoidosis

Fig. 9.34 Gold therapy for rheumatoid arthritis. 43-year-old female with high density material within non-enlarged axillary nodes (arrows) consistent with gold deposition

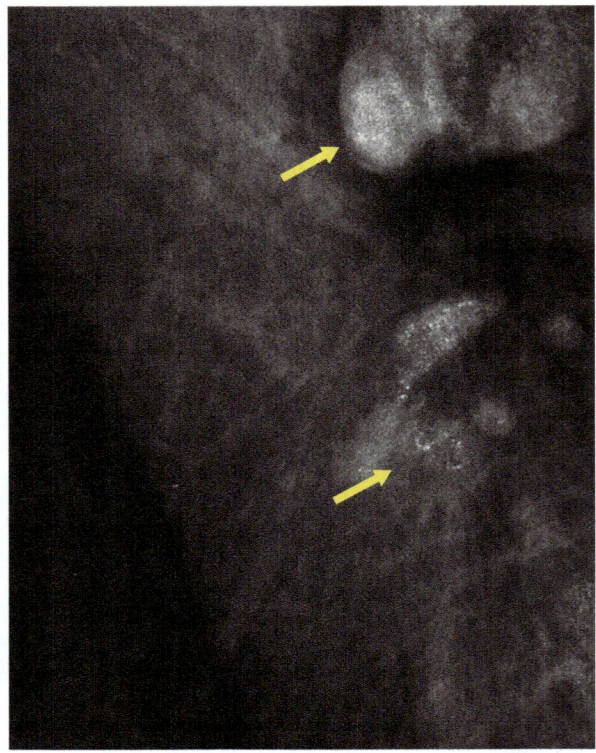

LYMPHOCYTIC MASTOPATHY (Aka. Diabetic Mastopathy)

- Sclerosing lymphocytic lobulitis with perivascular inflammation primarily affecting premenopausal women, many of whom have history of insulin-dependent diabetes mellitus
- Imaging shows focal asymmetry/asymmetries with hypovascular solid mass with posterior shadowing on US (Figs. 9.35 and e9.23)
- Diagnosed by core biopsy and managed conservatively

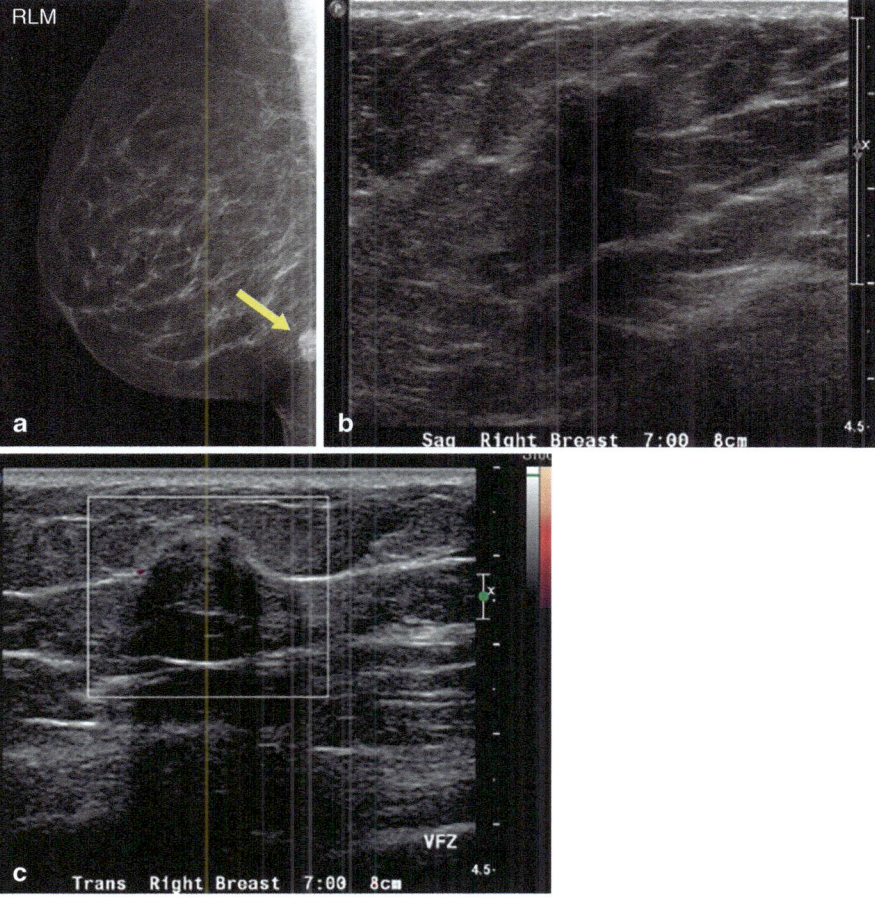

Fig. 9.35 **Lymphocytic mastopathy**. 43-year-old female. LM view (**a**) shows mass in the posterior inferior left breast (arrow). US (**b**, **c**) shows hypoechoic avascular mass with posterior acoustic shadowing. Biopsy confirmed lymphocytic mastopathy

DESMOID/FIBROMATOSIS

- Rare benign locally aggressive neoplasm characterized by low grade spindle cell proliferation
- May be associated with prior history of trauma, surgery, breast implants, or familial fibromatosis
- Most commonly present as palpable non-tender mass but can be painful if chest wall invasion

- Imaging
  - ○ Mammography—circumscribed to spiculated non-calcified mass (Fig. e9.24)
  - ○ Ultrasound—hypoechoic circumscribed to irregular mass
  - ○ MRI—enhancing mass with T1 hypointense to isointense signal and T2 hypointense to hyperintense signal (Fig. e9.25)
- Management—wide local excision given high risk of recurrence; if > 90% tumor volume T2 hyperintense on MR, may be followed on imaging

MYOFIBROBLASTOMA

- Uncommon benign stromal tumor comprised of spindle cells and hyalinized collagen that more commonly occurs in postmenopausal women and elderly men
- On imaging, circumscribed or irregular mass without calcifications (Fig. e9.26)
- Management—wide surgical excision to minimize chance of local recurrence

References

1. Agarwal M, Venkataraman S, Slanetz PJ. Infections in the breast—common imaging presentations and mimics. Semin Roentgenol. 2017;52(2):101–7.
2. Ferris-James DM, Iuanow E, Mehta TS, Shaheen RM, Slanetz PJ. Imaging approaches to diagnosis and management of common ductal abnormalities. Radiographics. 2012;32:1009–30.
3. Krishnamurthy S, Bevers T, Keurer H, Yang WT. Multidisciplinary considerations in the management of high-risk breast lesions. Am J Roentgenol. 2012;198:W132–40.
4. Kaneda HJ, Mack J, Kasales CJ, Schetter S. Pediatric and adolescent breast masses: a review of pathophysiology, imaging, diagnosis and treatment. Am J Roentgenol. 2013;200:W204–12.

Breast Malignancy

10

Danielle Del Re, Tom Soker, and Priscilla J. Slanetz

Includes primary breast cancer, extramammary metastatic disease to breast, and lymphoma/leukemia (primary and secondary).

PRIMARY BREAST CANCER

Heterogeneous disease originating from epithelial cells in the terminal duct lobular unit (TDLU)

- One in eight women will develop breast cancer in lifetime
  - Incidence increases with age (1:1000 age 40 to 5:1000 by age 80)
- Approximately 310,720 invasive carcinomas and 56,500 DCIS diagnosed annually in the USA (2024 estimate); men account for 1% of these diagnoses
- Early detection minimizes morbidity (e.g., less extensive surgery and less chemotherapy) and maximizes survival
  - 5-year survival 93–98% localized disease, 78–89% regional disease, 21–34% distant disease
  - Factors influencing survival: stage at diagnosis, tumor grade and receptor status, age at diagnosis, medical co-morbidities
  - Racial and ethnic minorities more likely diagnosed at later stage resulting in worse prognosis and higher morbidity

Supplementary Information The online version contains supplementary material available at https://doi.org/10.1007/978-3-031-56274-4_10.

D. Del Re · T. Soker · P. J. Slanetz (✉)
Division of Breast Imaging, Department of Radiology, Boston University Medical Center, Boston, MA, USA
e-mail: priscilla.slanetz@bmc.org

- Most commonly metastasizes to bones, lung, brain, and liver
- Risk factors: female gender, increasing age, family history of breast cancer (especially premenopausal first-degree relative), prior benign biopsy revealing atypia, BRCA-1 or 2 mutation carrier, early menarche, late menopause, dense breast tissue, Black race, late child-bearing (first child after age 30 years), nulliparity, obesity (high BMI), excessive alcohol intake

Detection and Diagnosis

- Imaging abnormality (mammography, ultrasound, or MRI) or symptomatic (palpable lump, discharge, nipple inversion, and focal pain)
  - Compare to prior exams, ideally 4–5 years prior
  - Look for mass (Fig. 10.1), asymmetry (Fig. 10.2), calcifications (Fig. 10.3), distortion (Fig. 10.4), nipple retraction/inversion, skin/trabecular thickening, enlarged axillary nodes
  - Pay extra attention to fat–glandular interfaces (Fig. 10.5), image edges (Fig. 10.6), nipple-areolar region (Fig. 10.7), retroglandular space, axilla
- Diagnose by percutaneous core needle biopsy
- Disease may be focal, multifocal (two or more tumors in <u>same</u> quadrant), or multicentric (two or more tumors in <u>different</u> quadrants) with or without axillary nodal involvement

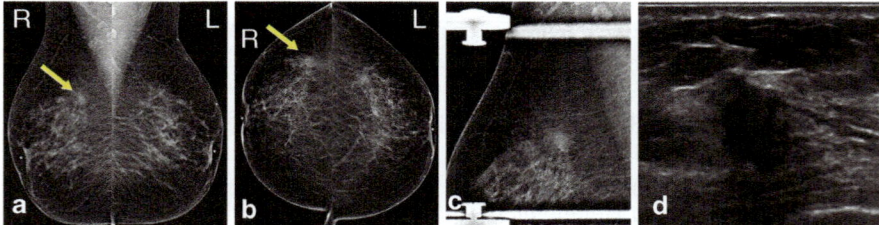

Fig. 10.1 **Invasive ductal cancer presenting as a mass**. 50-year-old female for screening. MLO (**a**) and CC (**b**) views show mass in upper outer right breast (yellow arrows). Spot compression MLO (**c**) confirms irregular mass with indistinct margins in the upper breast. US (**d**) shows irregular not parallel mass with posterior acoustic shadowing. Biopsy confirmed grade 2 invasive ductal cancer

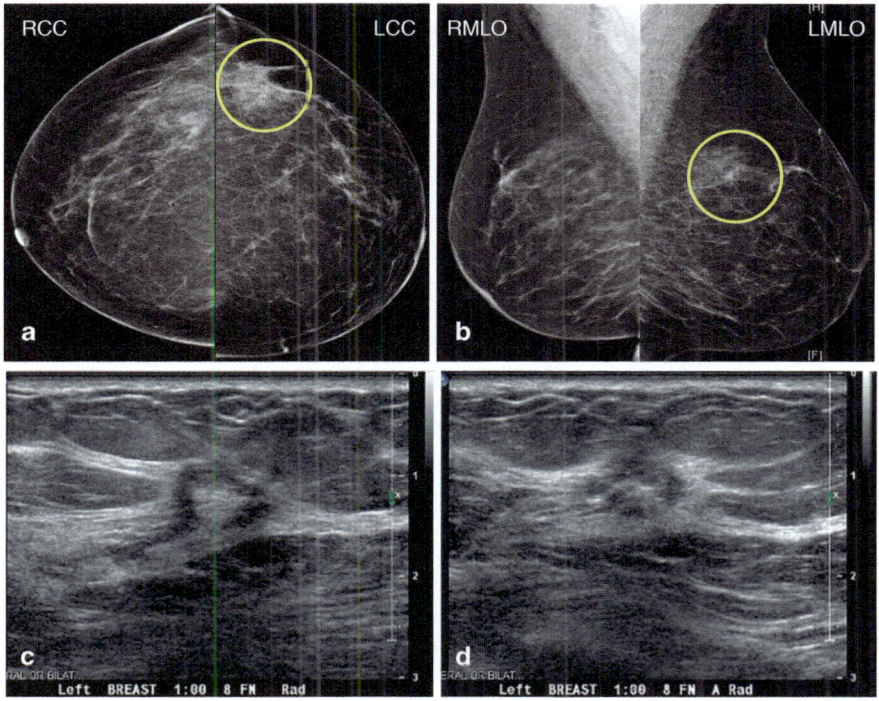

Fig. 10.2 Invasive ductal cancer as focal asymmetry. 47-year-old female with palpable left breast lump. CC (**a**) and MLO (**b**) views show focal asymmetry in upper outer left breast (yellow circles). US (**c**, **d**) shows an irregular mass with mixed echotexture. Biopsy confirmed grade 2 invasive ductal cancer

Fig. 10.3 Grade 2 DCIS presenting as grouped calcifications. A 68-year-old female with past history of left breast cancer with increasing calcifications inferior and lateral to biopsy bed (circle) on lateral (**a**) and CC (**b**) magnified views. Biopsy confirmed grade 2 DCIS

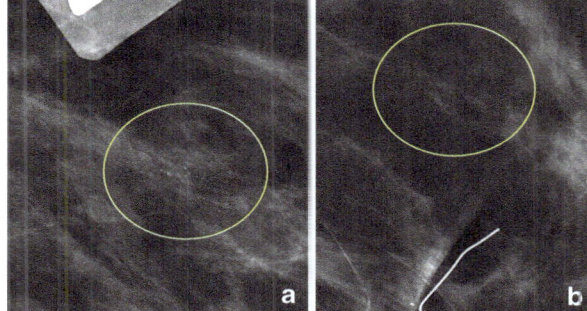

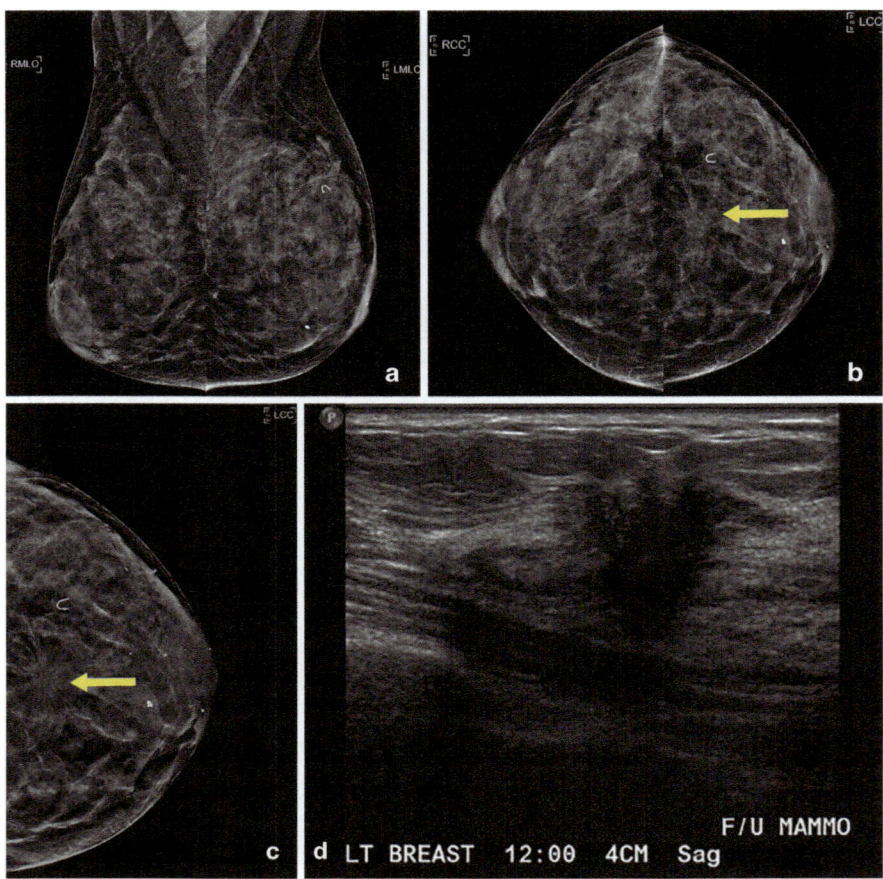

Fig. 10.4 **Invasive ductal cancer presenting as architectural distortion**. A 58-year-old female with history of benign left breast biopsy for screening. MLO (**a**) and CC (**b**) views show heterogeneously dense tissue and subtle area of distortion in the central left breast (arrow). CC Tomosynthesis slice (**c**) better shows distortion (arrow). Ultrasound (**d**) shows an irregular hypoechoic mass with posterior acoustic shadowing and ductal extension worrisome for malignancy. Biopsy confirmed grade 1 invasive ductal cancer

Fig. 10.5 Disruption of fat-glandular interface by invasive lobular cancer. A 47-year-old female for screening. Note how the fat glandular interface posteriorly is pulling in (arrows; **a**) when compared to the prior study (**b**). Biopsy confirmed invasive lobular cancer

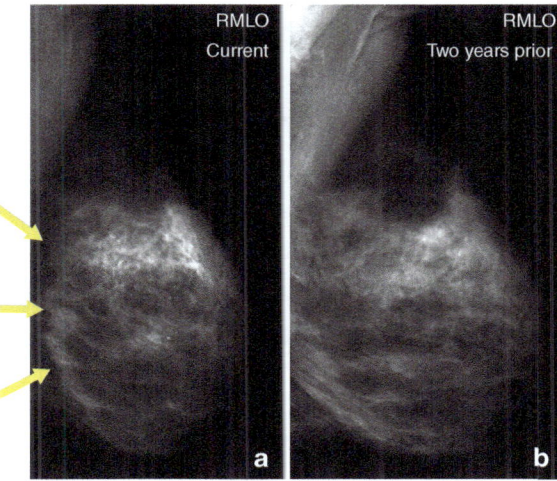

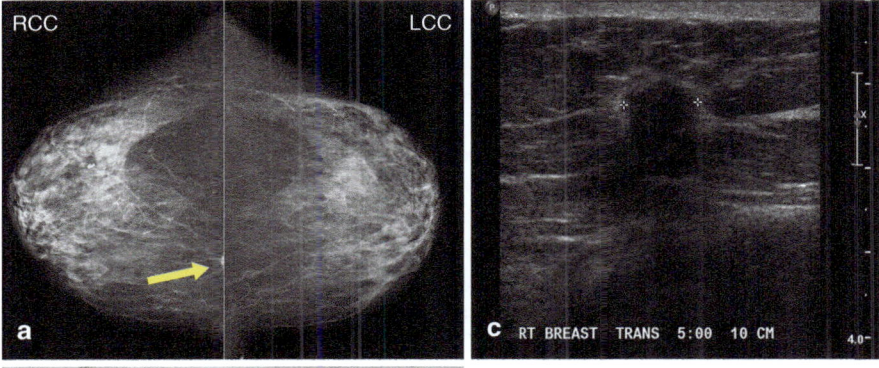

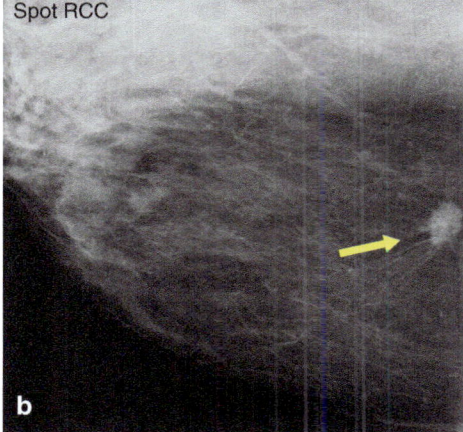

Fig. 10.6 Invasive ductal cancer on edge of image. 60-year-old female for screening. CC views (**a**) show dense asymmetry at edge of posterior medial right breast (arrow). Spot CC view (**b**) shows spiculated mass in posterior medial right breast (arrow). US (**c**) confirms an hypoechoic irregular mass with posterior acoustic shadowing. Biopsy confirmed grade 2 invasive ductal cancer

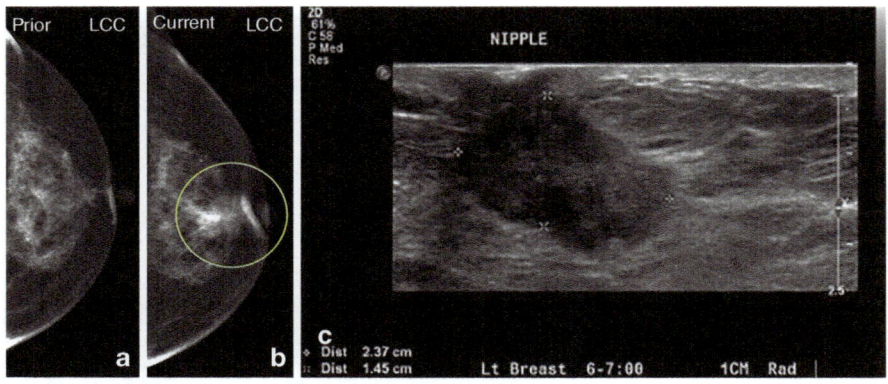

Fig. 10.7 **Nipple retraction due to malignancy**. 60-year-old female for screening. Comparing CC view from 2 years ago (**a**) to the current exam (**b**), there is retraction of the nipple and interval development of retroareolar density (circle). Ultrasound (**c**) confirms a solid irregular mass. Biopsy confirmed invasive ductal cancer

Histologic Subtypes

- **Ductal carcinoma in situ** (DCIS)—confined to duct with intact basement membrane (Fig. 10.8)
  - No risk of metastasis; 30–40% become invasive if untreated
  - Histologic grade 1–3 (low, intermediate, high)
  - Pathologic descriptors: comedo (central necrosis), solid, cribriform, papillary
  - Most commonly presents as calcifications (Figs. 10.9, e10.1, e10.2, and e10.3); mass seen in 10–14% (Fig. e10.4); rarely palpable
- **Invasive carcinoma**—tumor crosses basement membrane and "invades" stroma.
  - **Invasive ductal carcinoma** (IDC, approximately 85% of cases) (Fig. 10.10)
    - Most commonly presents as irregular spiculated mass ± calcifications, but can have benign features
    - Classification:
      - Classic, no special type (NST) (75%) (Figs. 10.11, e10.5, e10.6, e10.7, e10.8, e10.9, 10.12, and e10.10)
      - Invasive papillary (1–2%)—complex cystic mass, postmenopausal, good prognosis (Fig. e10.11)
      - Medullary (5%)—circumscribed mass, younger women, 25% are BRCA-1 positive, good prognosis
      - Tubular (1–2%)—associated with radial scars, good prognosis (Fig. e10.12)
      - Mucinous (2%)—circumscribed mass, high T2 signal on MRI, postmenopausal, good prognosis (Fig. e10.13)
      - Metaplastic (1%)—often have benign features, neoplastic epithelial cells differentiate into mesenchymal tissue, not chemosensitive, poor prognosis (Fig. e10.14)

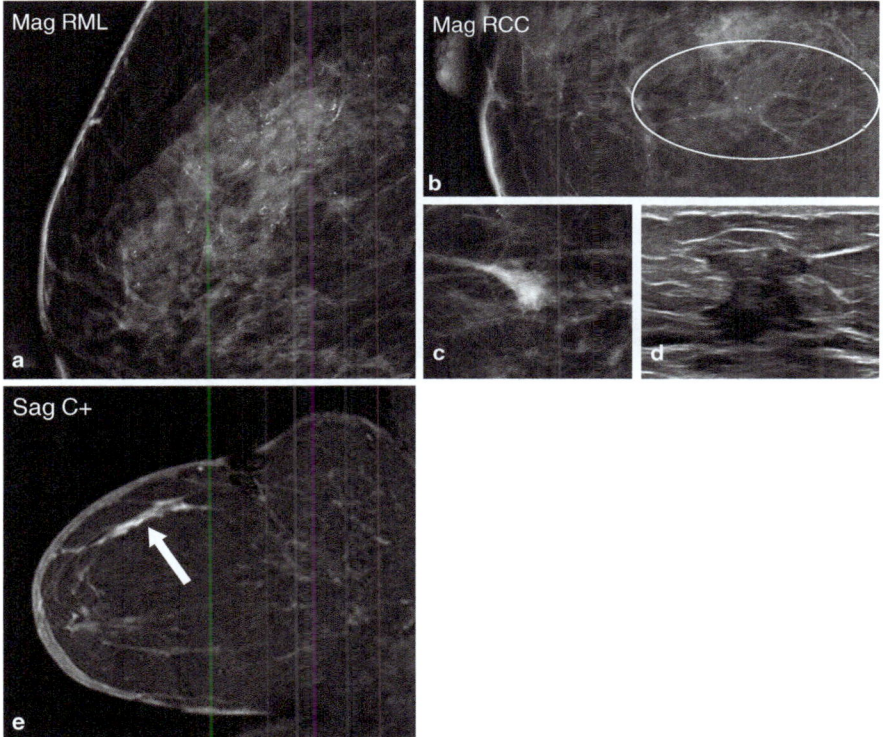

Fig. 10.8 Imaging appearance of DCIS. DCIS most commonly presents as calcifications, less likely a mass. (**a**) Screen-detected segmental pleomorphic and fine linear branching calcifications. (**b**) Screen-detected linear pleomorphic calcifications (white circle). (**c**) Screen-detected irregular mass on mammography with (**d**) corresponding mass on ultrasound with angular and indistinct margins. (**e**) Linear non-mass enhancement (arrow) on surveillance MRI in another patient previously treated for invasive ductal carcinoma

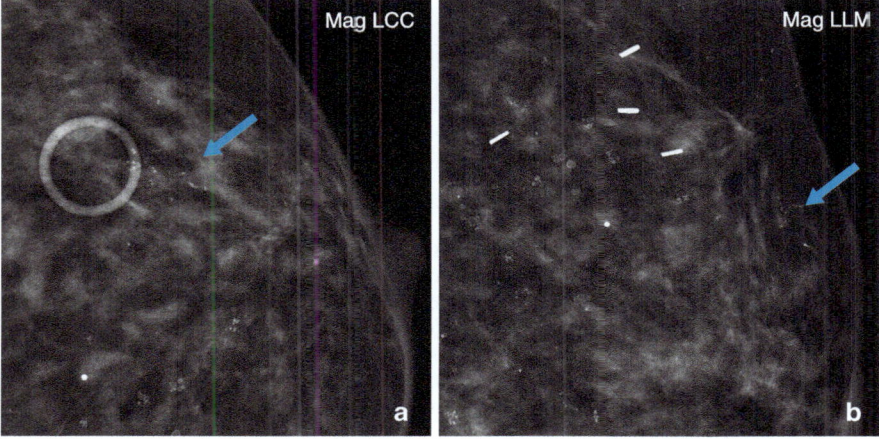

Fig. 10.9 Grade 3 DCIS. A 66-year-old female with linear branching calcifications on magnified CC (**a**) and lateral (**b**) views in a background of diffusely scattered dermal calcifications. Biopsy confirmed grade 3 DCIS with comedonecrosis

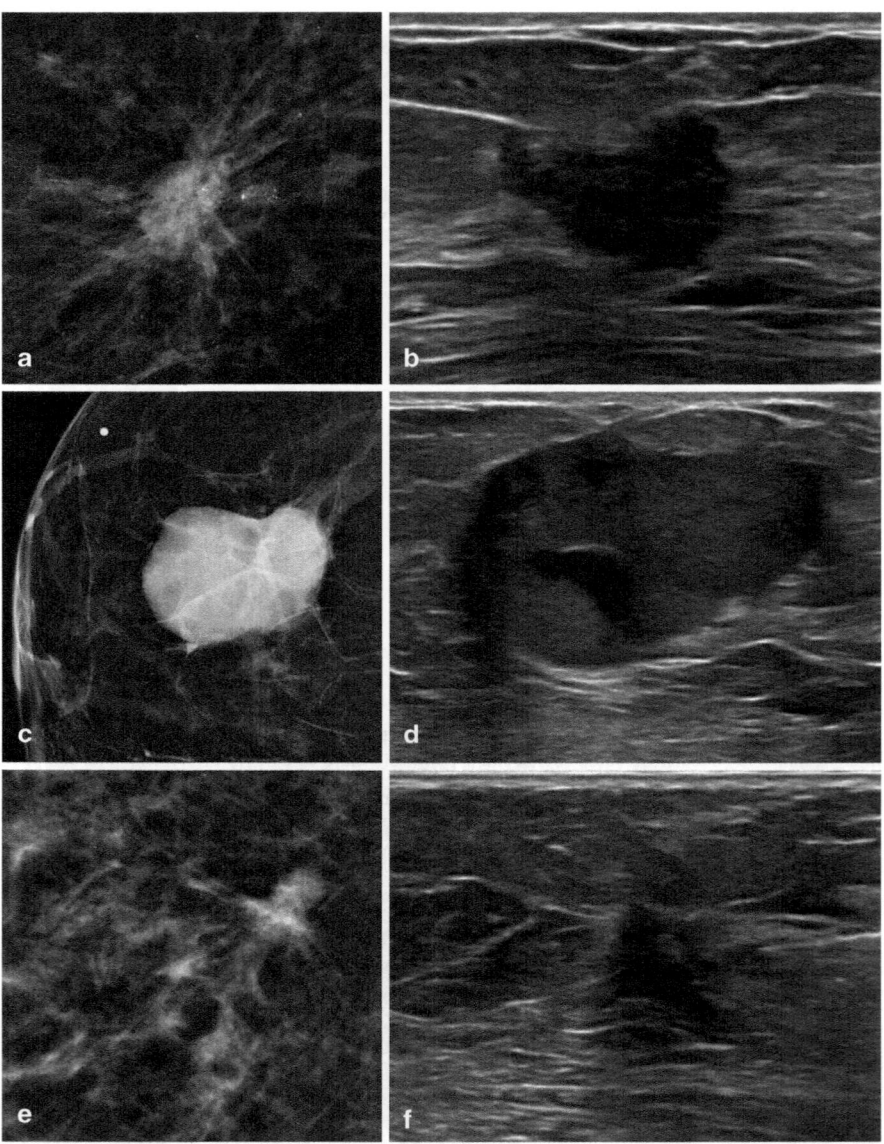

Fig. 10.10 Invasive ductal cancer (IDC) and its subtypes. (**a, b**) IDC, no specific type presenting as an irregular spiculated mass with associated pleomorphic calcifications. (**c, d**) Invasive papillary carcinoma presenting as a palpable circumscribed mass on mammography (**c**) with corresponding mixed cystic and solid mass on ultrasound (**d**). (**e, f**) Tubular carcinoma presenting as an irregular spiculated mass. (**g, h**) Mucinous carcinoma presenting as an irregular mass on mammography (**g**) with corresponding hypoechoic mass on ultrasound with circumscribed and indistinct margins (**h**). (**i, j**) Metaplastic carcinoma presenting as a palpable oval mass on mammography (**i**) with corresponding mixed cystic and solid mass on ultrasound (**j**)

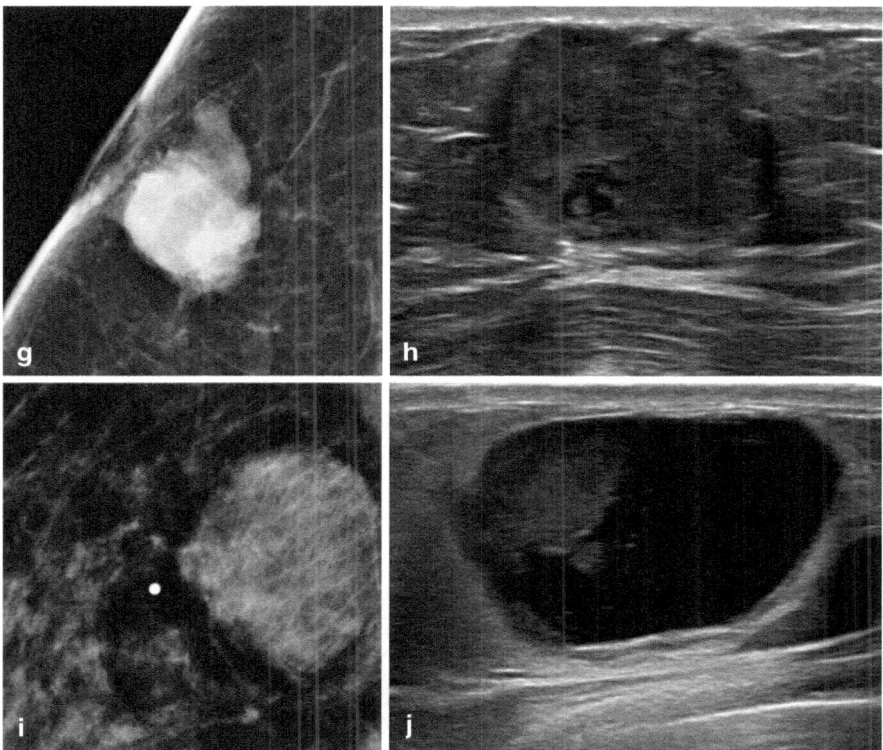

Fig. 10.10 (continued)

- o **Invasive lobular carcinoma** (ILC, approximately 15% of cases) (Figs. 10.13, 10.14, and 10.15)
  - • Infiltrate as single file of cells so more difficult to detect
  - • Often present at more advanced stage (larger mass) than invasive ductal cancers; more likely multifocal and multicentric
  - • MRI useful for preoperative staging
- • **Special cases**
  - o *Mammographically occult malignancy*—may present as metastatic axillary lymphadenopathy, be detected on screening MR or US, or as palpable finding; contrast-enhanced imaging can detect primary malignancy (Figs. 10.16 and e10.15)

○ *Inflammatory breast cancer*—rare invasive ductal or lobular carcinoma (1–5%) involving dermal lymphatics; see diffuse skin and trabecular thickening, often with underlying mass (Fig. 10.17)
  • Present with rapid onset of breast erythema, edema, "peau d'orange" skin
  • Skin punch biopsy may show tumor emboli in dermal lymphatics
  • Clinical diagnosis; imaging overlaps with locally advanced breast cancer (Fig. 10.18)
○ *Paget disease* of the nipple—tumor cells in epidermis, almost always associated with underlying DCIS (Fig. 10.19)
  • Present with red, scaly, ulcerated nipple/nipple-areolar complex
  • Mammogram normal in 15–50%; MR can often detect underlying malignancy

Molecular Classification

Four subtypes based on gene expression pattern; variable imaging, prognosis and response to therapy

• **Luminal (A and B)**—60–70% of invasive cancers; estrogen receptor (ER) and progesterone receptor (PR) receptor positive; treated with hormonal therapy; most often present as irregular mass without calcifications
  ○ **Luminal A**—ER/PR positive, HER2 negative; well-differentiated with good prognosis; less likely to have axillary involvement at diagnosis
  ○ **Luminal B**—ER/PR positive, usually HER2 negative but some HER2 positive; lower PR expression and higher Ki-67 (cell proliferation marker) than luminal A; less well-differentiated, more likely involving axillary nodes at diagnosis, and shorter overall survival than Luminal A
• **HER2-enriched**—12–20% of invasive cancers; ER/PR negative; human epidermal growth factor receptor 2 (HER2) positive
  ○ Present as calcifications or irregular mass with calcifications; > 50% multifocal/multicentric; poorer prognosis and more advanced stage at diagnosis compared to luminal cancers
  ○ Treat with trastuzumab (monoclonal antibody targeting Her2-neu receptor) yielding improved disease-free survival and overall survival
• **Basal-like**—15% of invasive cancers; majority triple negative (ER/PR/HER2 negative) with high Ki-67 and p53 mutation (Fig. 10.5)
  ○ Present as irregular mass, but up to 20% benign-appearing
  ○ More common in premenopausal and Black women; often high grade; increased risk of recurrence compared to luminal tumors
  ○ Often high grade with high proliferation rate and high rates of recurrence
  ○ Treat with neoadjuvant chemotherapy with 80% complete pathologic response

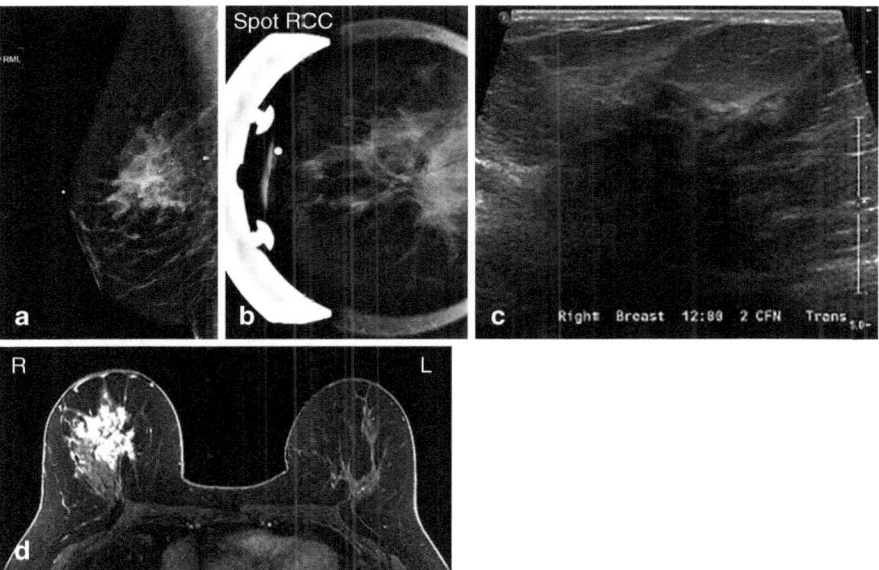

Fig. 10.11 **Invasive ductal cancer**. A 42-year-old female with palpable lump. MLO (**a**) and spot compression CC (**b**) views show dense irregular mass with associated distortion in the upper outer right breast. Ultrasound (**c**) shows an irregular hypoechoic mass with posterior acoustic shadowing. Initial core biopsy with a spring-loaded device revealed stromal fibrosis which was felt to be discordant. Axial T1-weighted postcontrast MR image (**d**) shows an irregular enhancing mass in the upper breast. Repeat biopsy using a vacuum-assisted device revealed invasive ductal cancer

Breast Cancer Staging

American Joint Committee on Cancer (AJCC) Staging System 8th edition uses traditional TNM anatomic staging combined with prognostic information from tumor grade, biomarkers, and gene expression profiling (see bibliography for details)

- **T**umor (T_{is} (DCIS)–T4)—size of the primary tumor; skin or chest wall involvement
- **N**ode (N0–N3)—extent of axillary nodal involvement
- **M**etastasis (M0 or M1)—presence (M1), absence (M0) of distant metastases
- TNM categories are combined to determine the disease stage (0–IV)

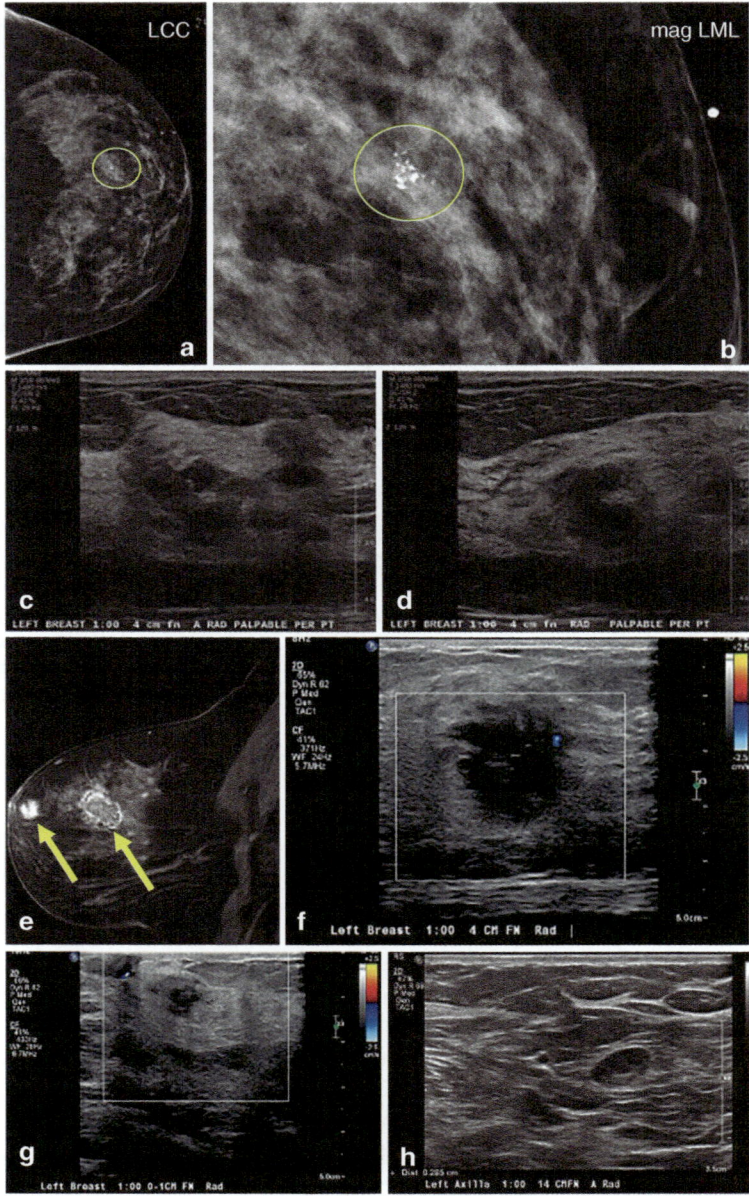

Fig. 10.12 **Multifocal invasive ductal cancer**. 36-year-old with left upper outer lump and strong family history of breast cancer in mother at age 38 years. CC (**a**) and magnified lateral (**b**) views show coarse heterogeneous grouped calcifications in the area of concern to the patient (yellow circle). Ultrasound (**c, d**) shows non-mass lesion with heterogeneous echotexture. Given family history, MRI was obtained six months later. Sagittal post contrast image (**e**) shows a rim-enhancing mass (arrow) and a second mass more anteriorly (arrow). Second look US (**f, g, h**) showed two solid suspicious masses and a borderline axillary node. Biopsy confirmed multifocal grade 3 invasive ductal cancer and metastatic axillary disease

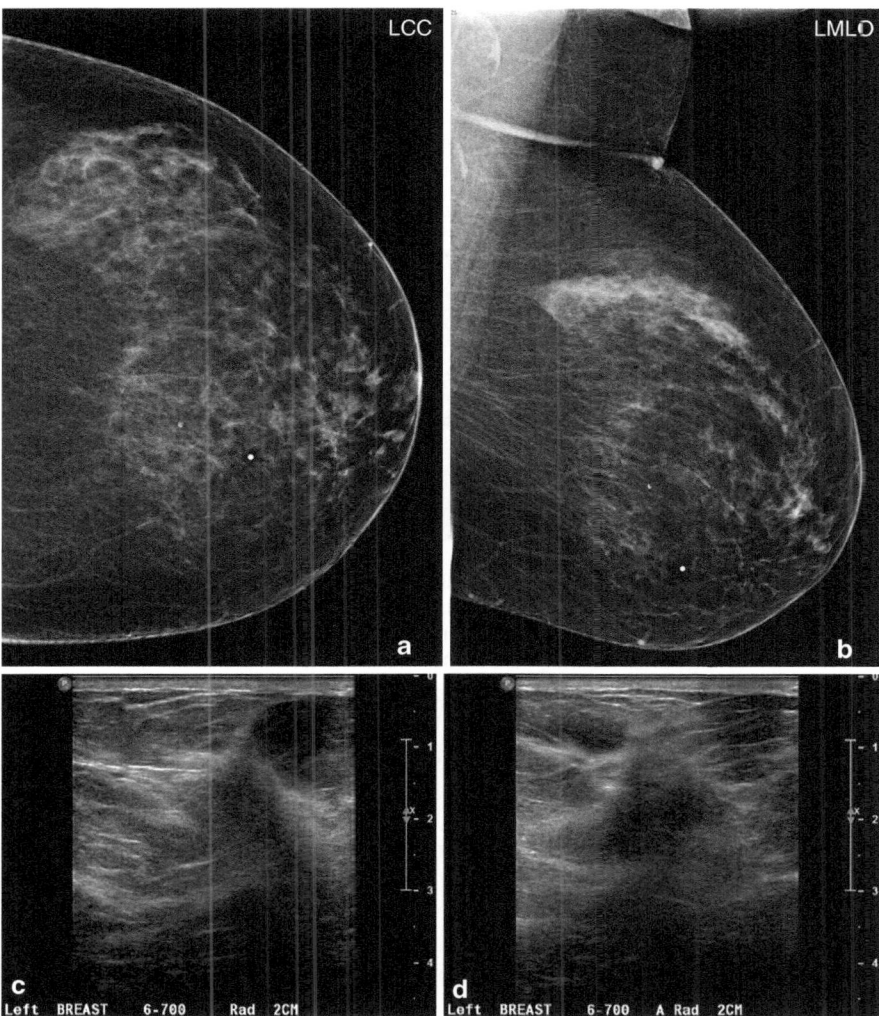

Fig. 10.13 Invasive lobular cancer. A 44-year-old female with persistent palpable left lump (BB) for 1.5 years. LCC (**a**) and LMLO (**b**) views show no definite finding. Ultrasound (**c, d**) shows subtle ill-defined shadowing at 6–7:00 in the area of concern to the patient. Biopsy confirmed grade 1 invasive lobular cancer

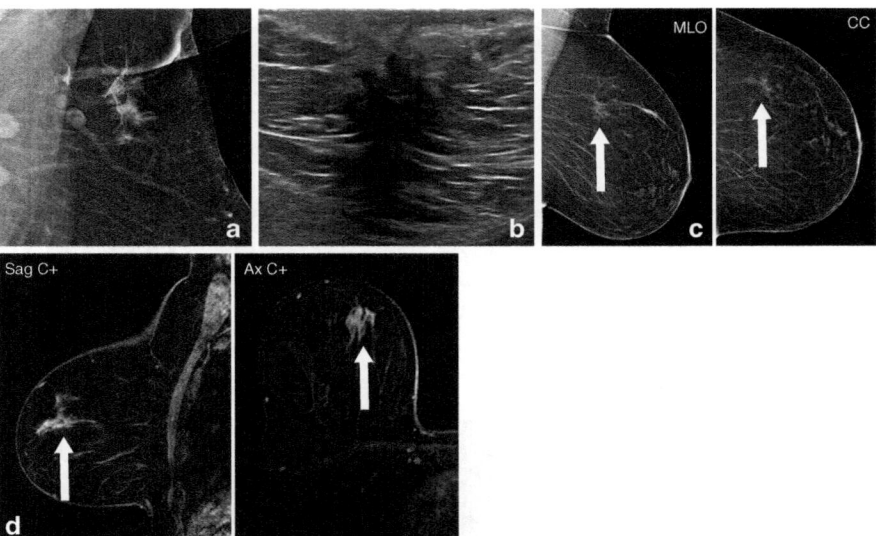

Fig. 10.14 **Invasive lobular carcinoma (ILC) presenting as an asymmetry in the axilla (a)** **corresponding to an irregular indistinct hypoechoic mass on US (b).** (**c**) ILC presenting as a focal asymmetry in the upper outer left breast (arrows). (**d**) Mammographically occult ILC identified as focal non-mass enhancement on MRI (arrows).

- **Tumor staging**—imaging determines tumor size and extent
  - Mammography ± ultrasound ± MRI
  - Pretreatment MRI indicated for young age (< 50 years), dense tissue (Fig. 10.20), invasive lobular cancer (Fig. 10.21), high-risk patient (elevated lifetime risk ≥ 20–25%), suspected multifocal or multicentric disease, mammographically occult tumor, discrepancy between clinical exam and imaging, intent of neoadjuvant chemotherapy to monitor response (Figs. 10.22 and e10.16)
- **Nodal staging**
  - Determined by location, size, number
    - Level I: lateral to pectoralis minor (Fig. e10.17)
    - Level II: posterior to pectoralis minor (including interpectoral Rotter nodes) (Fig. e10.18)
    - Level III: medial to pectoralis minor
    - Cervical and contralateral supraclavicular, axillary, and internal mammary nodes considered distant metastases
  - Axillary staging—targeted percutaneous biopsy, sentinel lymph node biopsy, full axillary node dissection
    - Routine axillary imaging varies by practice
    - US modality of choice to identify and biopsy nodes; clip if biopsy
    - Breast MRI and PET/CT for internal mammary nodes and distant disease

- **Distant Metastases**
  - No routine staging for stages 0–IIA; indicated for stage IIB or higher
  - Image with PET/CT <u>or</u> bone scan and CT chest, abdomen, pelvis

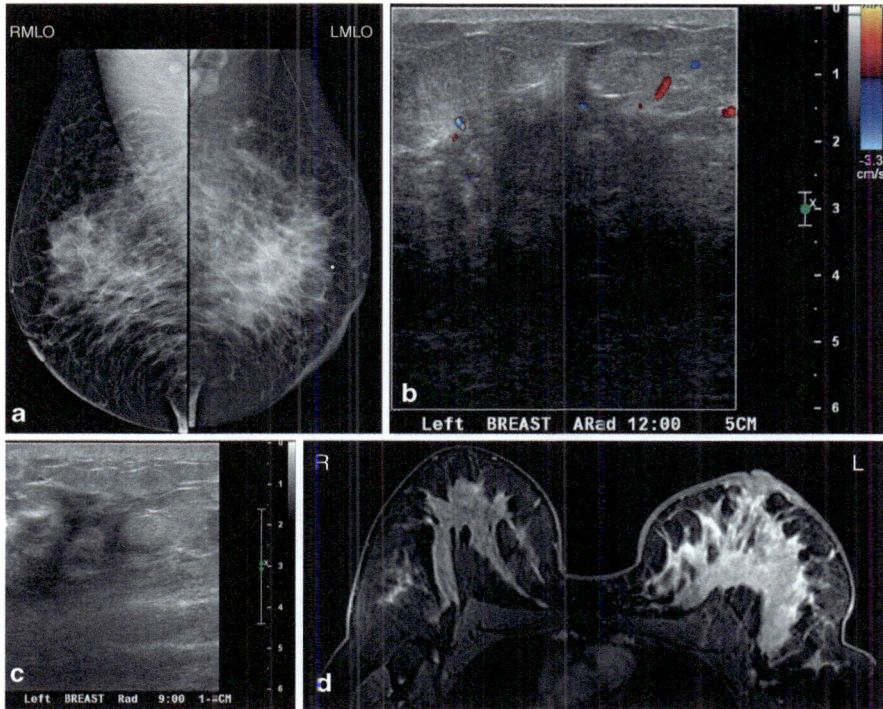

Fig. 10.15 48-year-old female with left breast enlargement after spontaneous abortion.
Bilateral MLO (**a**) views show diffuse increase density in the left breast with subtle distortion and
trabecular and skin thickening worrisome for an infiltrative process. Ultrasound (**b**, **c**) showed
multiple ill-defined hypoechoic areas with overlying skin thickening and minimally dilated lymphatics. Biopsy confirmed invasive lobular carcinoma. Axial T1-weighted postcontrast MR image
(**d**) shows enhancement of the entire left breast and no suspicious enhancement in the right breast.
The patient subsequently underwent neoadjuvant chemotherapy and ultimately left mastectomy.

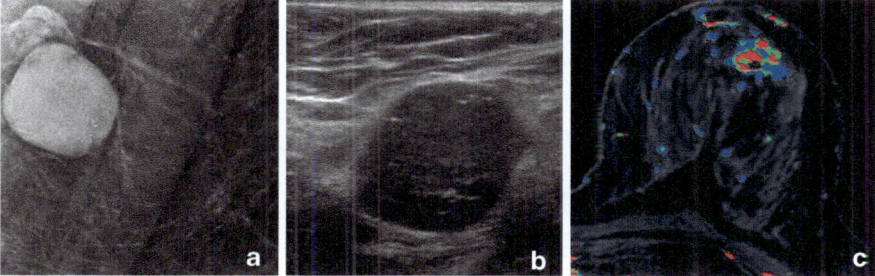

Fig. 10.16 Metastatic axillary node/mammographically occult malignancy. 56-year-old
female with multiple enlarged dense left axillary nodes with calcifications seen on the MLO view
(**a**). US shows a round solid axillary mass with a completely replaced hilum suspicious for malignancy (**b**). Biopsy revealed metastatic grade 3 invasive ductal carcinoma. MRI reveals mammographically occult malignancy with mixed kinetics in the outer central left breast (**c**)

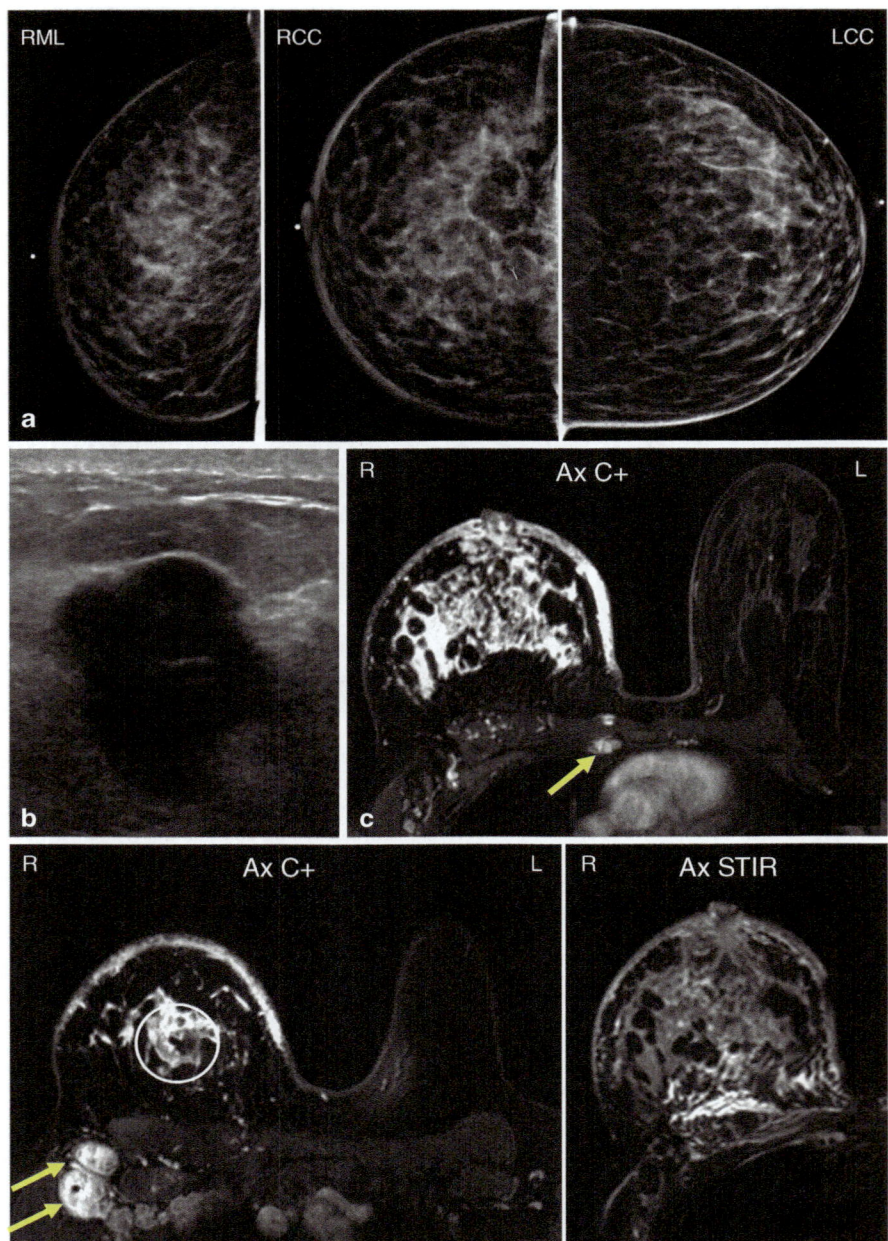

Fig. 10.17 (continued)

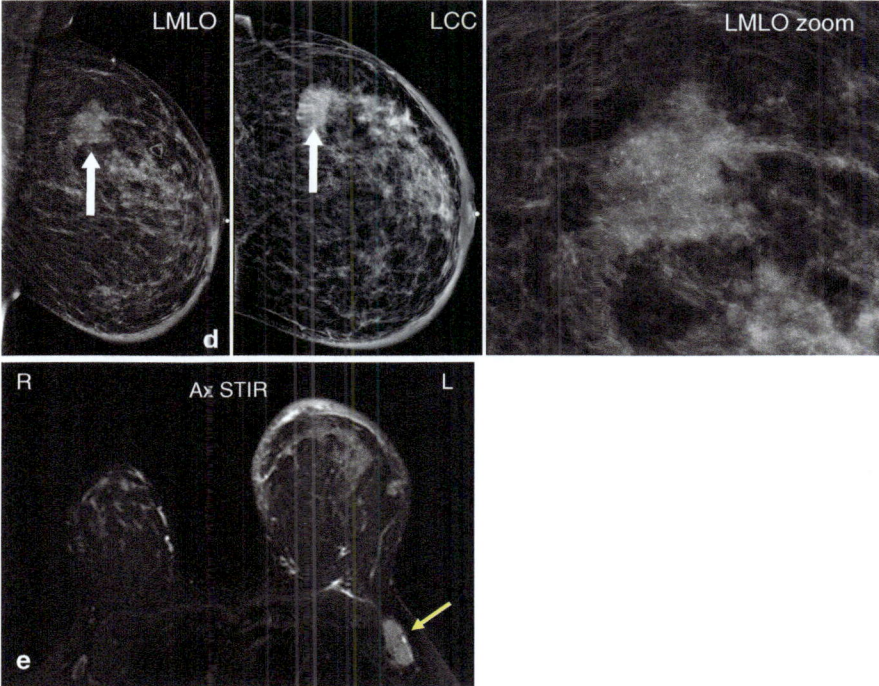

Fig. 10.17 Inflammatory breast cancer. (**a–c**) Inflammatory breast cancer (IBC) in a young woman with right breast lump, pain, swelling, and peau d'orange on exam. (**a**) Lateral and CC mammographic views show diffuse skin and trabecular thickening, more evident when compared to the normal LCC view. (**b**) Ultrasound at the site of palpable lump shows an irregular hypoechoic mass. (**c**) MRI shows diffuse non-mass enhancement and skin thickening with enhancement. The palpable mass is seen in the right upper breast (circle) along with extensive ipsilateral axillary and internal mammary lymphadenopathy (arrow). The STIR sequence shows skin and parenchymal edema typical of inflammation. (**d, e**) Locally advanced triple negative breast cancer can have a similar appearance, thus inflammatory breast cancer is a clinical diagnosis. (**d**) Left MLO, CC, and zoomed MLO views of a palpable mass shows an irregular mass with pleomorphic calcifications (arrows) and associated skin/trabecular thickening. (**e**) MRI STIR sequence shows skin and parenchymal edema, as well as ipsilateral adenopathy (arrow)

Management

- Combination of surgery, radiation therapy, and chemotherapy for local and distant control
- Surgery—lumpectomy, mastectomy; equivalent disease-free and overall survival; axillary nodal surgery for invasive cancers, provided eligible for chemotherapy
  - ○ Sentinel lymph node biopsy (SLNB; first draining nodes) vs. full (ALND; all nodes)
    - SLNB—T1–2 clinically node negative tumors clinically node negative status post neoadjuvant chemotherapy; risk of lymphedema 7–10%
      - Inject ^{99m}Tch-sulfur colloid and/or methylene blue dye around nipple/areolar complex or tumor bed; intraoperative probe identifies radioactive nodes and/or visibly "blue" nodes, both of which are excised

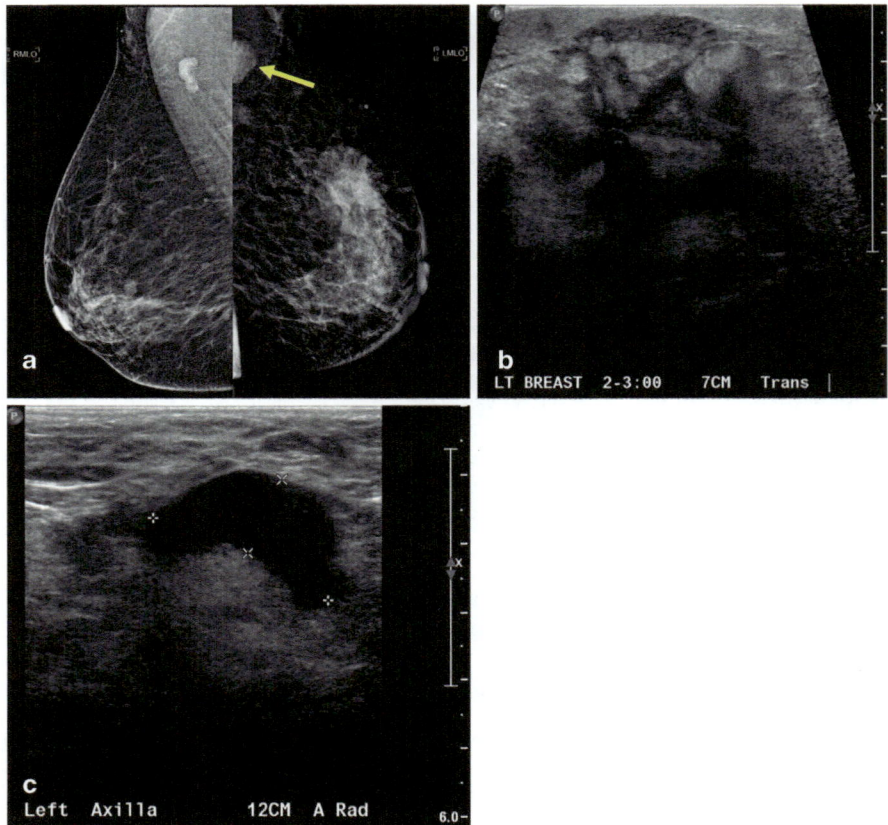

Fig. 10.18 Locally advanced breast cancer with metastatic node. 68-year-old female with 1-week history of left breast pain and warmth. Symptoms were unresponsive to antibiotics. Bilateral MLO views (**a**) show an irregular mass in upper left breast and an enlarged left axillary node (arrow). US (**b, c**) confirms non-mass finding with heterogeneous echotexture and abnormal left axillary node with 1.2 cm thickened cortex

- ALNB—clinically positive axilla, ≥ 3 sentinel nodes, inflammatory breast cancer; risk of lymphedema 25%
- ACOSOG Z0011 trial—no further surgery needed if 1–3 positive sentinel nodes and clinically node negative; systemic chemotherapy preferred

- US-guided core biopsy with clip placement of axillary node performed if clinical or imaging suspicion for nodal metastases; often localize clipped node for excision at time of surgery

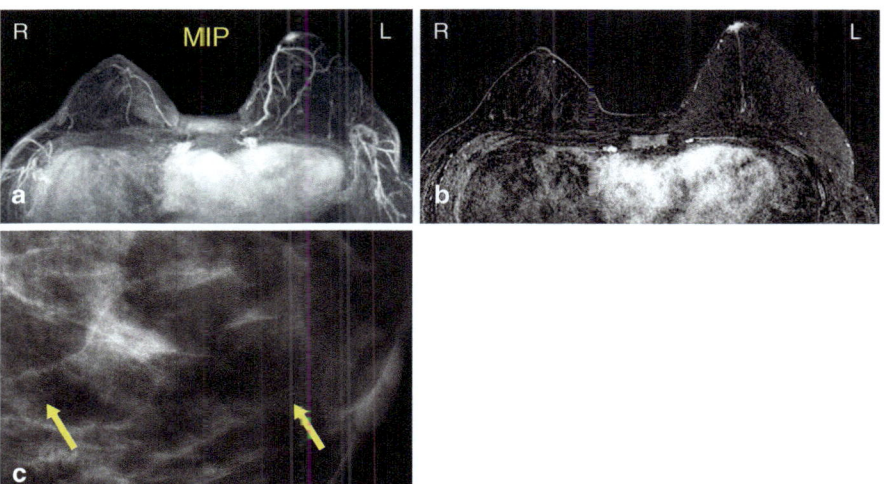

Fig. 10.19 **Paget's disease**. 33-year-old female with history of right lumpectomy 3 years ago now presenting with left intermittent clear discharge. MIP (**a**) and axial subtracted postcontrast (**b**) image from screening MRI show asymmetrically enhancing irregular nipple and linear non-mass enhancement in the central left breast with below threshold kinetics. Magnified lateral view (**c**) shows a few linear calcifications in ductal distribution. Biopsy confirmed high grade DCIS and Paget's disease

- Radiation—whole breast (4–6 weeks); other options include partial breast, chest wall (after mastectomy), regional lymph nodes
  - ○ Indicated for majority of DCIS and invasive cancers; surgical margins must be negative
  - ○ May be omitted for older (> 65 years) with ER/PR + tumors, minimal tumor burden
- Systemic therapy—preoperative (neoadjuvant) and/or postoperative (adjuvant)
  - ○ Agent used depends on breast cancer subtype/receptor status (hormone receptor+—endocrine therapy; HER2+—trastuzumab; triple negative tumors—systemic chemotherapy)
    - Endocrine (hormone) therapy—use for ≥ 5 years; tamoxifen if premenopausal, aromatase inhibitor (anastrozole, exemestane, letrozole) if postmenopausal; reduces risk of subsequent breast cancer by 30–50%
  - ○ Chemotherapy—(1) reduce tumor burden making breast conservation possible (neoadjuvant); (2) prevent recurrence; and (3) treat potential or known metastatic disease
    - Oncotype DX (21-gene genomic test) recurrence score (0–100)—predicts potential benefit of adjuvant chemotherapy in patients with early-stage HR+ HER2– cancers (stage I–IIIA); high score (≥ 26)—established benefit; intermediate (11–25) in women < 50 years—unclear benefit; low score (≤ 10)—not beneficial

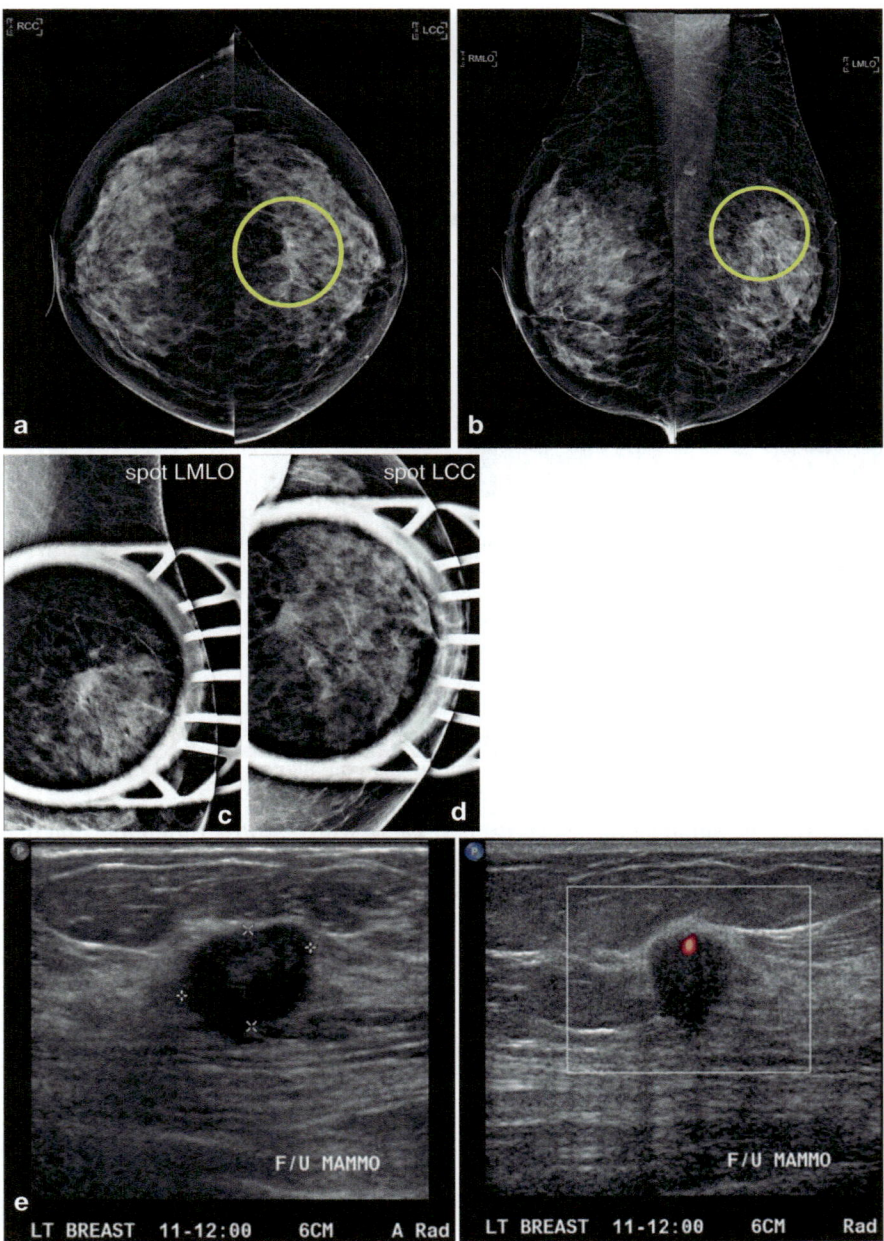

Fig. 10.20 Staging of invasive ductal cancer. 78-year-old female with history of prior benign right biopsy for screening. CC (**a**) and MLO (**b**) views show heterogeneously dense tissue with focal architectural distortion in the central upper left breast (circle). Spot compression MLO (**c**) and CC (**d**) views reveal persistence. Ultrasound (**e**) shows a solid mass with internal vascularity. Biopsy confirmed invasive ductal cancer. The patient was allergic to gadolinium so subsequently underwent contrast-enhanced mammography (CEM). CEM MLO (**f**) and CC (**g**) recombined images show the enhancing known left malignancy in the upper central breast (arrow) and an enhancing mass in the outer central right breast (circle). Second look US of the right breast (**h**) discovered an irregular hypoechoic mass at 9:00, which was biopsied revealing invasive ductal cancer

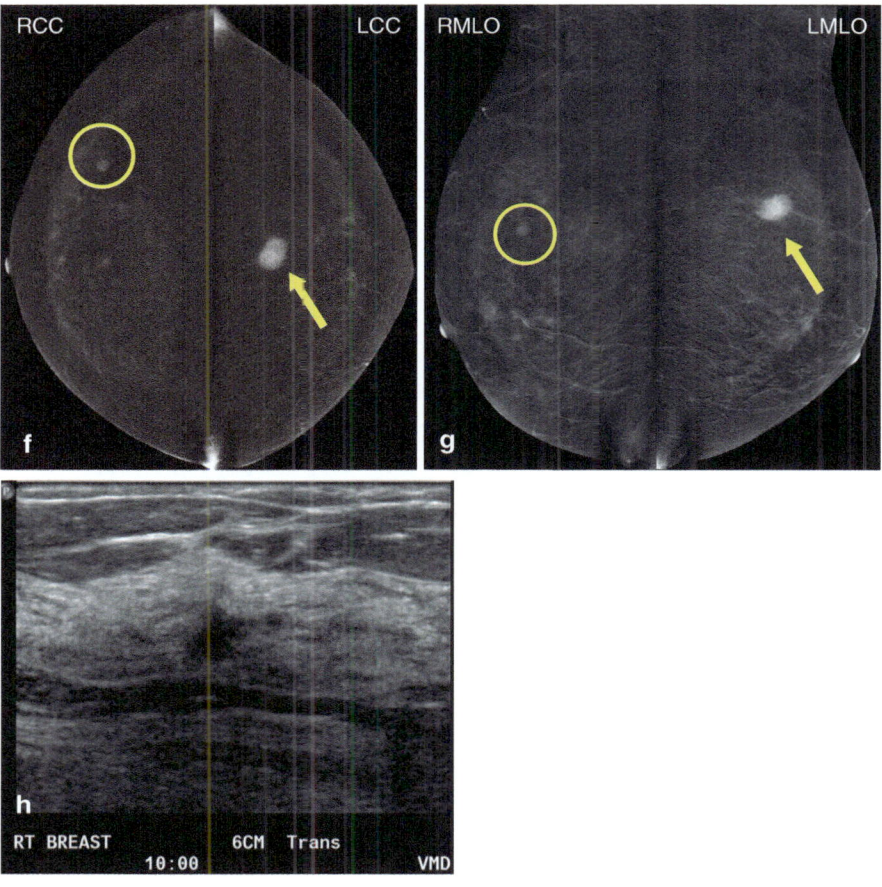

Fig. 10.20   (continued)

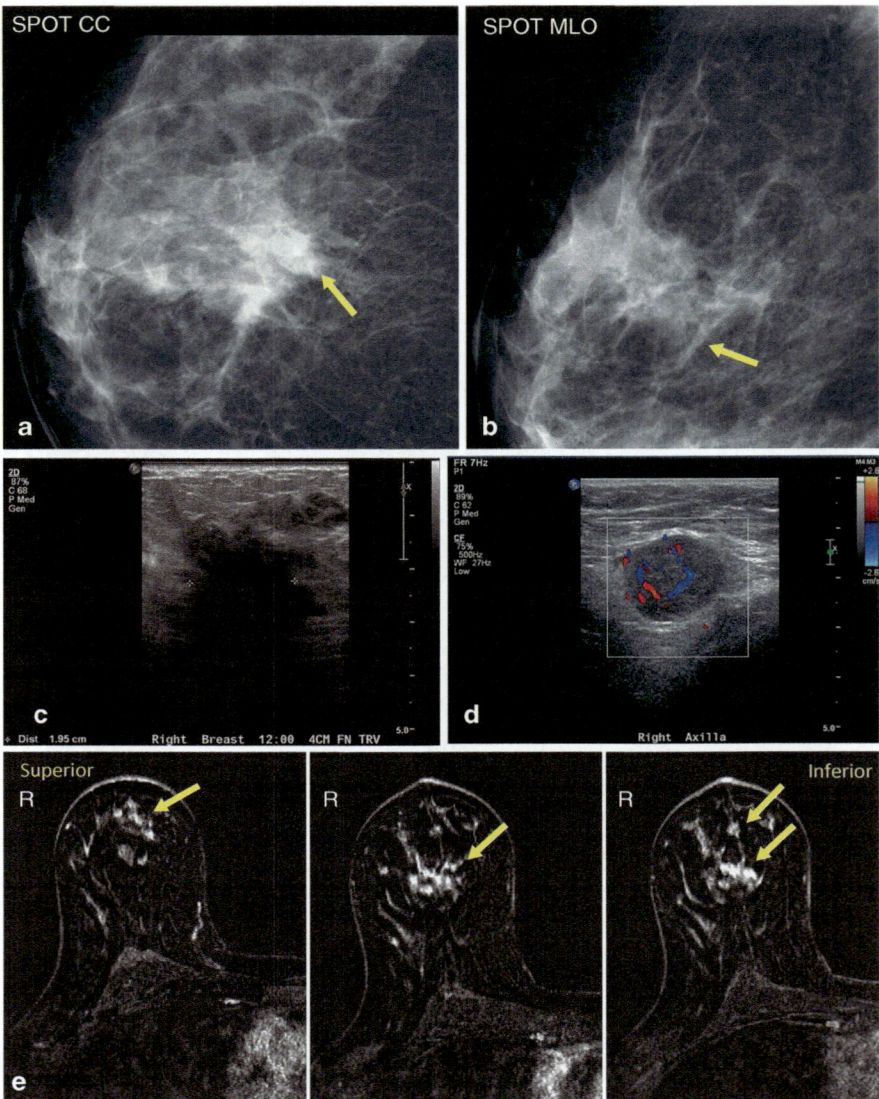

Fig. 10.21 **Staging of invasive lobular cancer**. 56-year-old female with questionable distortion in the central upper right breast on screening. Spot compression CC (**a**) and MLO (**b**) views demonstrate somewhat compressible tissue (arrows). Ultrasound (**c, d**) shows an irregular hypoechoic mass and a round axillary node with replacement of the fatty hilum. Biopsy showed grade 2 invasive lobular cancer with a metastatic axillary node. Axial T1-weighted postcontrast image (**e**) from superior to inferior shows multiple enhancing masses and non-mass enhancement in the upper and central right breast (arrows) consistent with multicentric and multifocal disease

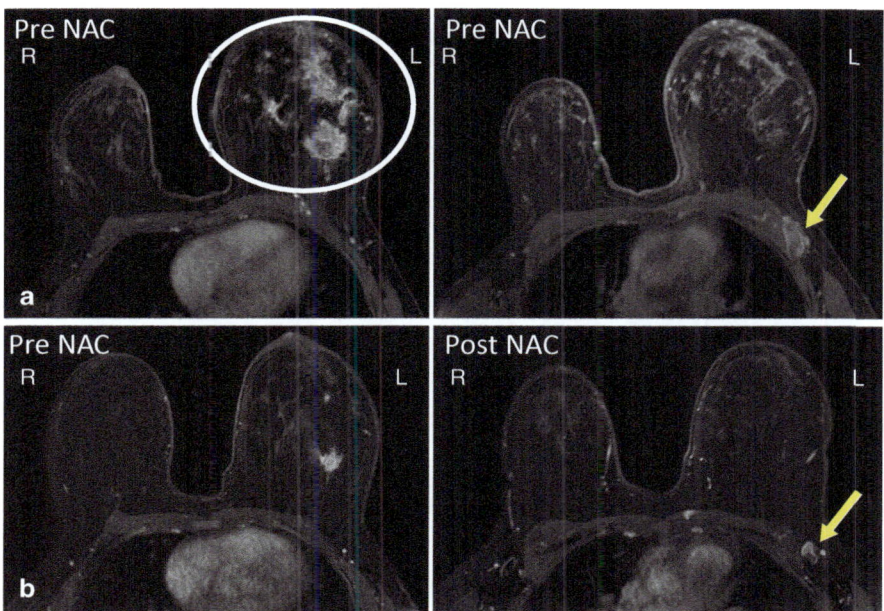

Fig. 10.22 MRI to evaluate response to neoadjuvant chemotherapy. Preoperative MRI is performed in breast cancer patients who will undergo neoadjuvant chemotherapy to monitor treatment response. (**a**) Preoperative MRI in a patient with locally advanced left breast cancer shows multiple irregular enhancing masses in the breast (circle), diffuse skin thickening, and an enlarged level I axillary lymph node (arrow). (**b**) Following neoadjuvant chemotherapy, there is significant reduction in the number and extent of the breast enhancement, improved skin thickening, and normalization of the previously enlarged node (arrow)

Imaging Post Conservation Breast

- Image with annual mammography, sometimes also MRI/CEM (if other risk factors); imaging of mastectomy side not routine
- Expected imaging findings (Fig. 10.23)
  - Post-op seroma (25% at 6 months; most resolve by 12–18 months)
  - Architectural distortion at lumpectomy bed (stable at 2 years)
  - Benign calcifications ± oil cysts in lumpectomy bed (up to 28% at 6–12 months, usually dystrophic (fat necrosis), coarsen over time)
  - Skin and trabecular thickening from radiation therapy (peaks at 6 months, stabilizes at 2 years)
- Breast cancer recurrence
  - Risk averages 1%/year with peak of 2.5% between years 2 and 6; typically occurs at or near lumpectomy bed due to treatment failure; after 10 years, likely new primary
  - Risk factors—close or positive surgical margins, inadequate radiation therapy, young age at diagnosis, multifocal or multicentric disease at diagnosis

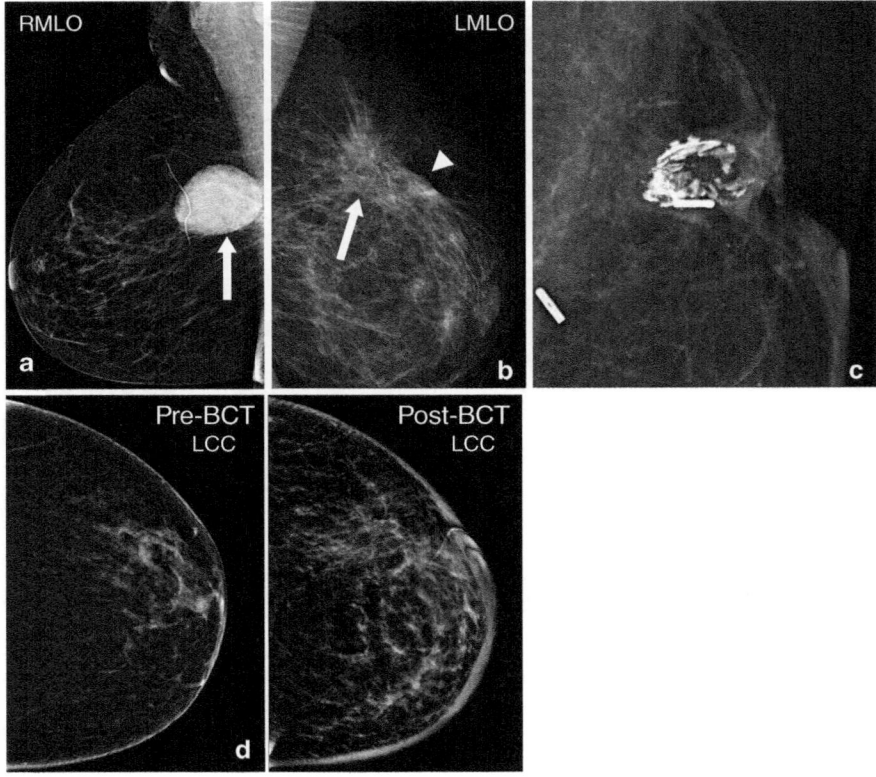

Fig. 10.23 **Expected findings after breast conservation**. (**a**) Postoperative seroma after lumpectomy (arrow). (**b**) Architectural distortion at the lumpectomy bed (arrow) with associated skin retraction (arrowhead). (**c**) Dystrophic coarse calcifications due to fat necrosis at the lumpectomy site. (**d**) Skin and trabecular thickening 6 months after completion of radiation therapy

- ○ Imaging findings (Figs. 10.24 and e10.19)
  - • New mass, asymmetry, or calcifications (Figs. e10.20 and e10.21)
  - • Increasing architectural distortion or density in lumpectomy bed
  - • Increasing skin or trabecular thickening
- • Radiation-induced angiosarcoma (Figs. 10.25, 10.26, and 10.27)
  - ○ Rare complication (0.05–0.3%) associated with poor prognosis; median time from diagnosis 7–8 years; present with erythematous skin lesions, focal skin thickening; may mimic bruising; treated with mastectomy ± chemotherapy

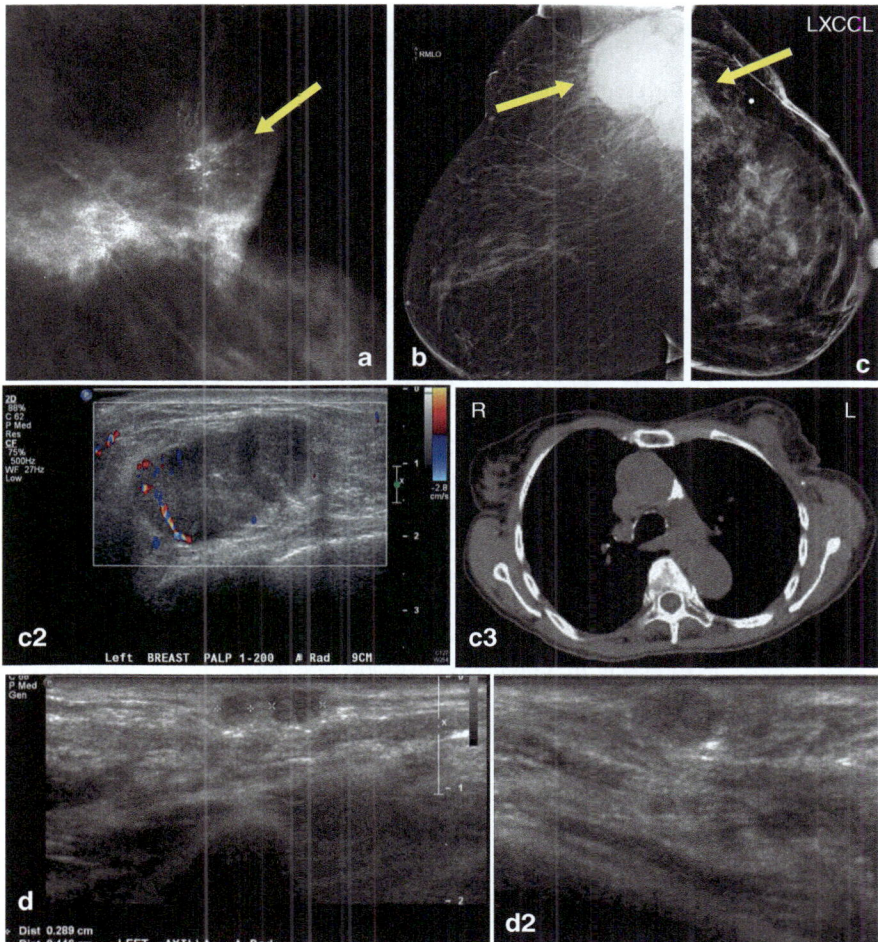

Fig. 10.24 Signs of recurrence following breast cancer treatment. (**a**) 55-year-old female who developed pleomorphic calcifications (**a**; arrow) adjacent to lumpectomy bed 3 years after completing treatment. Biopsy confirmed recurrent DCIS and invasive cancer. (**b**) 51-year-old female with axillary lump. RMLO view (**b**) shows enlarged dense axillary nodes (arrow) suspicious for metastatic disease. (**c**) 48-year-old female with palpable lump in lumpectomy bed 8 years after treatment. A dense mass (**c**; arrow) is incompletely visualized. Ultrasound confirms a solid hypoechoic mass (**c2**) which was biopsied and confirmed to be recurrent cancer. Axial CT shows the mass with invasion into underlying muscle (**c3**). (**d**) 36-year-o d female with palpable nodules in the axillary dissection scar. Ultrasound reveals multiple subcutaneous solid masses (**d, d2**). Biopsy confirmed recurrence

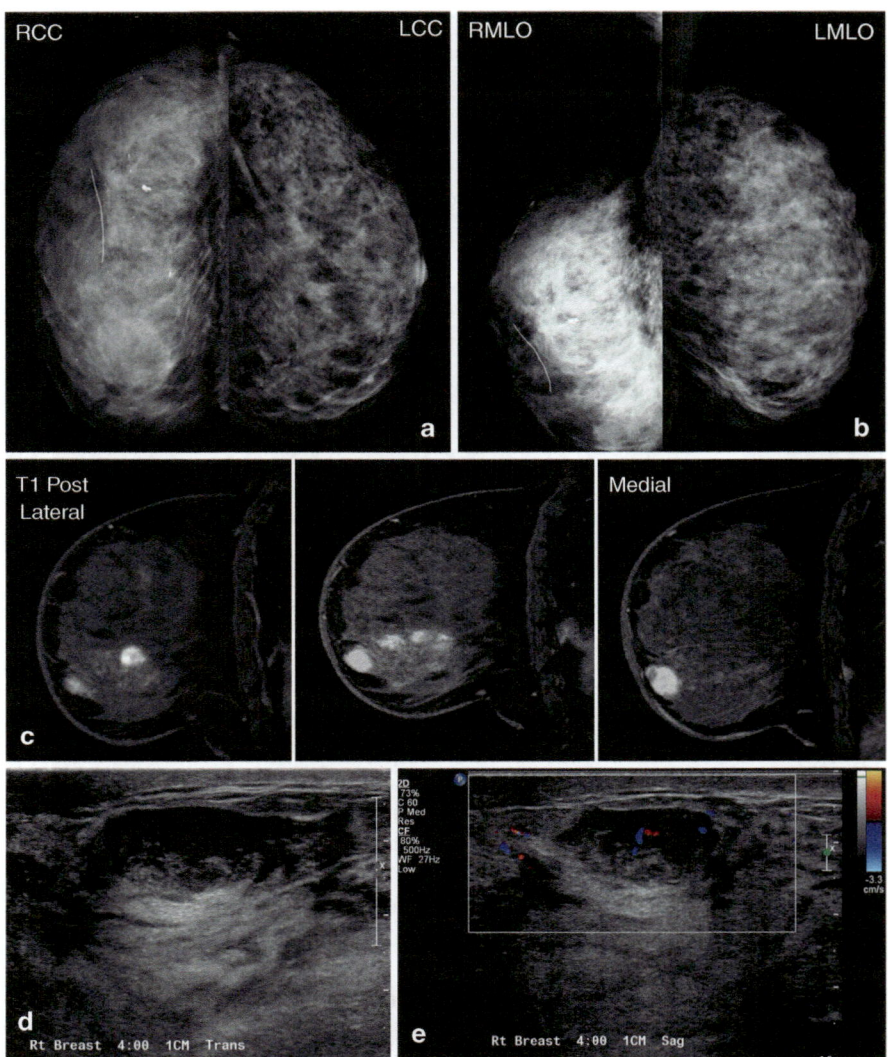

Fig. 10.25 **58-year-old status post right breast cancer 15 years ago treated with lumpectomy and radiation therapy.** CC (**a**) and MLO (**b**) views show global right asymmetry and the technologist noted that the right breast was less compressible. Sagittal T1-weighed postcontrast (**c**) images from lateral to medial show multiple enhancing masses in the right breast. Targeted ultrasound (**d, e**) shows multiple mixed cystic and solid lesions with internal vascularity. Biopsy revealed radiation-induced angiosarcoma

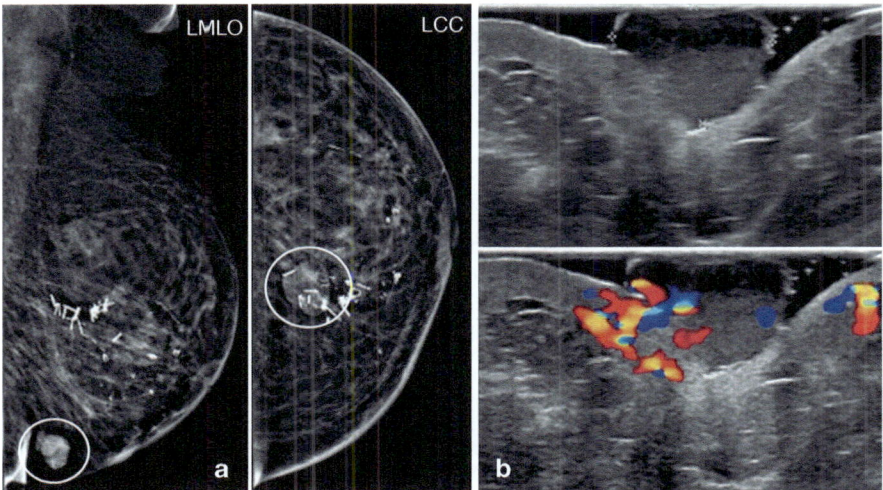

Fig. 10.26 Radiation-induced angiosarcoma. (a) Radiation-induced angiosarcoma presenting as a new lump (circles) in a patient with history of left breast cancer treated with lumpectomy and radiation 8 years earlier. (b) US shows a pedunculated exophytic skin lesion with marked vascular flow. Biopsy confirmed angiosarcoma

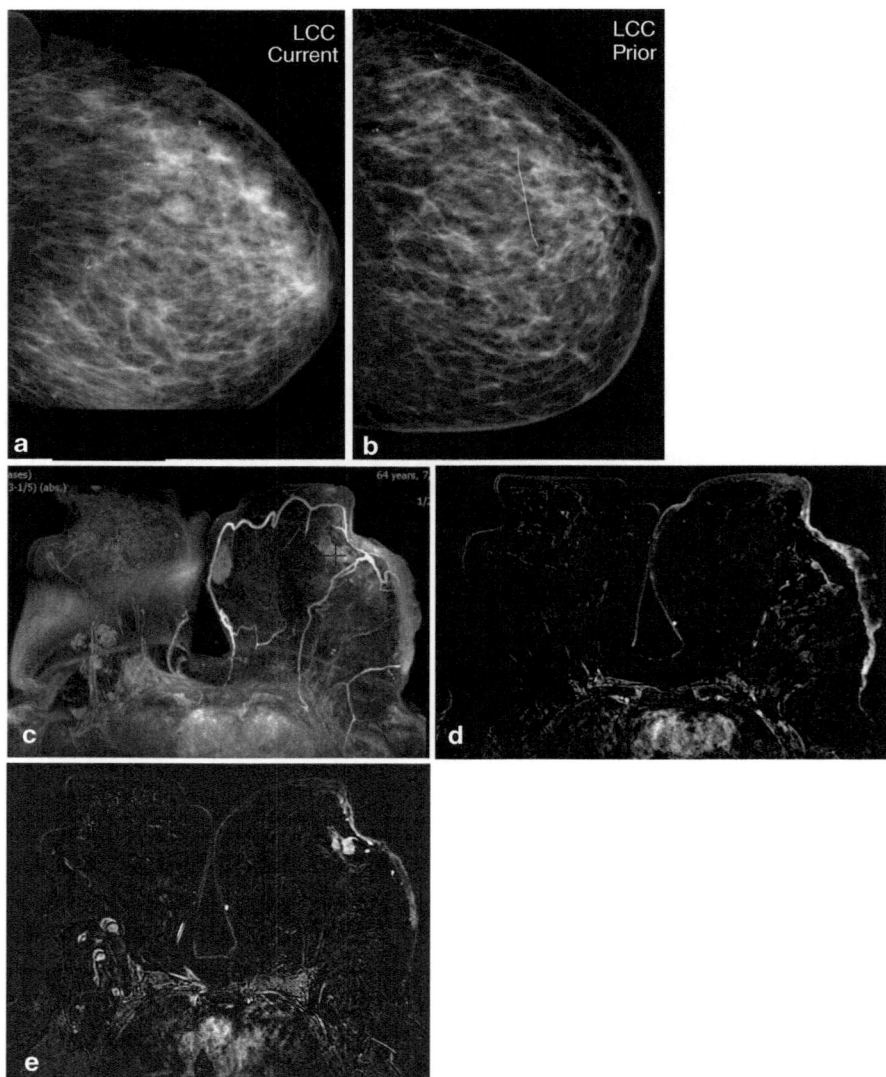

Fig. 10.27 Radiation-induced angiosarcoma. 64-year-old female with history of left breast cancer treated with breast conservation therapy 8 years ago presents with enlarging left bruise × 3 months. Increasing density and nodularity are seen on the CC view (**a**) when compared to a prior CC from 2 years prior (**b**). Axial MIP (**c**) and subtracted axial T1-weighted dynamic postcontrast (**d, e**) images show nodular skin thickening with areas of hypoenhancement and multiple enhancing parenchymal masses. Biopsy confirmed angiosarcoma

METASTATIC DISEASE TO THE BREAST

- Most commonly due to lymphoma/leukemia (Fig. 10.28), melanoma, sarcoma (Fig. 10.29), lung cancer, gastric cancer, and ovarian cancer; present as solitary mass or multiple masses with circumscribed/lobulated/indistinct margins; calcifications rare; tend to involve subcutaneous fat rather than glandular tissue

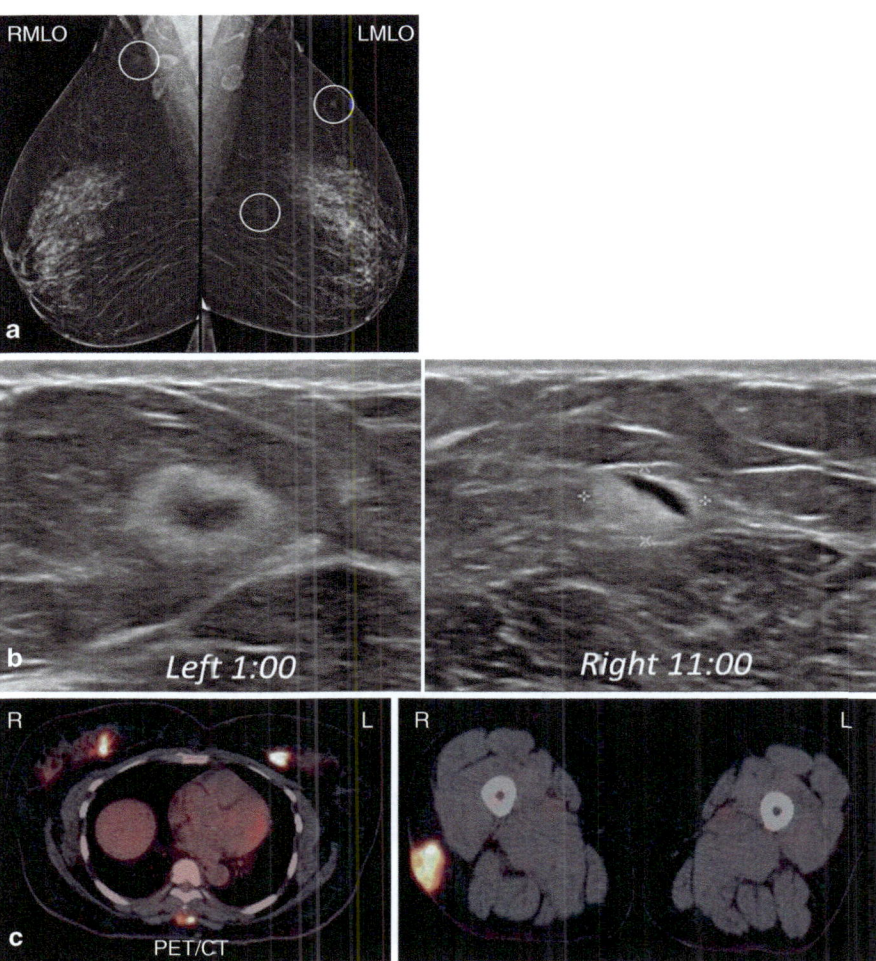

Fig. 10.28 Metastatic lymphoma to the breast. Peripheral T-cell lymphoma presenting as multiple bilateral indistinct masses on MG (**a**, circles). (**b**) US shows bilateral hypoechoic masses with an echogenic rind. (**c**) PET/CT performed after diagnosis reveals multiple subcutaneous hypermetabolic lesions involving the breasts, trunk, and extremities

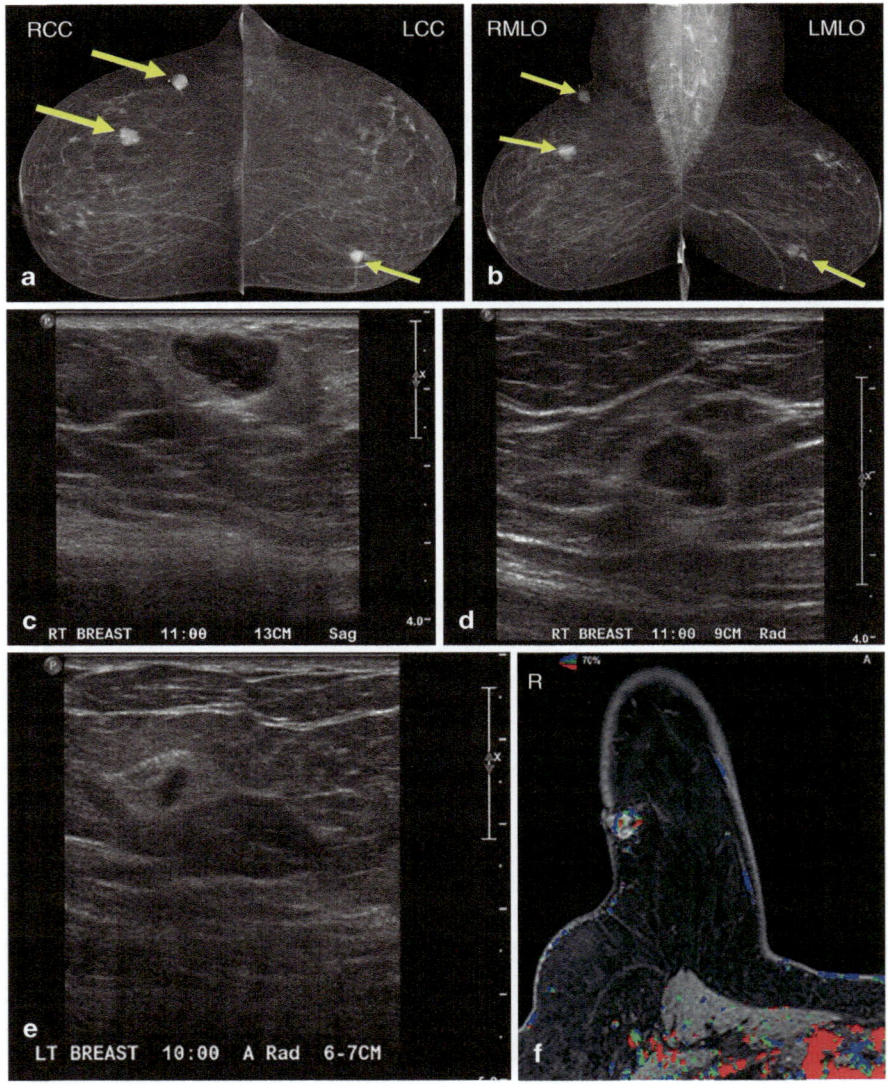

Fig. 10.29 **Metastatic disease from sarcoma**. 63-year-old female with palpable lump in upper outer right breast. Diagnostic CC (**a**) and MLO (**b**) views show multiple bilateral irregular and lobulated masses (arrows). Ultrasound identifies two solid hypoechoic masses in the right breast (**c, d**) and a hypoechoic mass with an echogenic rind in the left breast (**e**). Contrast enhanced MRI (**f–h**) showed enhancing masses with mixed kinetics. Biopsy confirmed metastatic sarcoma

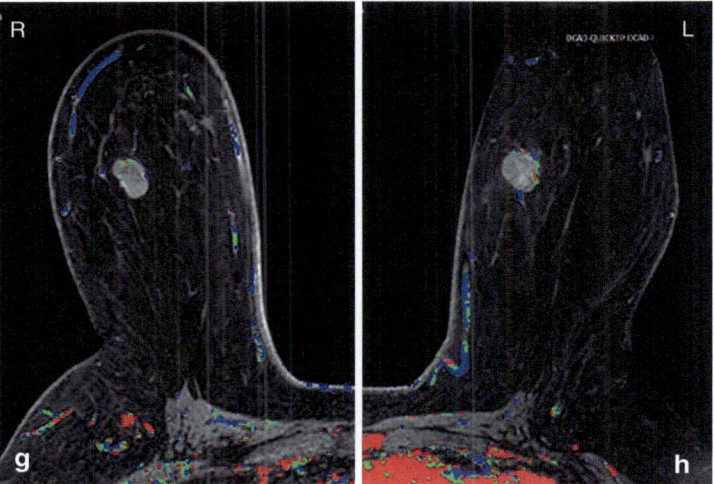

Fig. 10.29   (continued)

LYMPHOMA

- About 0.04–0.7% of all breast malignancies; more often secondary (metastatic) (Fig. e10.22) rather than primary (originating in the breast in the absence of prior or current extramammary lymphoma); treated with chemotherapy ± surgery

  - Primary breast lymphoma (Fig. e10.23)—most commonly B-cell origin
  - Secondary breast lymphoma—more likely multiple masses and bilateral involvement than primary (Fig. e10.24)

- Imaging findings overlap with primary breast cancer—solitary mass with circumscribed or indistinct margins, multiple masses, diffuse infiltrative process, axillary lymphadenopathy; calcifications and distortion rare
- Special subtype—breast implant-associated anaplastic large cell lymphoma (BIA-ALCL) (Figs. 10.30 and e10.25)

  - Rare; appears approximately 8–10 years after implant placement; any implant type at risk; most commonly presents as peri-implant effusion (60%), effusion + mass (20%), mass alone (17%); treat with surgical removal of implant and capsule + chemotherapy
  - Any implant-associated effusions > 1 year after placement in the absence of infection—US-guided aspiration with cytologic analysis

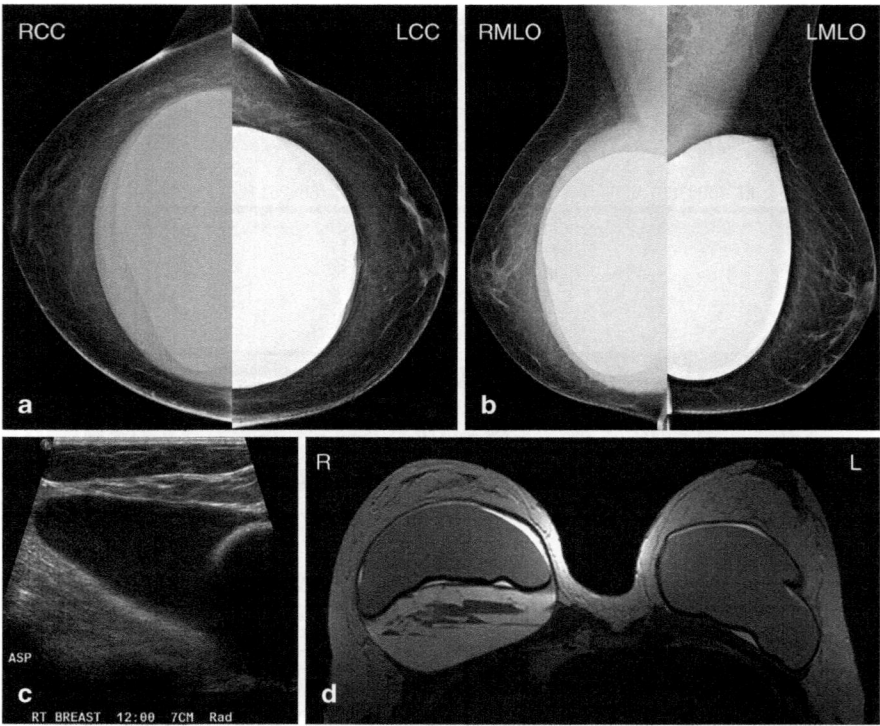

Fig. 10.30 Implant-associated lymphoma. 34-year-old transgender woman with acute onset of right breast swelling and pain with clinical concern for contracture. CC (**a**) and MLO (**b**) views show concentric density surrounding the right implant concerning for an effusion. Ultrasound (**c**) confirms fluid around the implant. MRI (**d**) shows a large collection with debris. Cytology of the fluid showed anaplastic large cell lymphoma

Further Readings

1. American College of Radiology Appropriateness Criteria. https://www.acr.org/ Clinical-Resources/ACR-Appropriateness-Criteria.
2. Makki J. Diversity of breast carcinoma: histologic subtypes and clinical relevance. Clin Med Insights Pathol. 2015;8:23–31.
3. Grimm LJ, Rabbar H, Abdelmalak M, et al. Ductal carcinoma in situ: state-of-the-art review. Radiology. 2022;302:246–55.
4. Yeh E, Jacene H, Bellon J, et al. What radiologists need to know about diagnosis and treatment of inflammatory breast cancer: a multidisciplinary approach. Radiographics. 2013;33:2003–17.
5. Johnson KS, Conant EF, Soo MS. Molecular subtypes of breast cancer: a review for breast radiologists. J Breast Imaging. 2021;3:12–24.
6. Teichgraeber DC, Guirguis MS, Whitman GJ. Breast cancer staging: updates in the *AJCC Cancer Staging Manual, 8th Edition*, and current challenges for radiologists. Am J Roentgenol. 2021;217:278–90.

7. Kalli S, Semine A, Cohen S, et al. American Joint Committee on Cancer's staging system for breast cancer: what the radiologist needs to know. Radiographics. 2018;38:1921–33.
8. Chang JM, Leung JW, Moy L, et al. Axillary nodal evaluation in breast cancer: state of the art. Radiology. 2020;295:500–15
9. Waks AG, Winer EP. Breast cancer treatment: a review. JAMA. 2019;321:288–300.
10. Chansakul T, Lai KC, Slanetz PJ. The post-conservation breast—Part 1, Expected imaging findings. Am J Roentgenol. 2012;198:321–30.
11. Chansakul T, Lai KC, Slanetz PJ. The post-conservation breast—Part 2, Unexpected imaging findings. Am J Roentgenol. 2012;198:331–43.
12. Sippo DA, Kulkarni K, Di Carlo P, et al. Metastatic disease to the breast from extramammary malignancies: a multimodality pictorial review. Curr Probl Diagn Radiol. 2016;45:225–32.

Pregnant and Lactating Patients

11

Kimberly Dao, Kitt Shaffer,
and Priscilla J. Slanetz

Hormonal changes of pregnancy and lactation lead to physiological changes in the breast.

Benign entities include galactocele, fibroadenoma, lactating adenoma, and puerperal mastitis.

Incidence of breast cancer in pregnant/lactating women = ~1 in 3000–10,000.

PHYSIOLOGIC CHANGES

- First trimester—develop lobular alveoli and lactiferous ducts
- Second trimester—proliferation and differentiation of alveolar epithelium into secretory epithelium
- Third trimester—differentiation of mild producing cells by prolactin with colostrum filling alveoli and ducts prior to delivery
- Postpartum—levels of estrogen and progesterone decrease resulting in greater lactogenic effect of prolactin on milk-producing cells
- Hormonal changes lead to increased breast size, tenderness, firmness, and nodularity which returns to baseline within 3 months after cessation of lactation

Supplementary Information The online version contains supplementary material available at https://doi.org/10.1007/978-3-031-66274-4_11.

K. Dao · K. Shaffer · P. J. Slanetz (✉)
Division of Breast Imaging, Department of Radiology, Boston University Medical Center, Boston, MA, USA
e-mail: kitt.shaffer@bmc.org; priscilla.slanetz@bmc.org

- Imaging
  - ○ Mammography—diffuse marked increase in overall breast density and breast size (Figs. 11.1, 11.2, and 11.3)
  - ○ US—diffuse hypoechogenicity due to enlargement of non-fatty fibroglandular tissues during pregnancy (Fig. 11.4); diffuse hyperechogenicity, prominent ducts, and increased vascularity during lactation (Fig. 11.5)
  - ○ MRI—diffuse increased T2 signal, prominent ducts, and bilateral enhancement if lactating; not performed during pregnancy as gadolinium is contraindicated given that it crosses placenta and safety not yet established

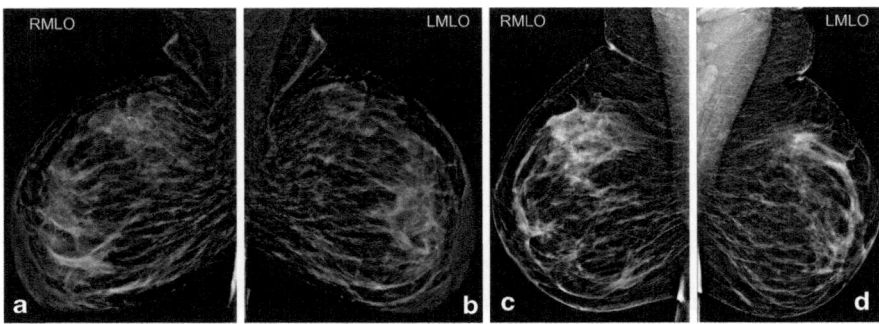

Fig. 11.1 31-year-old 21-week pregnant patient. Bilateral MLO views show enlarged breasts with increased glandular density and trabecular thickening (**a**, **b**), as compared to a prior mammogram (**c**, **d**) consistent with expected physiologic changes of pregnancy. A percutaneous biopsy clip in the upper right breast indicates the site of a prior benign biopsy

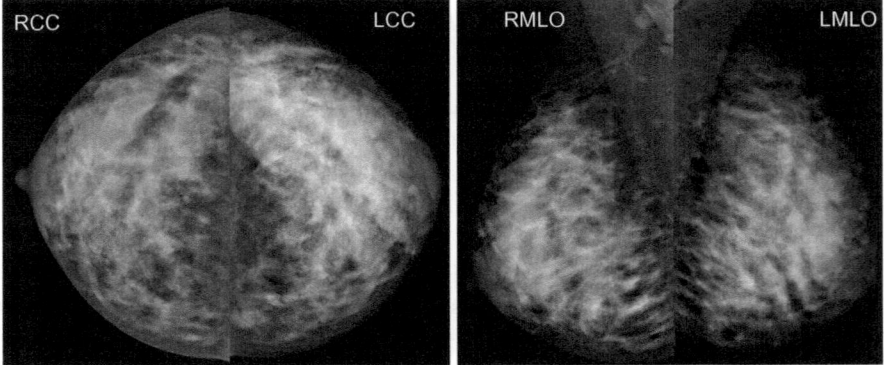

Fig. 11.2 35-year-old pregnant patient with a palpable lump in the right breast noted by her physician. Bilateral CC and MLO views revealed extremely dense breast tissues, an expected finding during pregnancy

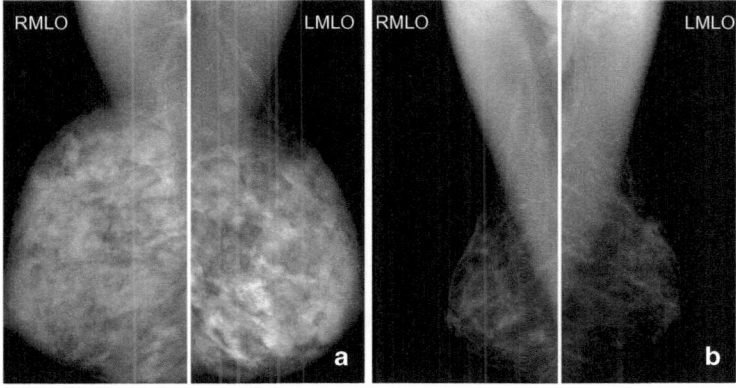

Fig. 11.3 **38-year-old lactating patient presenting with a palpable lump**. Bilateral MLO views (**a**) reveal extremely dense breast tissue and breast enlargement due to lactational state, as compared to (**b**) MLO views of same patient 2 years after cessation of breast-feeding

Fig. 11.4 38-year-old 16 weeks pregnant patient presenting with a right breast lump. Ultrasound at 12:00 shows heterogeneous predominantly hypoechoic breast tissue, typical of what is seen during pregnancy

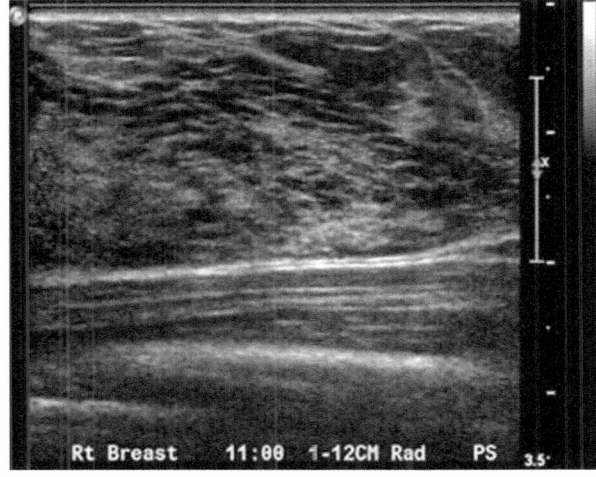

Fig. 11.5 29-year-old lactating patient presenting with a palpable left breast mass. Ultrasound of the left breast at 10:00 reveals prominent fluid-filled ducts and overall hyperechoic breast tissue, typical of what is seen during lactation

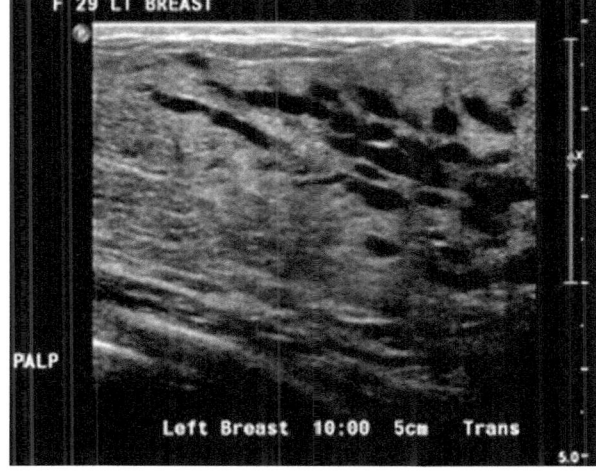

IMAGING

- Based on ACR Appropriateness Criteria*
- Screening—mammography not contraindicated but not routinely performed in practice
  - If high risk, annual mammography strongly advised; screening MRI contraindicated as gadolinium crosses placenta
  - If lactating, pump or nurse 1 hour prior to imaging; MRI can be performed safely if indicated but discard breast milk for 12–24 hours
- Pregnant with symptom (lump, pain, discharge)—start with US; if US suspicious, perform diagnostic mammography
  - Fetal radiation dose negligible (< 0.03 mGy for 4-view mammogram)
  - Radiation exposure comes from internal scatter so no shielding is indicated
- Lactating with symptom (lump, pain, discharge)—if < 30 years, start with US; otherwise perform diagnostic mammogram + US

BIOPSY CONSIDERATIONS

- Majority biopsied with ultrasound guidance
- Risks include bleeding, infection, and milk fistula (if lactating)
  - Milk fistula = tract between duct and skin created by biopsy needle that can close spontaneously but may necessitate cessation of lactation

BENIGN ENTITIES

OBSTRUCTED MILK DUCT

- Due to mechanical obstruction, change in infant feeding pattern, scarring from previous surgery, or infection
- Commonly presents as tender lump
- On US—non-compressible avascular tubular lesion, sometimes with surrounding edema (Fig. 11.6)
- Management—warm compresses and massage; frequent pumping; rarely antibiotics

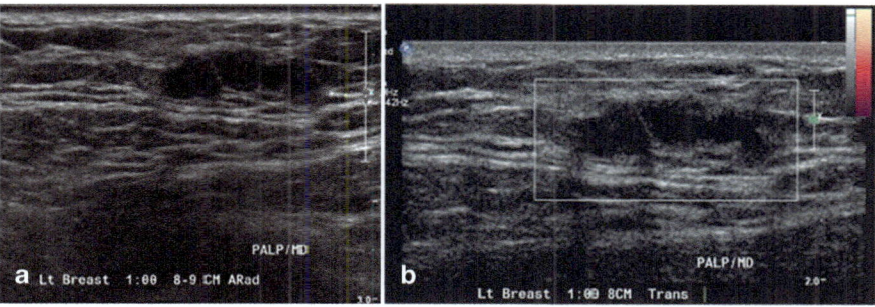

Fig. 11.6 (a, b) 32-year-old lactating patient with a palpable cord-like left breast mass. Ultrasound reveals a dilated tubular non-compressible avascular mass consistent with a blocked milk duct. The mass resolved spontaneously with conservative management

GALACTOCELE

- Most common benign breast lesion in lactating women that presents during late third trimester, after delivery or after cessation of lactation due to obstructed duct with distension of proximal lobular segments
- Variable contents of fat, protein, and water lead to varied appearance on imaging
- Imaging
  - Mammography—circumscribed mass with fat-fluid level (Fig. 11.7)
  - Ultrasound—circumscribed, oval or round anechoic to hypoechoic mass, often with a fat-fluid level, internal mobile debris, and posterior acoustic enhancement (Figs. 11.8, e11.1, and e11.2); no internal vascularity; can be mixed solid and cystic as lesion ages, may become hyperechoic
- Management—warm compresses and frequent pumping; drainage if symptomatic

LACTATING ADENOMA/LACTATIONAL CHANGES

- Lactational changes occur throughout the breast tissue due to lobular proliferation
  - May present as hypo- to iso-echoic mass or as round scattered or grouped calcifications (Figs. 11.9, 11.10, and e11.3)
- Lactating adenomas—benign neoplasm consisting of lobular aggregates with secretory changes
  - Occur during third trimester or lactation
  - May undergo infarction, regress after cessation of lactation, or recur with subsequent pregnancies

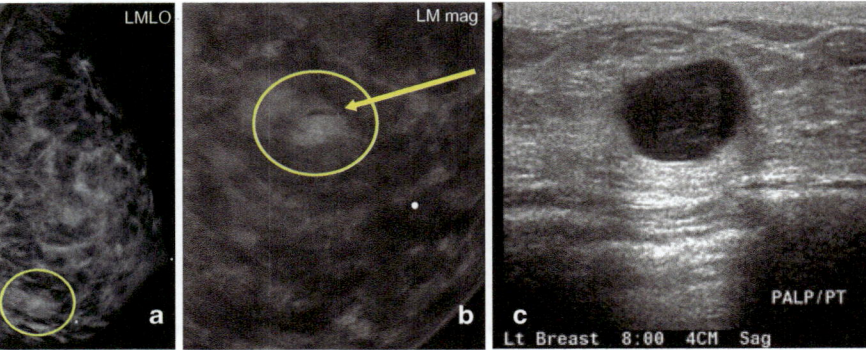

Fig. 11.7　34-year-old female presenting with a palpable left breast lump. MLO view (**a**) and magnified lateral view (**b**) show a circumscribed mass (circle) with a fat-fluid level (arrow) on the magnified lateral image which is diagnostic of a galactocele. Correlative ultrasound (**c**) shows a hypoechoic well-circumscribed mass with posterior acoustic enhancement

Fig. 11.8　30-year-old lactating patient who presents with a palpable left breast mass. Targeted ultrasound shows a circumscribed, oval, hypoechoic mass with layering internal debris, consistent with a galactocele

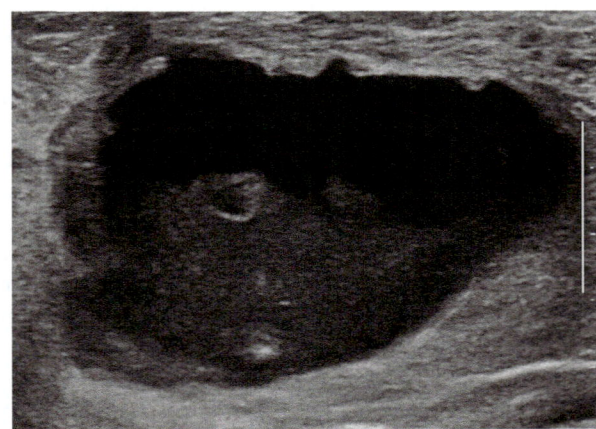

- Imaging
  - Mammography—circumscribed, oval or round mass ± radiolucent areas indicative of fatty content of milk; calcifications infrequent
  - Ultrasound—circumscribed, oval, hypoechoic mass with posterior acoustic enhancement (Figs. 11.11, e11.4, and e11.5)
- Management
  - Clinical and/or imaging follow-up to assess for stability
  - Image-guided biopsy is warranted if suspicious morphology features or enlarging

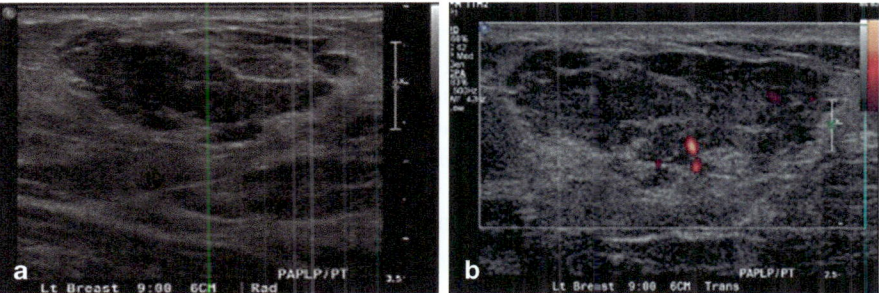

Fig. 11.9   24-year-old female with a palpable left breast mass. Ultrasound reveals a heterogeneous iso-echoic vascular mass (**a**, **b**), which on biopsy revealed lactational change

Fig. 11.10   28-year-old lactating patient presenting for screening. Bilateral MLO views show faint diffusely scattered round calcifications (arrows) consistent with lactational calcifications

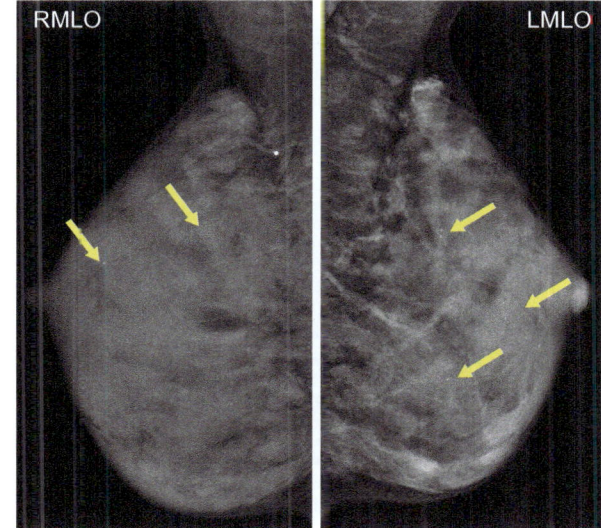

Fig. 11.11   34-year-old 28 weeks pregnant patient with right breast palpable finding. Right breast US shows a circumscribed, oval, hypoechoic mass with no posterior features. Ultrasound-guided core biopsy confirmed lactating adenoma

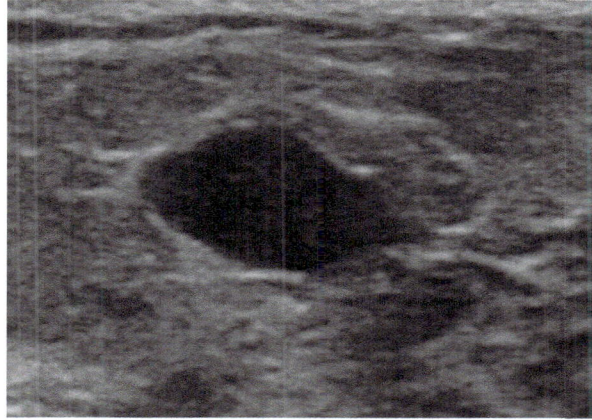

PUERPERAL MASTITIS/ABSCESS

- Breast infection with skin thickening and erythema most commonly seen with lactation 0–6 months postpartum sometimes complicated by abscess (4–11% of mastitis), focal collection of pus that requires drainage
- Most commonly due to *Staphylococcus aureus* and *Streptococcus* due to seeding of nipple-areolar complex by infant's nose/throat
- Ultrasound is first-line modality; mammography if suspicious US findings, not responsive to antibiotics, or recurrent
- Imaging
    - Ultrasound—skin thickening, soft tissue edema, hyperemia, dilated lymphatics, increased echogenicity (Figs. 11.12 and e11.6); ductal debris with ductal wall thickening, focal heterogeneous complex cystic collection with posterior acoustic enhancement = abscess (Fig. 11.13)
    - Mammography—increased density, trabecular and skin thickening, reactive axillary lymph nodes; often mass if there is an abscess
- Management—antibiotics, percutaneous drainage of abscess with aspirate sent for culture and sensitivity, frequent pumping/nursing, warm compresses

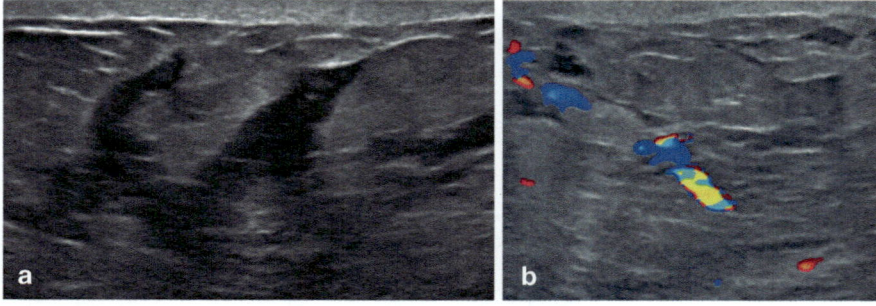

Fig. 11.12 28-year-old lactating patient with focal right breast pain, swelling, erythema, and fever. Right breast US shows skin thickening, subcutaneous soft tissue edema, and inflammatory changes (**a**). There is increased vascularity in the tissues on color Doppler (**b**). Findings are consistent with puerperal mastitis. No drainable collection was seen

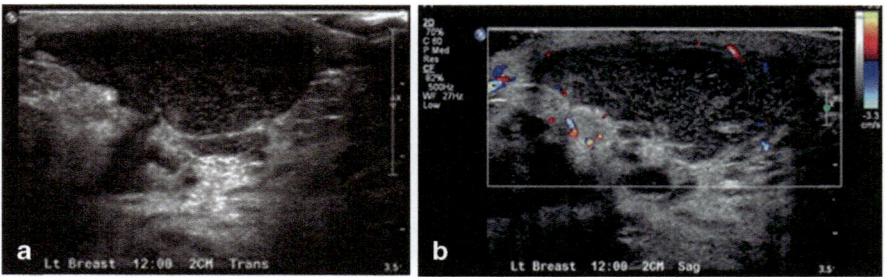

Fig. 11.13 28-year-old lactating patient with focal breast tenderness and erythema for 3 days with fever and chills. Ultrasound shows a complicated fluid collection (**a**) with peripheral vascularity (**b**) and overlying skin thickening consistent with abscess

FIBROADENOMA

- Most common benign mass in young women presenting as firm mobile mass that often enlarges due to elevated circulating estrogen levels during pregnancy
  - May appear atypical on imaging being heterogeneous with microcystic changes, increased vascularity and prominent ducts
  - Can undergo infarction due to rapid growth presenting as painful mass on exam
- Imaging
  - Ultrasound—circumscribed, oval hypo- to iso-echoic mass (Figs. 11.14 and e11.7); may have heterogeneous internal echotexture, increased vascularity, and lobulations
  - Mammography—circumscribed, oval or round mass with or without coarse calcifications
- Management
  - Percutaneous biopsy if suspicious morphology or enlarging

Fig. 11.14   34-year-old pregnant patient presenting for 2-year follow-up of probable benign palpable mass. Right breast ultrasound shows a stable circumscribed, oval, hypoechoic mass without internal vascularity, consistent with a fibroadenoma

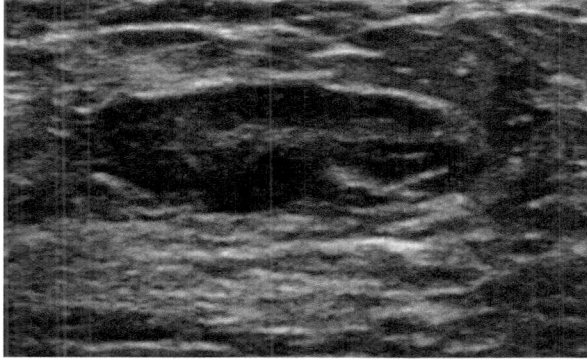

HYPERPLASTIC LYMPH NODES

- Enlarged intramammary and axillary reactive nodes due to lactation not infrequently found on imaging
- Imaging
  - ○ Mammography—smooth oval or bean-shaped mass with fatty central hilum in upper outer breast or axilla (Fig. 11.15)
  - ○ Ultrasound—oval hypoechoic mass with <0.3 cm cortical thickness
- Management—clinical or imaging follow-up reasonable; percutaneous biopsy if suspicious (> 0.3 cm cortical thickness)

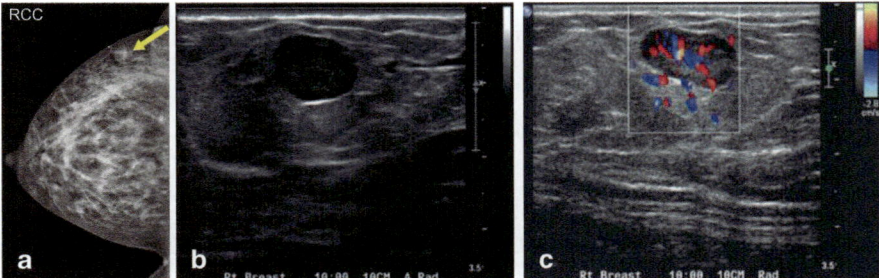

Fig. 11.15 **38-year-old lactating patient with a right breast lump**. CC view (**a**) shows a circumscribed mass (arrow) in the outer upper right breast corresponding to the area of concern. US (**b**, **c**) shows a well circumscribed mass with a hypoechoic cortex and echogenic center and prominent internal vascularity. Findings are consistent with a reactive intramammary lymph node

HIDRADENITIS SUPPURATIVA

- Infected sweat gland due to obstruction of epidermal gland
- Presents as superficial swollen painful axillary mass complicated by sinus tracts, scarring, and cellulitis (Fig. 11.16)
- Management—warm compresses, antibiotics

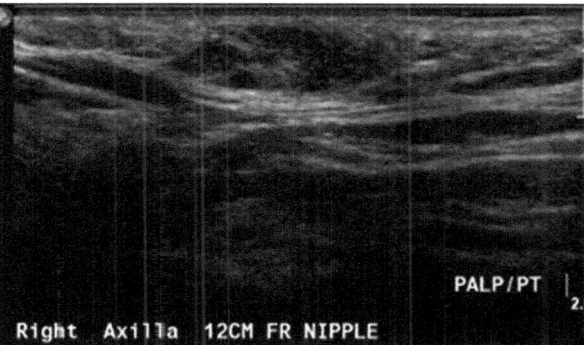

Fig. 11.16   29-year-old pregnant patient with a palpable right axillary lump. Ultrasound reveals a superficial indeterminate hypoechoic heterogeneous mass with peripheral vascularity. Biopsy confirmed benign fibroadipose tissue with eccrine ducts and glands and a single hair follicle consistent with hidradenitis suppurativa

GRANULOMATOUS MASTITIS

- Rare inflammatory disease of unknown etiology affecting women within 6 years of pregnancy characterized by non-caseating, non-vasculitic granulomatous changes, and infrequent sinus tract to skin
- Presents as distinct firm hard mass that tends to spare subareolar area
- Imaging
  - Mammography—may be normal or show mass with variable shape and margins; can mimic breast malignancy (Figs. 11.17 and 11.18)
  - Ultrasound—variable ranging from multiple tubular hypoechoic areas to large irregular hypoechoic mass (Figs. e11.8 and e11.9)
- Diagnosis often requires percutaneous biopsy with specimens sent to pathology and microbiology (specifically, *Corynebacterium*)
- Management—steroids/immunosuppressants; antibiotics if cystic neutrophilic variant; rarely surgery

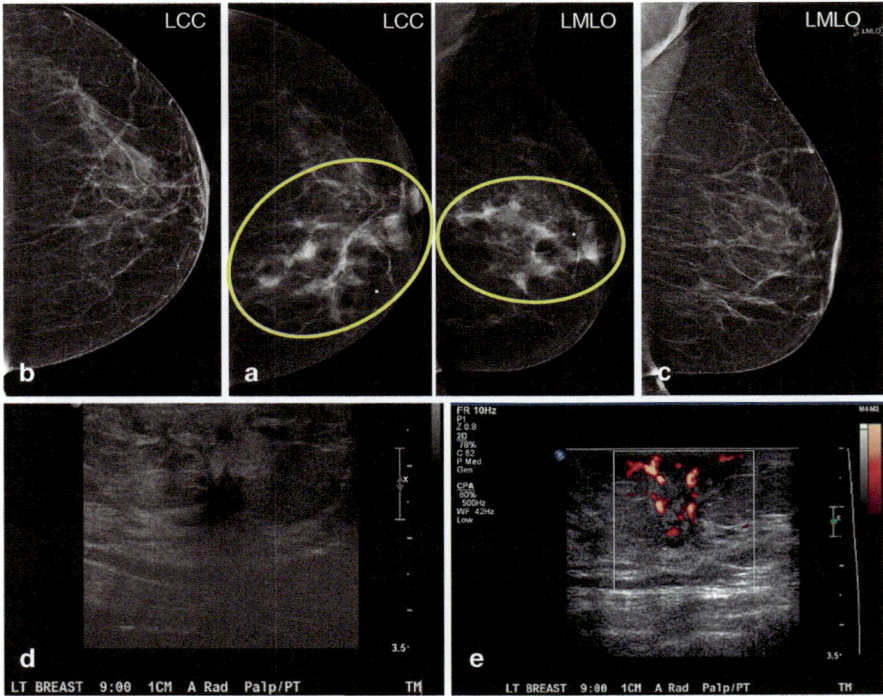

Fig. 11.17 43-year-old patient 2 years postpartum presenting with increasing left breast firmness for 2 months. Left CC and MLO (**a**) views show multiple irregular masses in a segmental distribution (oval) which developed since a normal mammogram 5 months prior (**b**, **c**). Ultrasound shows one of the irregular hypoechoic masses (**d**) with posterior acoustic shadowing, prominent internal vascularity (**e**), and overlying skin thickening. Findings are concerning for inflammatory breast cancer. Biopsy confirmed cystic neutrophilic granulomatous mastitis, a variant that is associated with *Corynebacterium*. The patient was treated with antibiotics and systemic steroids

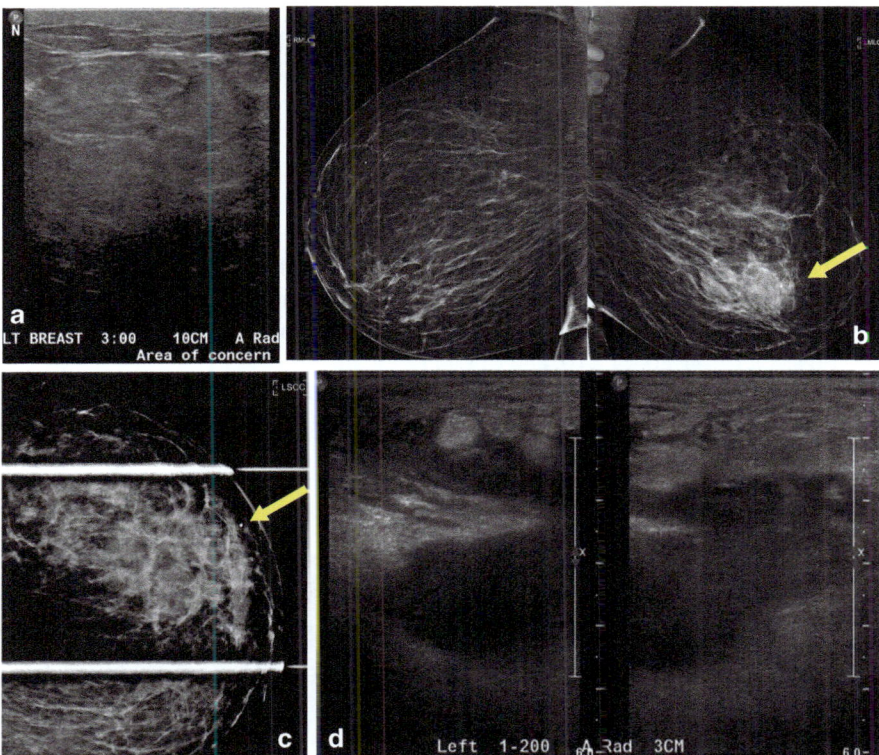

Fig. 11.18 **40-year-old patient 1-year postpartum with breast swelling, tenderness, and firmness**. Ultrasound (**a**) shows breast edema and skin thickening consistent with mastitis. The patient was treated with antibiotics. Her symptoms somewhat improved but waxed and waned over the next 6 months. Bilateral MLO views (**b**) and spot compression left CC view (**c**) show an irregular mass (arrow) in the central outer left breast. Ultrasound (**d**) shows diffuse skin thickening, dilated lymphatics, and a hypoechoic irregular mass. Findings were concerning for locally advanced breast cancer. Biopsy confirmed granulomatous mastitis

PREGNANCY-ASSOCIATED BREAST CARCINOMA (PABC)

- Defined as breast cancer occurring during pregnancy or within first year after delivery
- Accounts for 1–2% all newly diagnosed cancers
- Occurs 1 in 3000–10,000 pregnancies
- Presents as a painless, palpable mass, sometimes with nipple discharge or lymphadenopathy
  - Tend to be diagnosed at more advanced stage, higher grade, ER/PR negative, HER2 positive, and worse overall prognosis than non-PABC
- Imaging findings on mammography and ultrasound identical to non-PABC (Figs. 11.19, 11.20, e11.10, and e11.11)
  - Central necrosis more likely due to rapid growth (Fig. e11.12)
  - Mammography used to evaluate extent of disease and screen contralateral breast

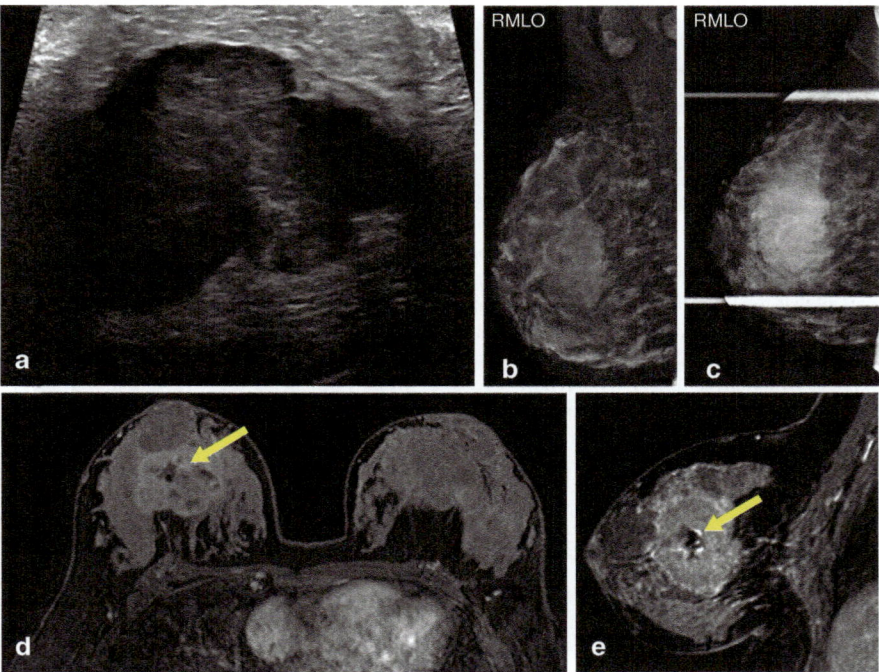

Fig. 11.19 37-year-old lactating patient 6 months postpartum presenting with palpable finding in the right breast. Right breast US (**a**) shows a large, irregular, hypoechoic mass with indistinct margins. Right MLO (**b**) and spot compression MLO (**c**) views show a partially obscured, irregular mass and axillary lymphadenopathy. Subsequent axial (**d**) and sagittal (**e**) contrast-enhanced MR images confirm an irregular, enhancing mass with mixed enhancement kinetics. Susceptibility artifact corresponds to the biopsy clip (arrow). Ultrasound-guided core biopsy confirmed invasive ductal carcinoma

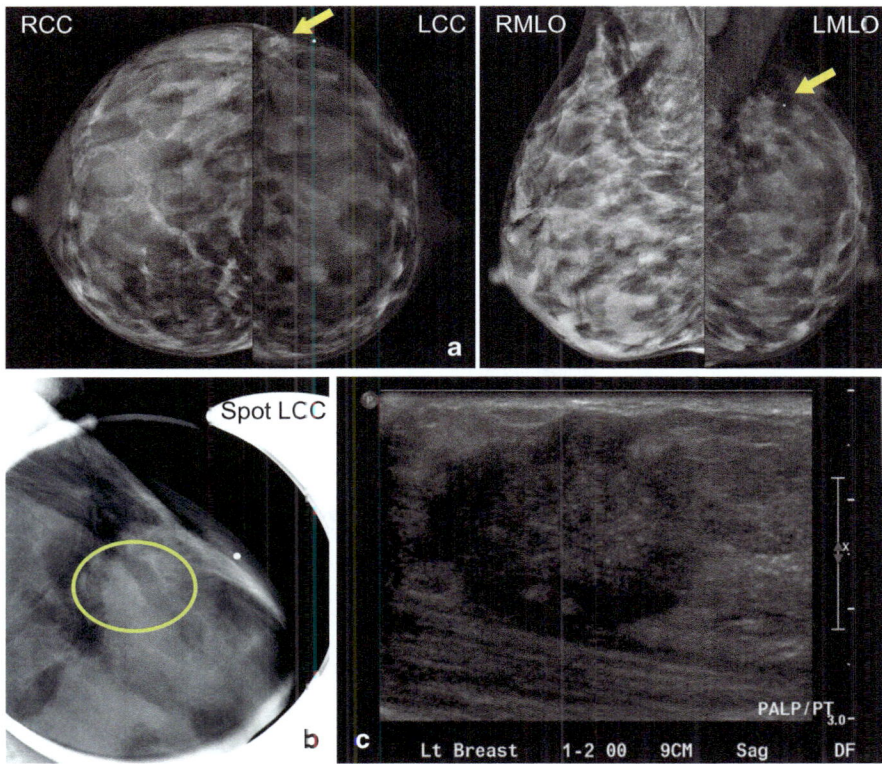

Fig. 11.20 40-year-old lactating patient with a palpable left upper outer breast mass for 1 month. Bilateral CC and MLO views (**a**) confirm an irregular obscured mass (arrow) in the area of concern. Spot compression CC view (**b**) shows focal skin retraction with an underlying obscured mass with associated fine microcalcifications (circle). Ultrasound (**c**) shows an irregular hypoechoic mass with internal echogenic foci consistent with calcifications. Biopsy confirmed high grade invasive ductal cancer and ductal carcinoma in situ

- ○ MRI contraindicated during pregnancy as gadolinium crosses placenta; limited value during lactation due to marked background parenchymal enhancement
- Management—prompt percutaneous biopsy to establish diagnosis
  - ○ Chemotherapy and surgery safe during pregnancy; radiation delayed until after delivery
  - ○ Therapeutic abortion does not improve prognosis

OTHER MALIGNANCIES

- Most commonly metastatic due to lymphoma/leukemia, melanoma, or lung cancer
- Primary breast lymphoma can also occur, but is rare (Fig. e11.13)

Further Readings

1. Expert Panel on Breast Imaging, di Florio-Alexander RM, Slanetz PJ, et al. ACR Appropriateness Criteria® breast imaging of pregnant and lactating women. J Am Coll Radiol. 2018;15:S263–75.
2. Parker S, Saettele M, Morgan M, Stein M, Winkler N. Spectrum of pregnancy- and lactation-related benign breast findings. Curr Probl Diagn Radiol. 2017;46:432–40.
3. Vashi R, Hooley R, Butler R, Geisel J, Philpotts L. Breast imaging of the pregnant and lactating patient: imaging modalities and pregnancy-associated breast cancer. AJR Am J Roentgenol. 2013;200:321–8.
4. Vashi R, Hooley R, Butler R, Geisel J, Philpotts L. Breast imaging of the pregnant and lactating patient: physiologic changes and common benign entities. AJR Am J Roentgenol. 2013;200:329–36.

Breast Augmentation and Breast Reconstruction

12

Priscilla J. Slanetz
and Vandana Dialani

Performed most commonly for cosmetic purposes or after mastectomy for breast cancer; less commonly for congenital breast hypoplasia

Involves placement of breast implant or autologous flap (most commonly deep inferior epigastric perforator flap (DIEP) or transverse rectus abdominis flap (TRAM)); less commonly, implant with latissimus dorsi flap

Rarely, free injection of silicone or other materials into breast (e.g., fat, poly-acrylamide gel (PAAG), hyaluronic acid, paraffin)

BREAST IMPLANTS

Material

- Typically composed of silicone (Fig. 12.1) or saline (Fig. 12.2); very rarely, PAAG (Fig. 12.3) or fat (Fig. 12.4)
- Most often consists of a foreign material encapsulated by an envelope (single lumen); less commonly, double lumen (typically outer saline and inner silicone) (Fig. 12.5)

Supplementary Information The online version contains supplementary material available at https://doi.org/10.1007/978-3-031-66274-4_12.

P. J. Slanetz (✉)
Division of Breast Imaging, Department of Radiology, Boston University Medical Center, Boston, MA, USA
e-mail: Priscilla.slanetz@bmc.org

V. Dialani
Division of Breast Imaging, Department of Radiology, Beth Israel Deaconess Medical Center, Boston, MA, USA
e-mail: vdialani@bidmc.harvard.edu

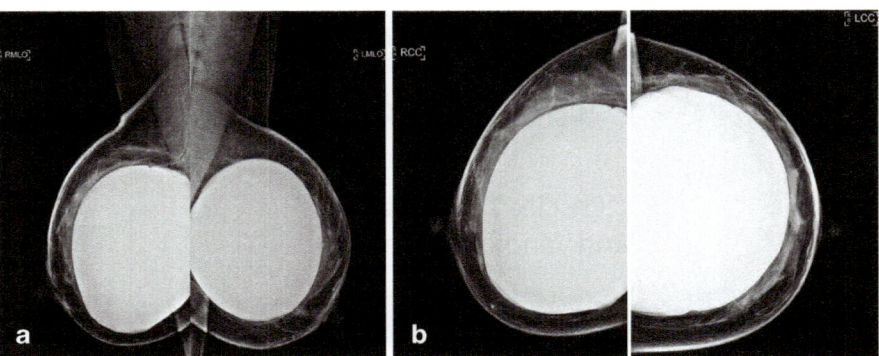

Fig. 12.1 Silicone implants: 56-year-old woman presenting for screening mammography. (**a**) Bilateral MLO and (**b**) CC views show prepectoral silicone implants. Notice the high x-ray attenuation of the silicone

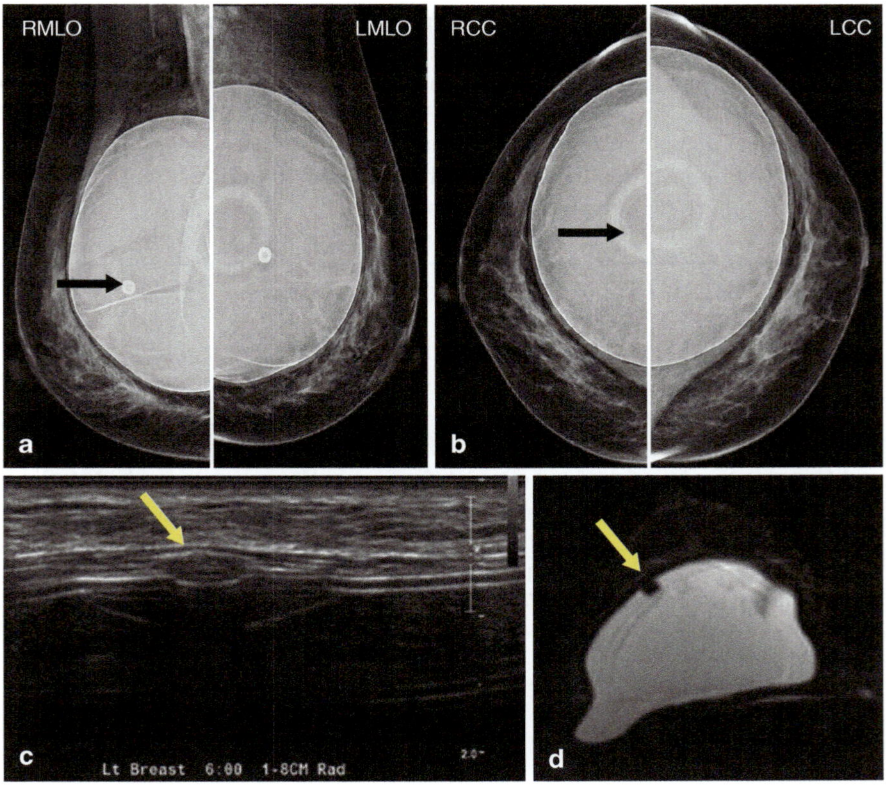

Fig. 12.2 Saline implants: 45-year-old woman presenting for screening mammography. (**a**) Bilateral MLO and (**b**) CC views show intact retropectoral saline implants. As saline implants are relatively radiolucent, the valve (arrow) and even folds of the implant envelope may be seen. Note the appearance of the valve on US (**c**) and on MRI (**d**)

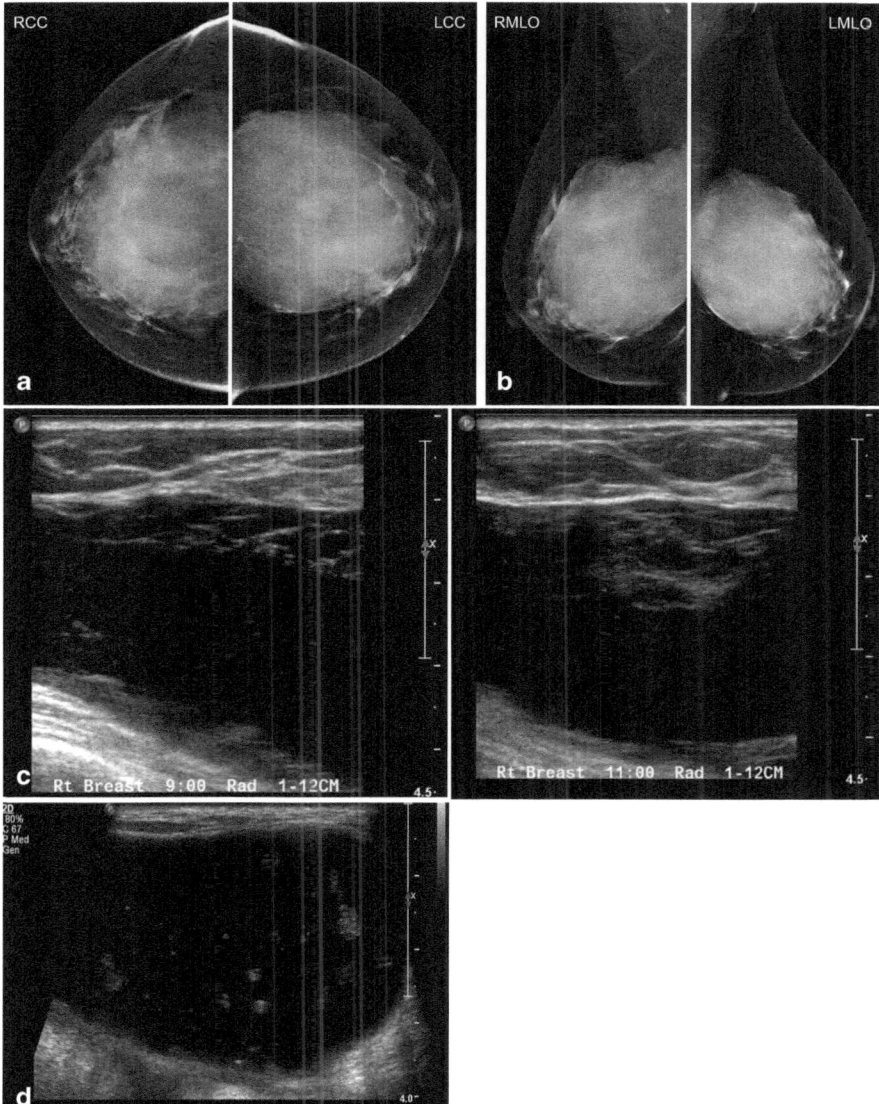

Fig. 12.3 PAAG implants: 55-year-old woman presenting for screening mammography. Notice how the homogeneous gel has similar attenuation to the overlying dense breast tissue on the CC (**a**) and MLO (**b**) views. Ultrasound shows hypoechoic collection, sometimes with a thick wall (**c**). On real-time imaging, floating echogenic debris (**d**) may be seen

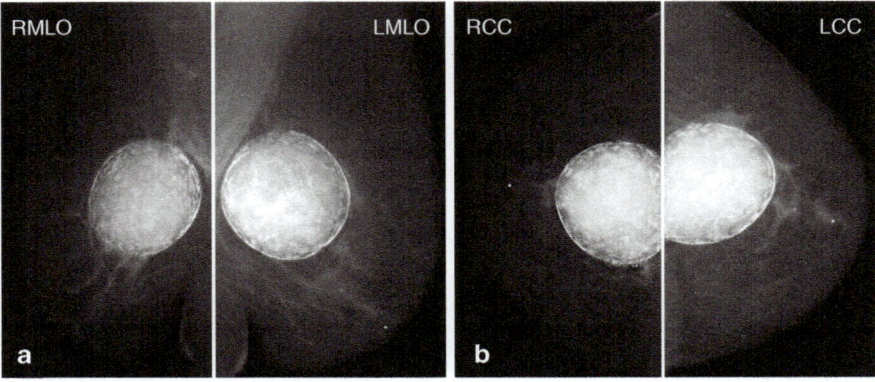

Fig. 12.4 Fat injections: 68-year-old woman with bilateral fat injections. Bilateral MLO (**a**) and CC views (**b**) show calcified fat necrosis

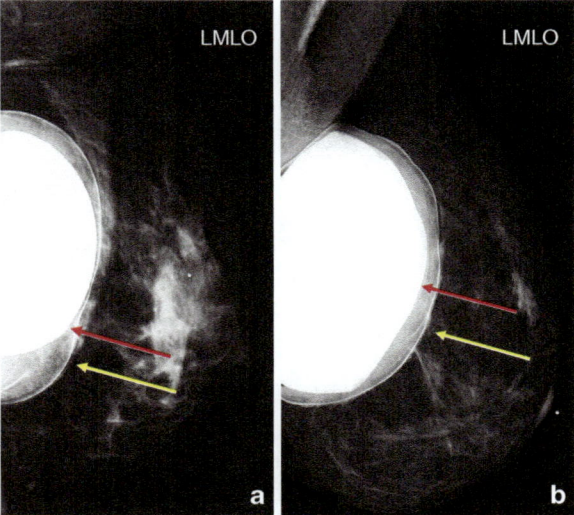

Fig. 12.5 Double lumen breast implants. (**a**) Retropectoral double lumen implant. (**b**) Prepectoral double lumen implant. Notice the outer lucent component filled with saline (yellow arrows) and the inner lumen filled with dense silicone (red arrows)

Location

- Prepectoral (within the breast tissue) (Fig. 12.6a) or retropectoral/subpectoral (beneath the pectoral muscle) (Fig. 12.6b)
- When placed, the body forms a capsule around the implant envelope to "wall it off" (foreign body reaction)

Normal Appearance and Potential Complications

- Radial folds—infoldings of envelope that appear as curvilinear low signal lines that extend into but not across implant (Fig. 12.7)
- Rupture
  ○ Intracapsular—the elastomere shell is no longer intact and the implant contents are now only contained by the capsule which is intact (Figs. 12.8 and e12.1)
  ○ Extracapsular—the capsule has ruptured, and the implant contents extrude into the surrounding breast tissue (Fig. 12.9)

    - Silicone implant—most often not detectable on exam; sometimes may have palpable lump f extracapsular (Fig. 12.10)
    - Saline implant—on exam, smaller breast size on side of collapse (Fig. 12.11); can confirm on imaging with mammography or US
    - Double lumen implant—outer saline component collapses; detect as single this lumen on affected side (Fig. e12.2)
- Herniation—envelope is intact but herniates through a defect in the capsule; no need to intervene unless cosmetic deformity (Fig. e12.3)
- Peri-implant fluid collection — most often reactive, but large collection raises this concern for implant-associated lymphoma (Fig. e12.4)
- Capsular calcification—relatively common and can lead to firmness, immobility, and ultimately contracture (Fig. 12.12)
- Capsular contraction—implant becomes round, firm, and immobile (Figs. 12.13 and e12.5); very rarely, implant infection can occur (Figs. 12.14 and e12.6)
- Implant-associated masses—fat necrosis (Fig. e12.7), fibromatosis/desmoid tumor (Fig. 12.15), anaplastic large cell lymphoma (Fig. 12.15), sarcoma (Fig. e12.8)

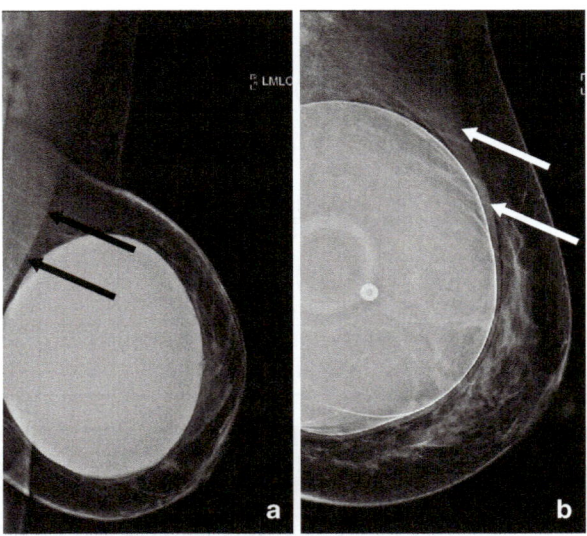

Fig. 12.6 (**a**) **Prepectoral implant:** The implant is within the glandular tissue and the pectoralis muscle (black arrows) is behind the implant. (**b**) **Retropectoral implant**. The implant is under the pectoralis muscle (white arrows) and the glandular tissue is free from the implant

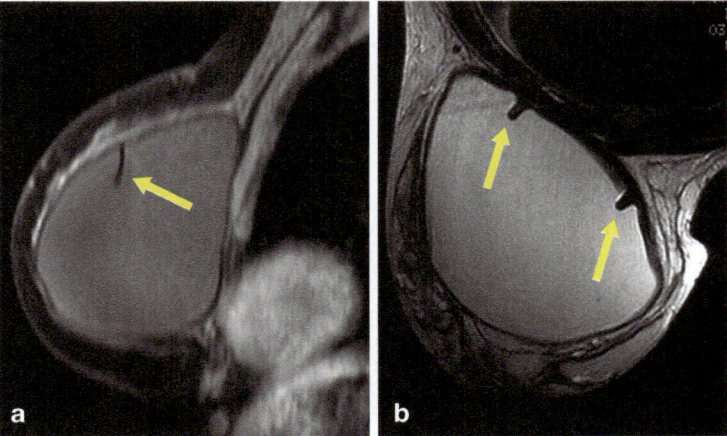

Fig. 12.7 **Radial folds**. (**a**) Sagittal and (**b**) axial images of silicone implant shows typical radial folds of envelope (yellow arrows) appearing as low signal curvilinear lines that extend into the lumen but not entirely across implant

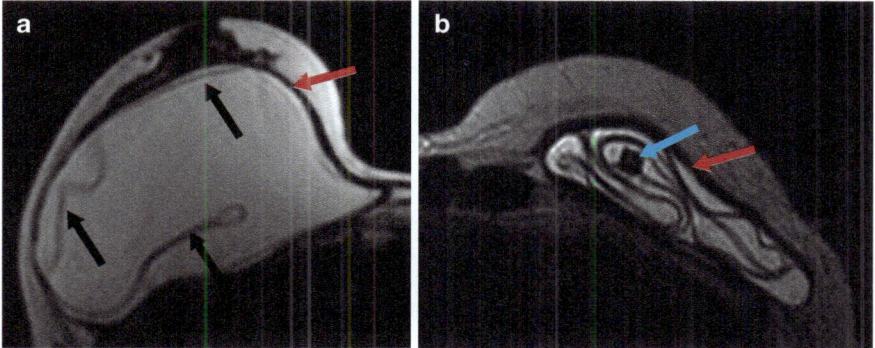

Fig. 12.8 Intracapsular rupture. (a) Folded elastomere shell of silicone implant (black arrows) contained within an intact capsule (red arrow) consistent with *linguine sign*, and (b) saline implant rupture contained by capsule. Notice the valve of collapsed saline implant (blue arrow). Remember that MRI is not indicated for saline implant rupture as such rupture is evident on physical exam and can be easily confirmed on mammography or ultrasound

Fig. 12.9 Bilateral MLO views with extracapsular rupture on the left. (a) Extrusion of silicone into surrounding tissues (white arrow) - notice the irregular contour to the superior aspect of the left prepectoral silicone implant. (b) Another patient with silicone granulomas (red arrows) from prior extracapsular rupture (c) Third patient with post-inflammatory reaction around extruded silicone related to prior extracapsular rupture (blue arrows)

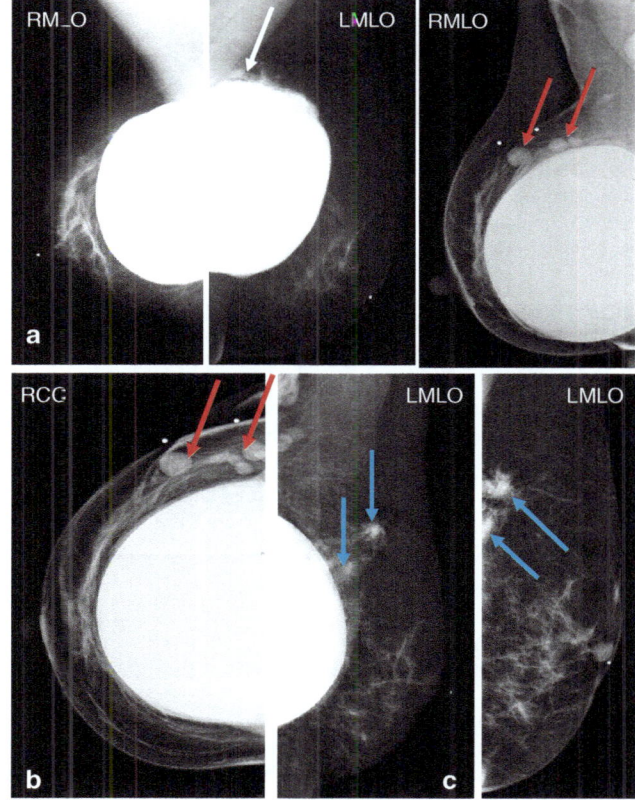

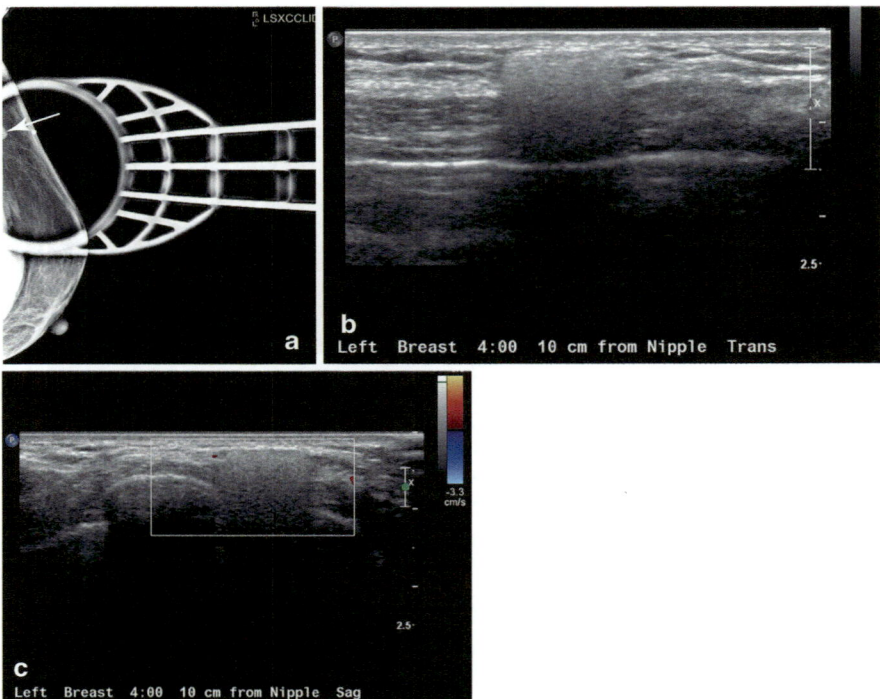

Fig. 12.10 Silicone granuloma. 61-year-old with palpable left breast lump at 4:00. (**a**) Spot compression CC view shows dense incompletely visualized mass in the far outer posterior breast (arrow). Implant is displaced posteriorly and inferiorly. (**b**, **c**) Ultrasound shows a hyperechoic shadowing avascular mass consistent with silicone granuloma

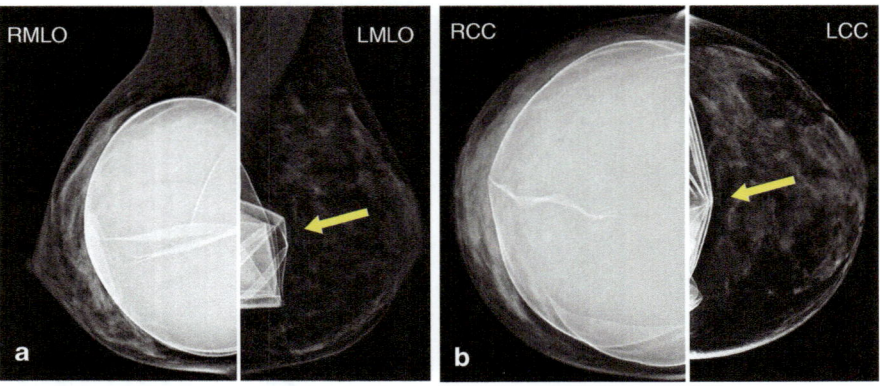

Fig. 12.11 Ruptured saline implant. 44-year-old for screening. Bilateral MLO (**a**) and CC (**b**) views reveal intact right saline implant and ruptured left saline implant (yellow arrow). The envelope is collapsed as saline was resorbed by body after rupture

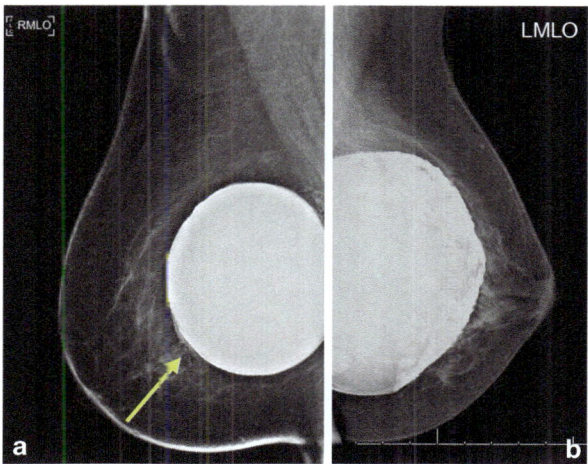

Fig. 12.12 Capsular calcifications. RMLO (**a**) view shows thin rim of calcification along the implant surface (yellow arrow). LMLO view (**b**) in another patient shows more extensive coarse calcification overlying implant surface

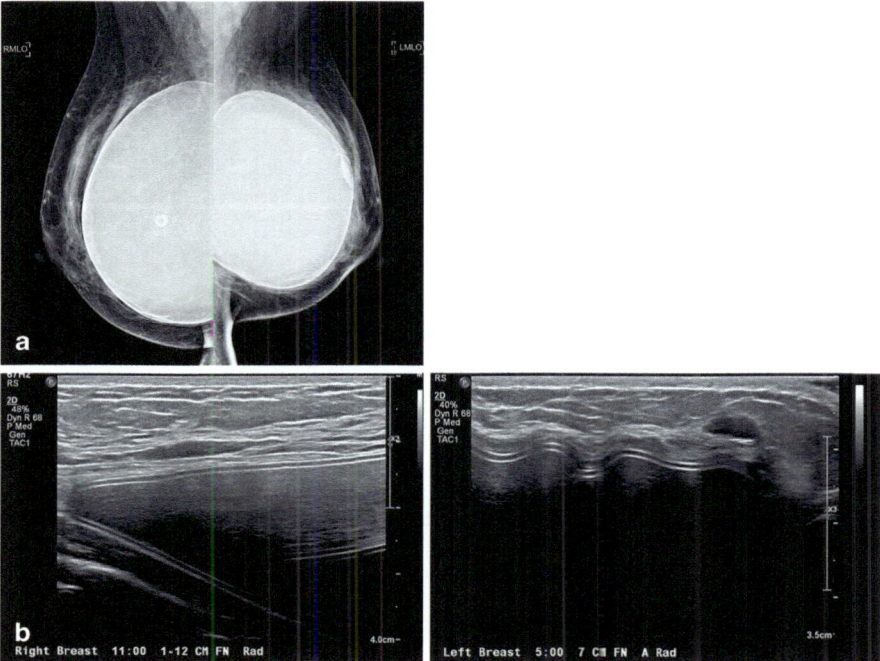

Fig. 12.13 Left implant contracture. 44-year-old woman with immobile right implant 8 months after placement. (**a**) Bilateral MLO views show rounded left subpectoral implant as compared to right. (**b**) Ultrasound shows increased undulations of the left implant envelope as compared to the right consistent with implant contracture

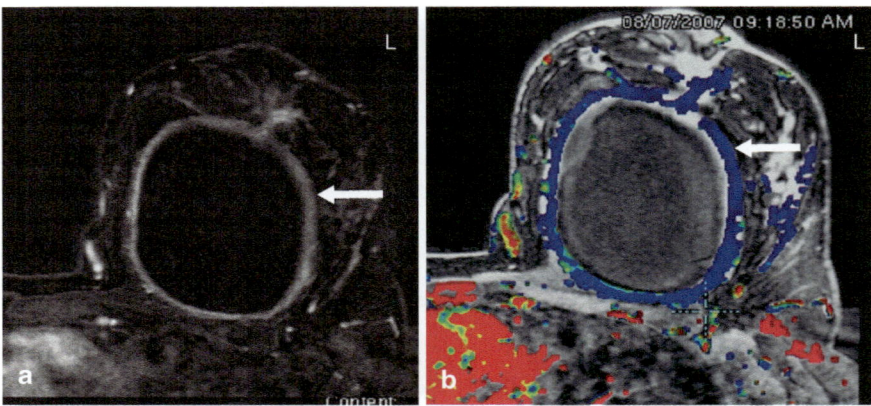

Fig. 12.14 Infected implant. 48-year-old with fever and acute tenderness. (**a**) Axial postcontrast MRI and (**b**) kinetic color map shows enhancement of implant capsule consistent with inflammation (white arrows)

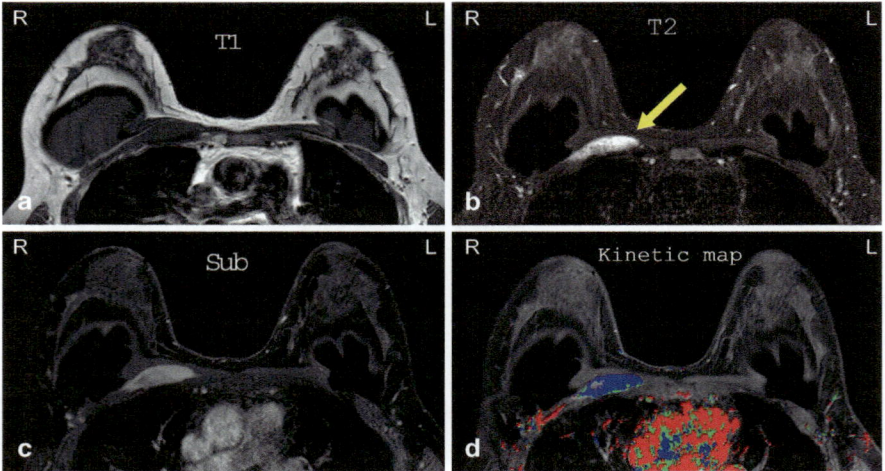

Fig. 12.15 44-year-old with enlarging lump along medial aspect of right implant. Axial T1-weighted (**a**), T2-weighted (**b**), postcontrast-subtracted dynamic (**c**) and kinetic map (**d**) show T1 hypointense T2 hyperintense progressively enhancing mass (arrow) contiguous with postero-medial aspect of the implant. Biopsy confirmed desmoid tumor

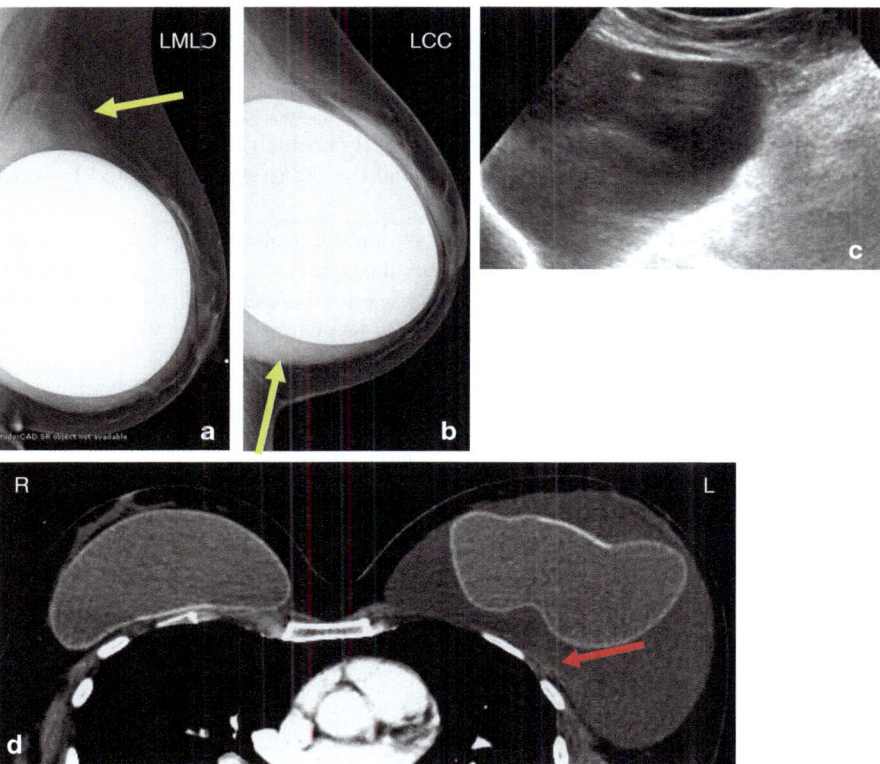

Fig. 12.16 **Implant-associated lymphoma**. 44-year-old with progressive left breast enlargement over 3 months. MLO (**a**) and CC (**b**) views show diffuse abnormal density around prepectoral silicone implant (yellow arrows). Ultrasound (**c**) shows a large fluid collection. Axial CT (**d**) shows large fluid collection surrounding the implant with subtle enhancing foci along the left chest wall (red arrow). Cytology from aspiration was concerning for malignancy. Surgical pathology confirmed pericapsular anaplastic large-cell lymphoma

Imaging

- Mammography
  - Views—conventional CC and MLO views including implant and CC and MLO implant-displaced (Eklund) (Fig. 12.17), which better images the breast tissue as the implant is pushed back and the breast tissue is pulled forward onto the image
  - Intact implant—smooth contour and symmetric in shape; capsule may calcify
    - Silicone—very dense; unable to see through
    - Saline—relatively radiolucent; can see implant valve and folds of envelope; breast tissue behind implant may be visible

- Ultrasound
  - Performed to confirm rupture suspected on mammography or to evaluate a palpable lump
  - Intact implant—thin echogenic line of the envelope containing primarily anechoic material; envelope may have undulations or folds
  - Saline—valve appears as focal area of capsular thickening
  - Ruptured implant

    - Silicone
      - Intracapsular rupture—parallel thin white lines that are arranged at multiple levels similar to climbing a ladder (*stepladder* sign) (Fig. 12.18)
      - Extracapsular rupture—focal echogenic area with posterior shadowing (*snowstorm* sign) (Fig. 12.19)
    - Saline—visible collapsed envelope
- MRI
  - Most sensitive and specific test to detect silicone implant rupture; **not** indicated for assessing integrity of saline implants
  - Intact implant
    - Silicone—T2 intermediate-to-high signal, low signal on silicone suppressed sequence or high signal on silicone selective sequence; often see radial folds (infoldings of the envelope)
  - Ruptured implant
    - Intracapsular rupture (Fig. 12.18)—curvilinear low signal lines within the silicone representing collapsed envelope (*linguine* sign); focal collection of silicone between envelope and capsule (*teardrop or key-hole* sign) or thin line of silicone between implant envelope and fibrous capsule (*subcapsular line sign*) indicates early rupture
    - Extracapsular rupture (Fig. 12.19)—silicone extruding into surrounding breast tissue; often see silicone within axillary lymph nodes; *linguine* sign may or may not be seen

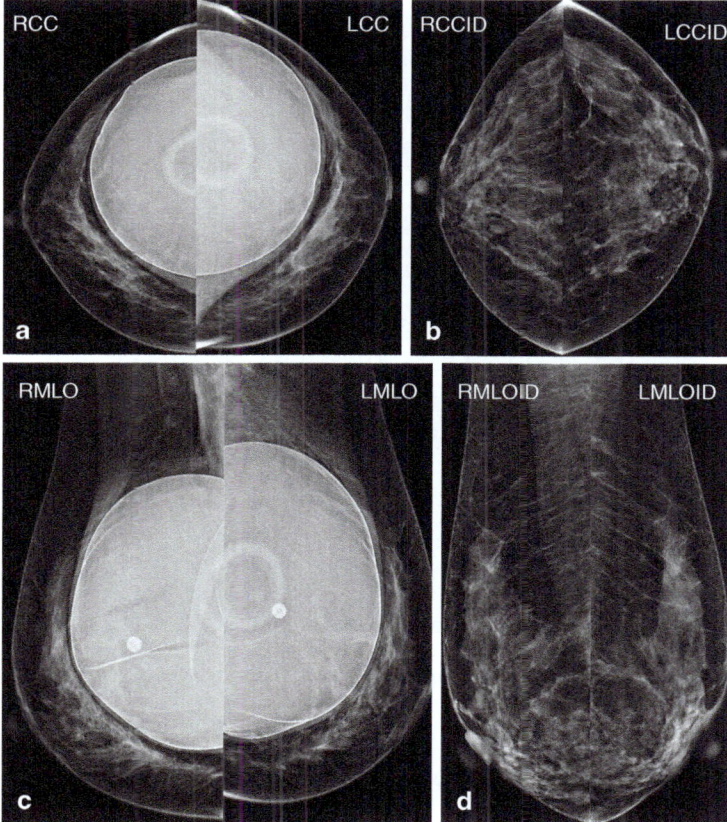

Fig. 12.17 (**a**) **45-year-old woman presented for screening**. Bilateral CC views show retropectoral saline implant with valve and (**b**) Bilateral implant displaced CC views show heterogeneously
dense tissue. (**c**) Bilateral MLO views show the retropectoral saline implant with valve and (**d**)
Bilateral implant displaced MLO views show the glandular tissue separate from the implant as the
implant is pushed back during imaging and not in the field of view improving visualization of the
glandular tissue

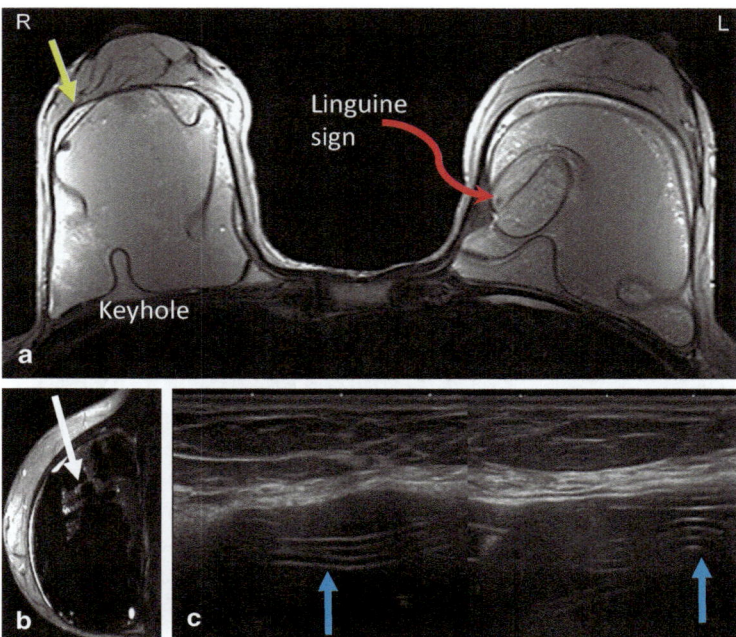

Fig. 12.18 **Bilateral intracapsular rupture**. Axial STIR image shows the dark intact fibrous capsule (yellow arrow) and the *linguine* and *keyhole* signs consistent with intracapsular rupture. *Linguine* sign (red arrow) - wavy line made by the collapsed implant shell. *Keyhole* and *Teardrop* signs - appearance of silicone on both sides of the ruptured implant. (**b**) Sagittal silicone-suppressed images reveal "salad oil" sign (white arrow). (**c**) Ultrasound shows intracapsular rupture as a step-ladder sign (blue arrows)

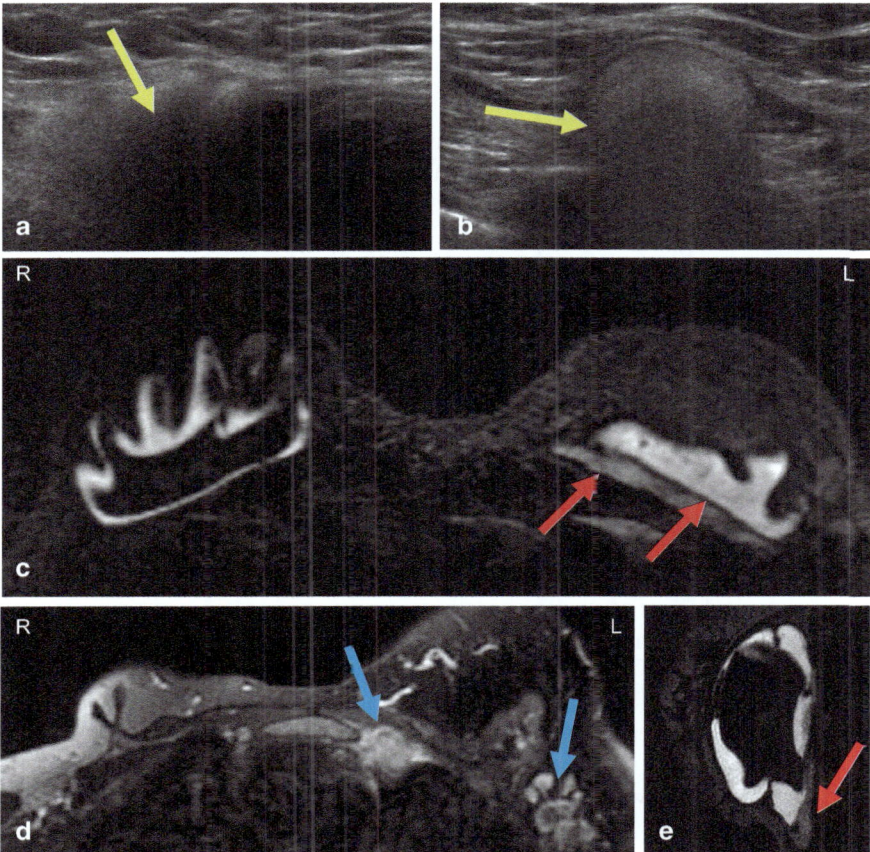

Fig. 12.19 **Extracapsular rupture with silicone lymphadenopathy**. 42-year-old woman with pain in the left axilla and inner lower left breast and history of bilateral double lumen (inner silicone, outer saline) implants. (**a, b**) Ultrasound shows "snowstorm" appearance of free silicone in tissues adjacent to the implant (arrow). (**c**) Axial STIR, (**d**) axial silicone suppressed and (**e**) sagittal silicone-suppressed MR images show left breast implant extracapsular rupture (red arrows) and free silicone (*drop of signal*) in enlarged internal mammary and left axillary lymph nodes (blue arrows)

FREE SILICONE INJECTIONS

Material and Location

- Free injection of silicone into breast tissue resulting in foreign body reaction
- Performed in Asia and South America; illegal in USA, although may be seen in transgender population

Potential Complications

- Painful palpable lumps secondary to silicone granulomas
- Calcifications due to foreign body reaction

Imaging (Figs. 12.20 and e12.9)

- Mammography
  - Multiple high-density nodular densities and masses; may see coarse calcifications
  - Reduced mammographic sensitivity; if high risk, may also screen with MRI
- Ultrasound
  - Multiple mixed-echogenicity, hyperechoic, hypoechoic, or anechoic masses with heterogeneous posterior acoustic shadowing (*snowstorm*)
- MRI
  - Masses with low T1 signal and high T2 high signal, which suppress on silicone sequences and are non-enhancing
  - If enhancement, consider silicone granuloma with fat necrosis or malignancy

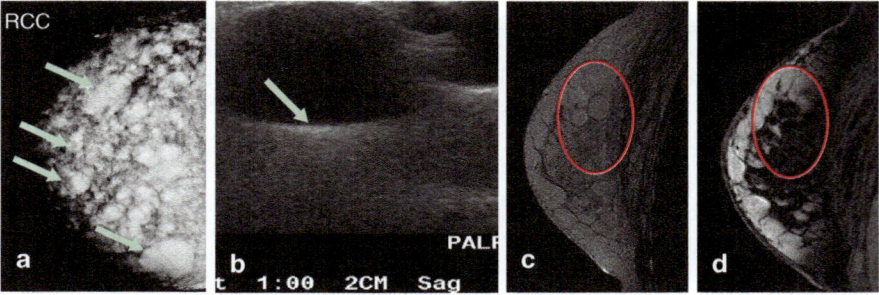

Fig. 12.20 Free silicone injections. 46-year-old transgender woman with history of bilateral free silicone injections. (**a**) CC view shows multiple, well-circumscribed hyperdense silicone granulomas (green arrows). (**b**) Ultrasound shows innumerable homogenous, hypoechoic, well-circumscribed masses with posterior acoustic enhancement (green arrow) consistent with silicone granulomas. (**c**) Sagittal non-fat-saturated T2-weighted MRI image and (**d**) sagittal T1-weighted silicone-suppressed image show non-enhancing round masses with T2 intermediate signal and T1 low signal consistent with free silicone (red circles)

BREAST RECONSTRUCTION

Material

- Comprised of implant and/or autologous flaps (deep inferior epigastric perforator (DIEP) (Fig. 12.21), transverse rectus abdominis muscle (TRAM) (Figs. 12.22 and e12.10) or latissimus dorsi (LAT) (Figs. 12.23 and e12.11))
- Free-fat injections into the lumpectomy bed for improved cosmesis

Potential Complications

- Infection/abscess and recurrence within flap (Fig. 12.24)

Imaging

- Mammography
  - Although not routinely imaged, the appearance depends on the flap (combination of fat and possibly muscle)
  - There may be calcifications related to fat necrosis, but if indeterminate may require biopsy
- Ultrasound—typically performed for palpable lump
- MRI—appearance depends on the specific flap; muscular pedicle enhances; often fat necrosis present

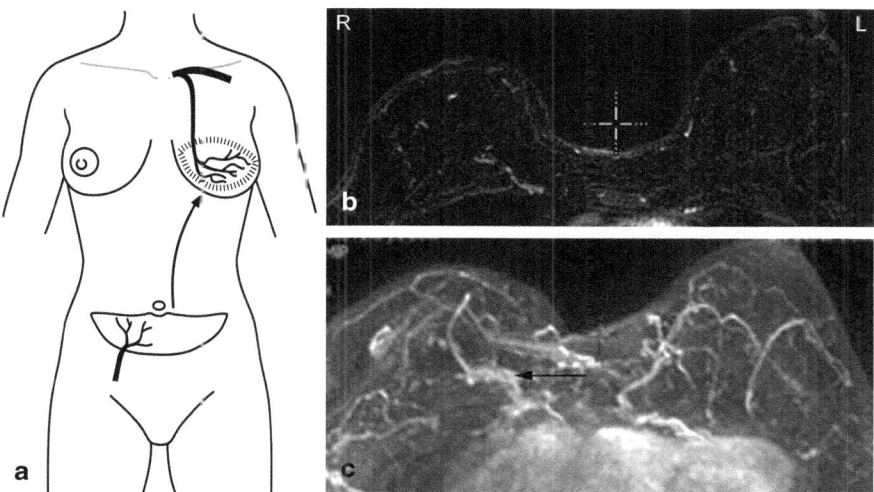

Fig. 12.21 **The DIEP flap is supplied by intramuscular perforators from the deep inferior epigastric artery and vein.** (a) During flap harvest, these perforators are meticulously dissected free from the surrounding muscle and preserved intact and the pedicle is anastomosed to the internal mammary vessels in the chest. (b) Axial fat-saturated T1W images with postcontrast gadolinium injection and (c) 3D reformatted axial images show replacement of the normal glandular tissue of the breast with lower abdominal fat and the anastomosis of the vascular pedicle (black arrow) to internal mammary artery

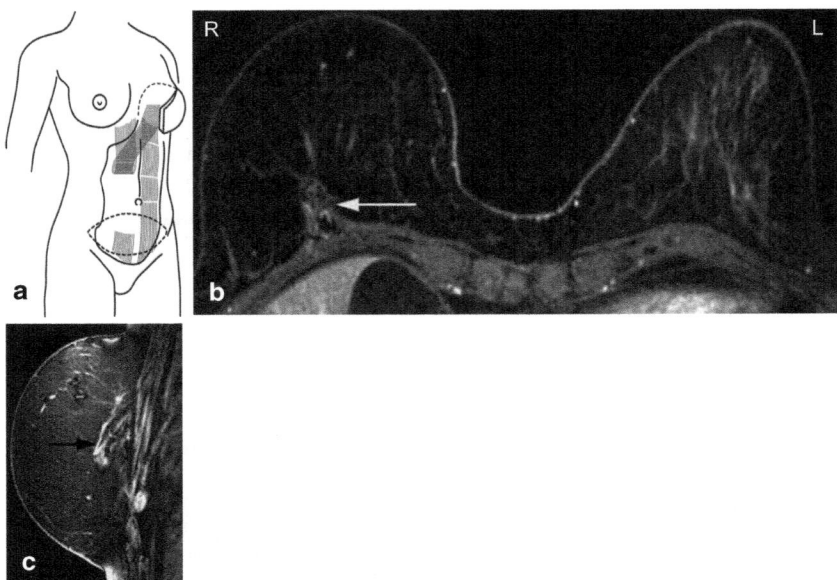

Fig. 12.22 (**a**) **Transverse rectus abdominis muscle (TRAM) is rotated up to the chest for flap breast reconstruction.** (**b**) Fat-saturated T1-weighted axial image and (**c**) sagittal image show replacement of the normal glandular tissue of the breast with lower abdominal fat and the presence of atrophied rectus abdominis muscle along the anterior chest wall (arrows)

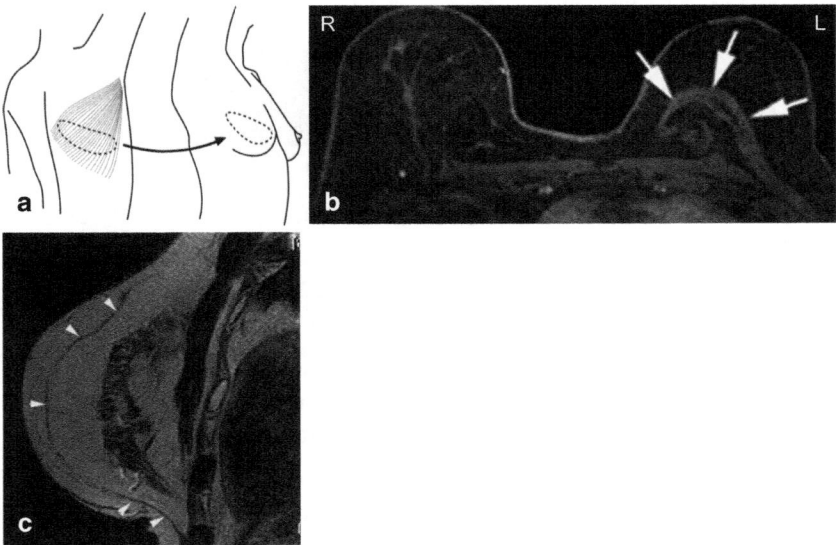

Fig. 12.23 Reconstruction with latissimus dorsi myocutaneous flap—(**a**) **Latissimus dorsi muscle, fat, and skin are rotated to reconstruct the breast with or without implant placement** (**b**) Axial fat-saturated T1-weighted image with postcontrast gadolinium injection and (**c**) axial sagittal non fat-saturated T1-weighted image show latissimus dorsi muscle flipped anteriorly for reconstruction (white arrows) and the denuded dermal layer is seen parallel to the chest wall (white arrowheads)

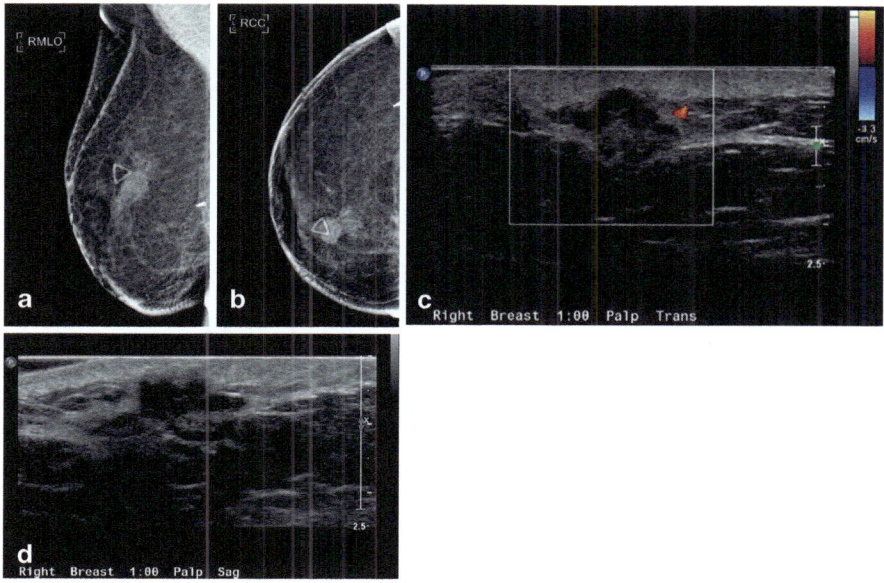

Fig. 12.24 Cancer recurrence within TRAM flap. Invasive ductal carcinoma. 51-year-old with history of right breast DCIS status post mastectomy with TRAM flap reconstruction 15 years ago presents with palpable right breast lump. MLO (**a**) and CC (**b**) views show irregular mass in the inner upper right breast. Ultrasound (**c**, **d**) reveals an irregular hypoechoic mass with minimal peripheral vascularity. Biopsy confirmed invasive ductal cancer

BREAST REDUCTION

Surgical procedure to reduce the size of the breasts, which results in bilateral post-surgical changes with a "swirling" pattern of the remaining breast tissue (Figs. 12.25 and e12.12). Often associated dermal and periareolar calcifications, fibrotic bands, nipple elevation, and changes of fat necrosis often seen.

Potential Complications

- Infection/abscess
- Scar carcinoma

Imaging

- Mammography—bilateral postsurgical changes and possibly calcifications sug-gestive of fat necrosis
- Ultrasound—not typically performed, unless palpable lump or discharge
- MRI—bilateral postsurgical changes

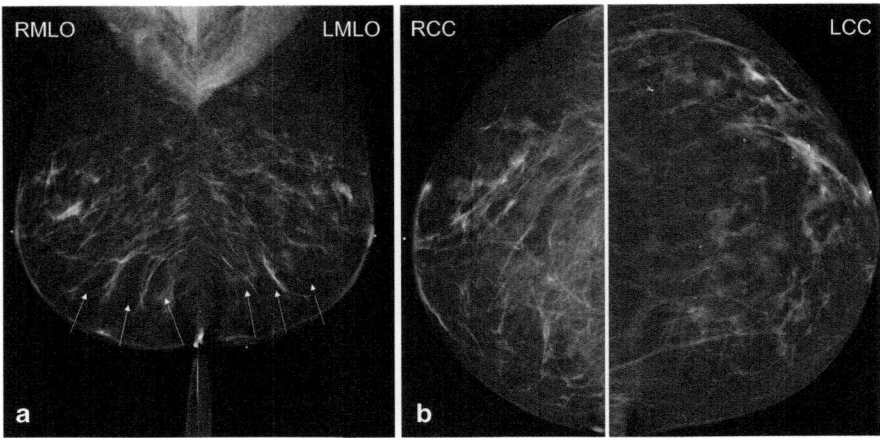

Fig. 12.25 Bilateral reduction mammoplasty. (a) Bilateral MLO and (b) bilateral CC views of a 53-year-old show a swirling pattern in the inferior breast (arrows) typical of reduction surgery

Further Readings

1. Lourenco AP, Moy L, Baron P, et al. ACR Appropriateness Criteria breast implant evaluation. J Am Coll Radiol. 2018;15:S13–25.
2. Juanperre S, Perez E, Huc O, Motos N, Pont J, Pedraza S. Imaging of breast implants—a pictorial review. Insights Imaging. 2011;2(6):653–70.
3. Venkataraman S, Hines N, Slanetz PJ. Challenges in mammography: Part 2, Multimodality review of breast augmentation—imaging findings and complications. Am J Roentgenol. 2011;197(6):W1301–45.
4. Dialani V, Lai KC, Slanetz PJ. MR imaging of the reconstructed breast: what the radiologist needs to know. Insights Imaging. 2012;3(3):201–13.
5. Raj SD, Karimova EJ, Fishman MDC, Fein-Zachary V, Phillips J, Dialani V, Slanetz PJ. Imaging of breast implant associated complications and pathologic conditions. Radiographics. 2017;37(5):1603–4.

Male Patients

13

Kimberly Dao, Kitt Shaffer,
and Priscilla J. Slanetz

Most common symptomatic entity is gynecomastia; other benign entities include sebaceous cysts/epidermoid inclusion cysts, hematoma, fat necrosis, lipoma, mastitis/abscess, PASH, and myofibroblastoma.

Male breast cancer uncommon representing approximately 1% of all new cancer diagnoses.

May rarely see metastatic disease or lymphoma.

ANATOMY

- Similar structure to female breast up until puberty
- Androgen secretion during puberty inhibits ductal and lobule development
- Mature male breast consists of mainly fat, primitive subareolar ducts, minimal stroma, and skin
- May have intramammary and axillary lymph nodes but due to absent lobules, rarely see cysts, fibroadenomas, phyllodes, lobular neoplasia, or lobular carcinoma

Supplementary Information The online version contains supplementary material available at https://doi.org/10.1007/978-3-031-66274-4_13.

K. Dao · K. Shaffer · P. J. Slanetz (✉)
Division of Breast Imaging, Department of Radiology, Boston University Medical Center, Boston, MA, USA
e-mail: kitt.shaffer@bmc.org; priscilla.slanetz@bmc.org

IMAGING

- Based on ACR Appropriateness Criteria®
  o Suspect gynecomastia or pseudo-gynecomastia—No imaging needed
  o Palpable mass < 25 years, start with ultrasound; ≥ 25 years, start with bilateral diagnostic mammography
  o Exam suspicious of breast cancer (axillary nodes, nipple discharge, nipple retraction, etc.)—bilateral diagnostic mammography and ultrasound

COMMON BENIGN ENTITIES

GYNECOMASTIA

- Unilateral or bilateral breast enlargement due to stromal and ductal proliferation (Figs. 13.1 and 13.2)
- Causes include: idiopathic; physiologic (maternal hormones during infancy, puberty, senescence); drugs (alcohol, marijuana, opioids, anabolic steroids); medications (chemotherapeutic agents, estrogen therapy, antihypertensives, antidepressants, cimetidine, anti-psychotics, digitalis, spironolactone); hypogonadism (pituitary hormone deficiency, Klinefelter syndrome); hyperthyroidism; cirrhosis; neoplasm (hepatocellular carcinoma, adrenal carcinoma, testicular tumors); and chronic renal disease
- On physical exam, unilateral or bilateral breast enlargement, tenderness, swelling, and/or subareolar soft, mobile, palpable mass
- Imaging types
  o Nodular—most common type; usually < 1 year in duration
    - On mammography, fan-shaped subareolar stromal tissue with indistinct borders that blend into the surrounding tissue (Fig. 13.3)
    - On US, subcutaneous edema and prominent subareolar ducts
  o Dendritic—chronic gynecomastia; usually ≥ 1 year in duration; fibrotic and most often irreversible
    - On mammography, flame-shaped subareolar stromal tissue that branches into surrounding tissue (Figs. 13.4 and e13.1)
    - On US, subareolar fibroglandular tissue and small ducts (Fig. e13.2)
  o Diffuse glandular—associated with exogenous estrogen therapy
    - On mammography, similar to female breast; heterogeneously dense breast tissue containing both nodular and dendritic patterns (Fig. e13.3)
    - On US, dense breast tissue with both nodular and dendritic patterns, subareolar hypoechoic tissue that may mimic cancer
- Management
  o Identify possible physiologic or pharmacologic causes to remove triggering agent
  o May resolve spontaneously
  o If refractory and symptomatic, may require treatment with androgens or selective estrogen-receptor modulators and even surgery

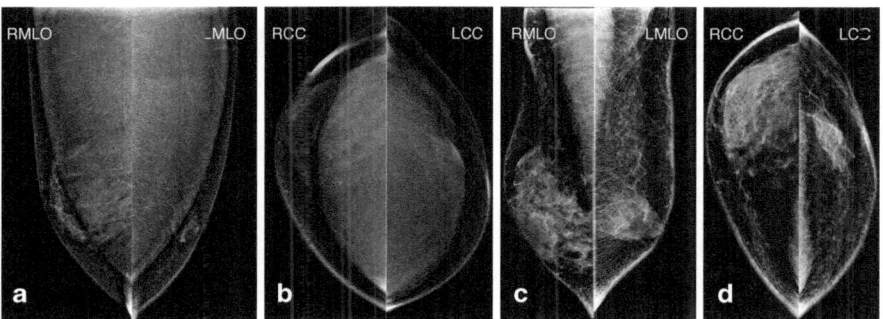

Fig. 13.1 32-year-old man with breast pain. Bilateral MLO (**a**) and CC views (**b**) show prominent pectoralis muscles and retroareolar breast tissue consistent with gynecomastia. Pectoralis displaced MLO (**c**) and CC (**d**) views better visualize the degree of gynecomastia

Fig. 13.2 25-year-old man presenting with asymmetric left breast enlargement. Bilateral MLO (**a**) and CC (**b**) views reveal unilateral left gynecomastia. The patient opted for surgical excision

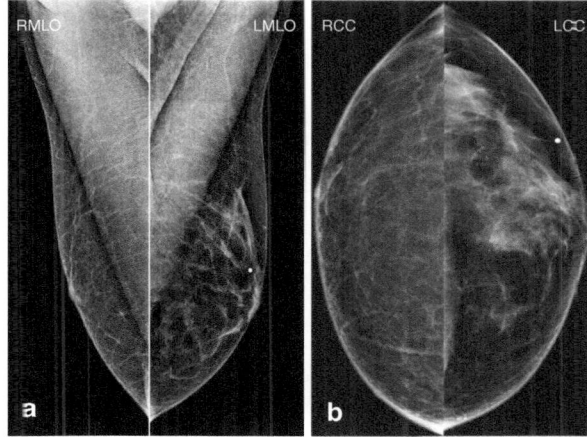

Fig. 13.3 **35-year-old man with a palpable right breast subareolar mass**. Bilateral MLO views show right greater than left subareolar stromal tissue that blends into the surrounding subcutaneous fat (arrows) consistent with nodular gynecomastia

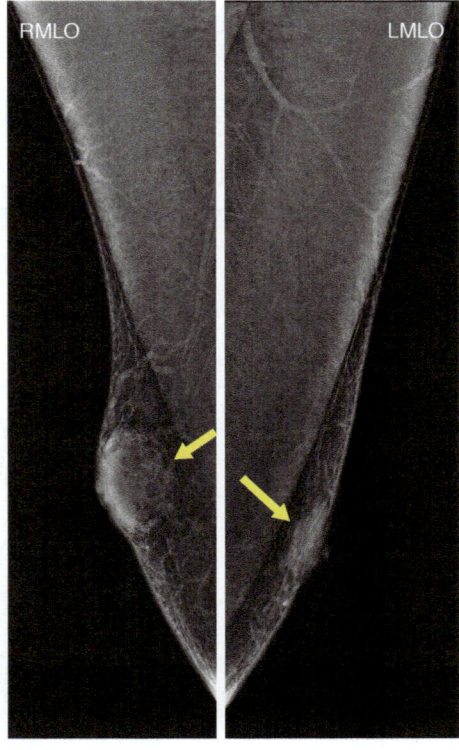

Fig. 13.4 **34-year-old man with left nipple pain**. Bilateral MLO views show left greater than right subareolar flame-shaped stromal tissue that branches into the surrounding subcutaneous tissue consistent dendritic gynecomastia

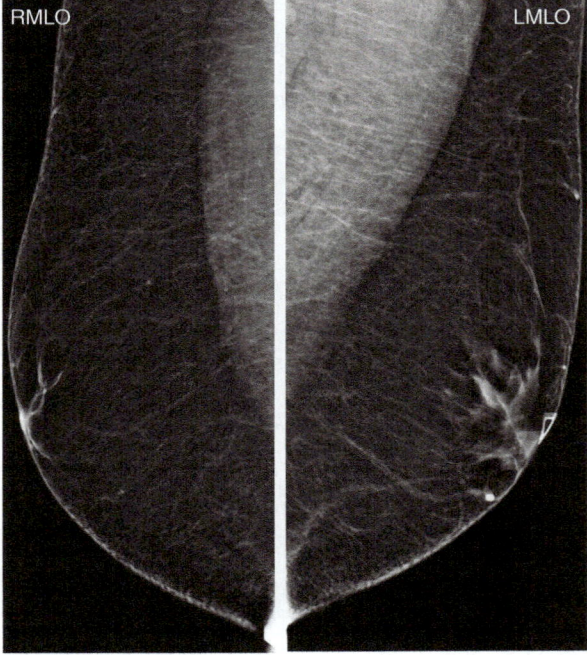

PSEUDO-GYNECOMASTIA

- Increased subcutaneous fat without increase in fibroglandular tissue
- On exam, diffuse enlargement without discrete palpable mass
- On mammography, diffusely increased fatty tissue (Fig. 13.5)
- Management: conservative; weight loss

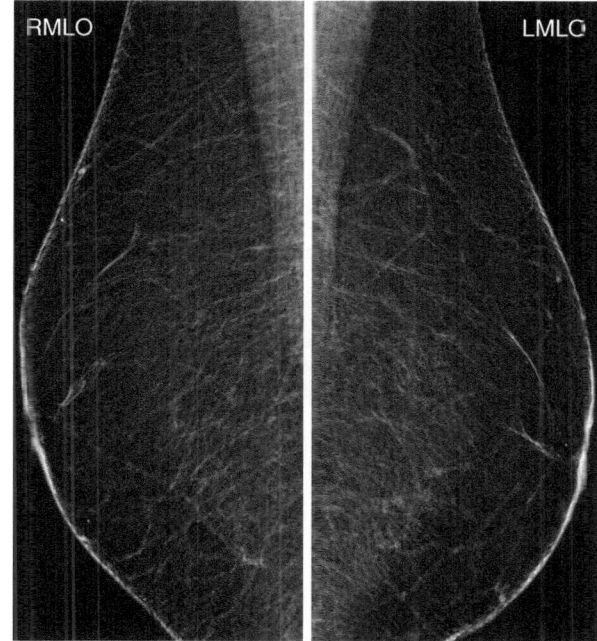

Fig. 13.5   43-year-old man who presents for work up of "excess breast tissue." Bilateral MLO views show diffusely increased fatty tissue without substantial subareolar fibroglandular tissue resulting in enlarged breasts. Findings are consistent with pseudogynecomastia

SKIN LESIONS

- Sebaceous or epidermoid inclusion cyst can occur
- Circumscribed superficial low attenuation mass arising from obstructed follicles or sebaceous glands with variable echogenicity on US (Fig. 13.6)
- Management—surgical excision if symptomatic

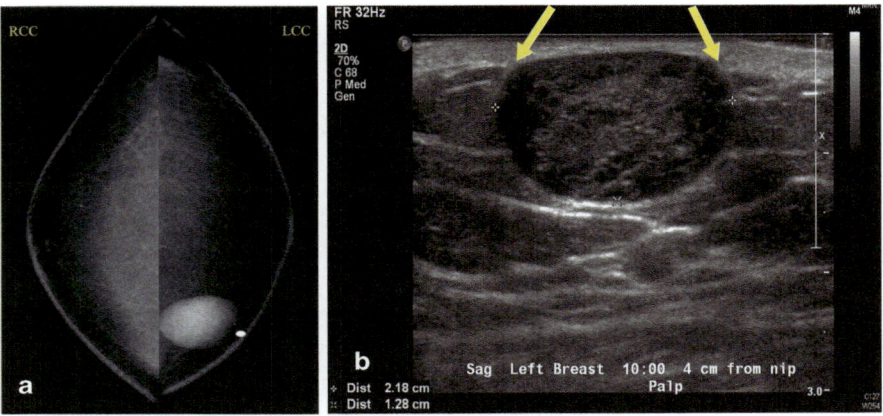

Fig. 13.6 **61-year-old man with a right breast lump**. Left CC view (**a**) shows a superficial circumscribed oval mass. Targeted ultrasound (**b**) reveals a well-circumscribed hypoechoic mass in the subcutaneous tissue with a claw sign (arrows), indicative of an epidermoid inclusion cyst

TRAUMA

- Hematoma or fat necrosis occur secondary to recent or remote trauma, respectively
- Imaging
  - Hematomas—circumscribed or irregular masses with variable echogenicity on US (most commonly echogenic) (Figs. 13.7 and e13.4)
  - Fat necrosis—circumscribed radiolucent mass with variable echogenicity or as ill-defined mass with dystrophic coarse calcifications (Fig. e13.5)
- Management—conservative, NSAIDS if painful

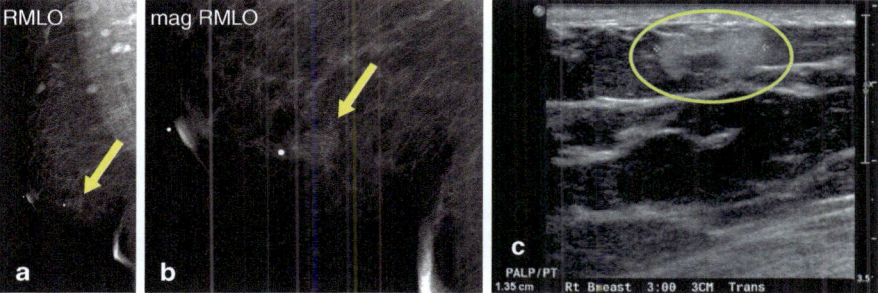

Fig. 13.7   45-year-old man with a painful palpable right breast lump. Right MLO view (**a**) and magnified MLO view (**b**) show an irregular superficial mass (arrows). Targeted ultrasound (**c**) reveals a predominantly echogenic mass with central hypoechogenicity (circle). The patient subsequently reported breast trauma. Imaging was consistent with a hematoma. On follow-up imaging (not shown), the findings resolved

LIPOMA

- Benign tumor consisting of mature fat cells often presenting as painless, soft palpable mass
- Often multiple and bilateral
- On mammography, encapsulated, radiolucent lesion containing fat (Fig. 13.8)
- On US, most often hyperechoic circumscribed mass without internal vascularity (Figs. e13.6 and e13.7)
- Management—conservative, surgical excision if enlarges

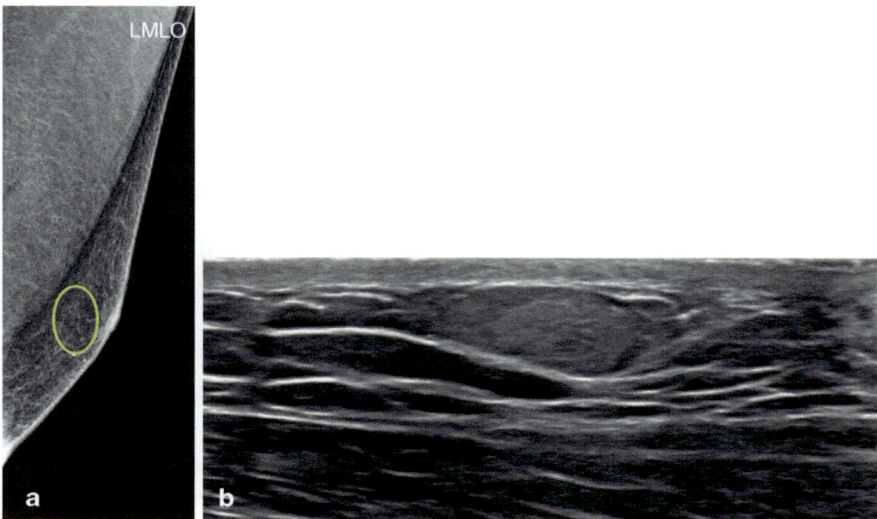

Fig. 13.8 53-year-old man with palpable left breast mass for 5 years. Left MLO view (**a**) shows a metallic BB placed in the area of palpable finding with a suggestion of a circumscribed, oval, radiolucent mass (circle). Targeted left breast ultrasound (**b**) shows a corresponding circumscribed, oval, slightly hyperechoic mass with no posterior features, and no internal vascularity. Findings are consistent with a lipoma

MASTITIS/ABSCESS

- Breast infection ± abscess presenting as tender erythematous enlarged breast or lump (Fig. 13.9)
- Management—antibiotics ± percutaneous drainage

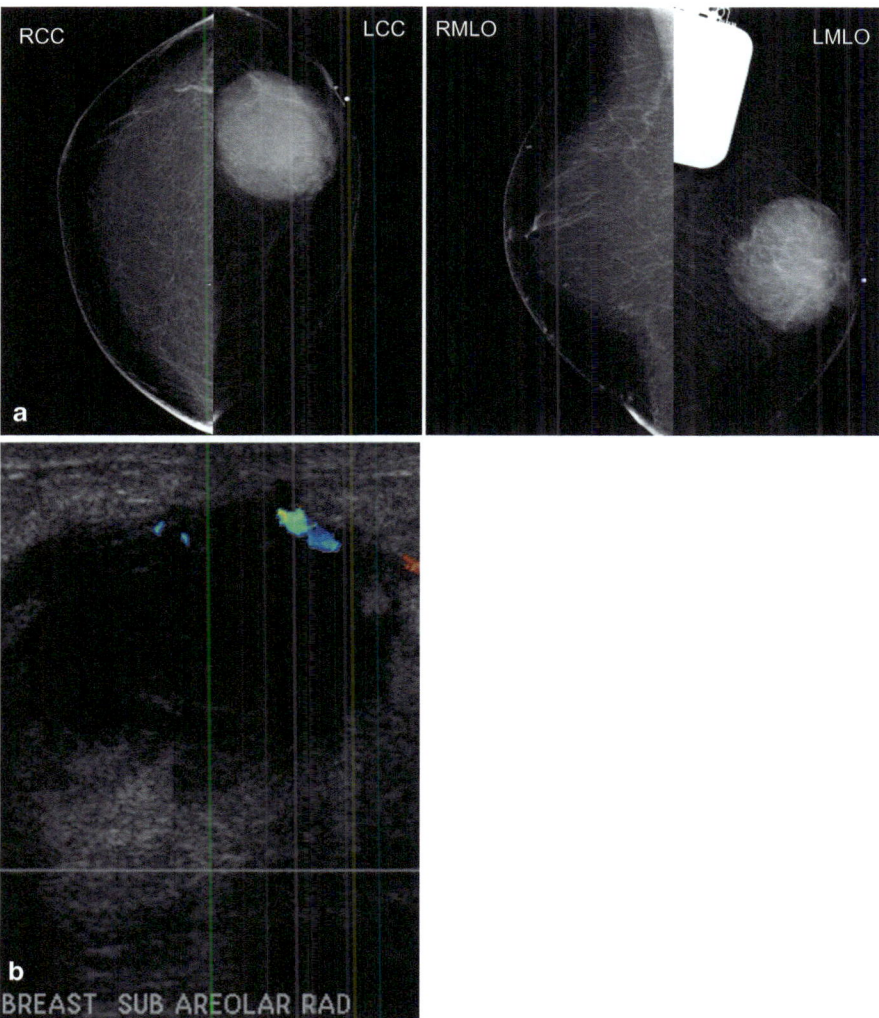

Fig. 13.9 67-year-old man presenting with a left breast mass accompanied by fever and chills 1 week after placement of a pacemaker. Bilateral CC and MLO views (**a**) show a large circumscribed mass in the outer central left breast corresponding to the area of concern. Targeted ultrasound (**b**) shows an irregular hypoechoic mass with peripheral vascularity. Percutaneous drainage revealed purulent material consistent with abscess

PASH

- Benign proliferative lesion presenting as palpable mass
- On imaging, circumscribed oval hypoechoic mass (Fig. e13.8)
- Management—conservative

MYOFIBROBLASTOMA

- Uncommon benign stromal tumor comprised of spindle cells and hyalinized collagen that more commonly occurs in postmenopausal women and elderly men
- On imaging, circumscribed or irregular mass without calcifications (Fig. e13.9)
- Management—wide surgical excision to minimize chance of local recurrence

MALIGNANCY

PRIMARY BREAST CANCER

- Presents ~ 5–10 years later and at more advanced stages, most likely due to delay in diagnosis
- On exam, unilateral, painless, palpable mass often eccentric to the nipple. Nipple discharge, nipple retraction, skin thickening, and axillary lymphadenopathy may be present
- Risk factors
  - Genetic—BRCA2 > BRCA1 mutations, family history of breast cancer in a first-degree male or female relative, Klinefelter syndrome
  - Increased estrogen exposure—exogenous estrogen therapy, obesity, finasteride therapy for prostate cancer
  - Prior radiation therapy to the chest
- Most common histologic subtype is infiltrating ductal carcinoma not otherwise specified (80%), followed by ductal carcinoma in situ (5%)
- Imaging
  - MG—irregular, spiculated mass with or without calcifications, most often located eccentric to the nipple (Fig. 13.10); skin thickening, nipple retraction, axillary lymphadenopathy may be present (Figs. e13.10–e13.12 and 13.11)
  - US—irregular, solid, hypoechoic mass, located eccentric to the nipple with internal vascularity and posterior shadowing (Figs. e13.10–e13.12 and 13.11)
- Management
  - Image-guided core biopsy for any finding with suspicious features
  - Depending on the stage of the cancer, treatment will include a combination of surgery, radiation therapy, and/or chemotherapy

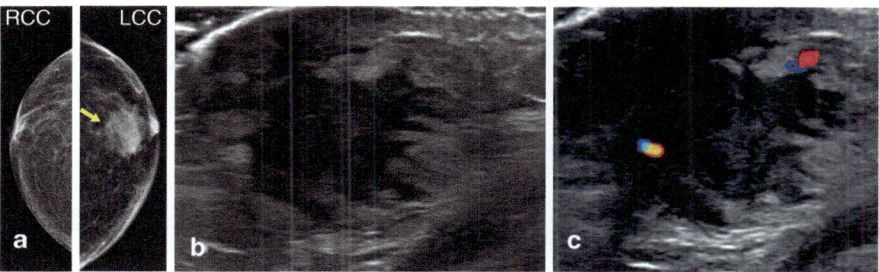

Fig. 13.10 88-year-old man with a palpable left subareolar mass associated with bloody nipple discharge. Bilateral CC views (**a**) show an irregular mass in the subareolar left breast (arrow) corresponding to the palpable finding. Subsequent targeted left breast ultrasound (**b, c**) shows an irregular, hypoechoic mass with heterogeneous internal echotexture and prominent internal and peripheral vascularity. Ultrasound-guided core biopsy confirmed invasive ductal carcinoma

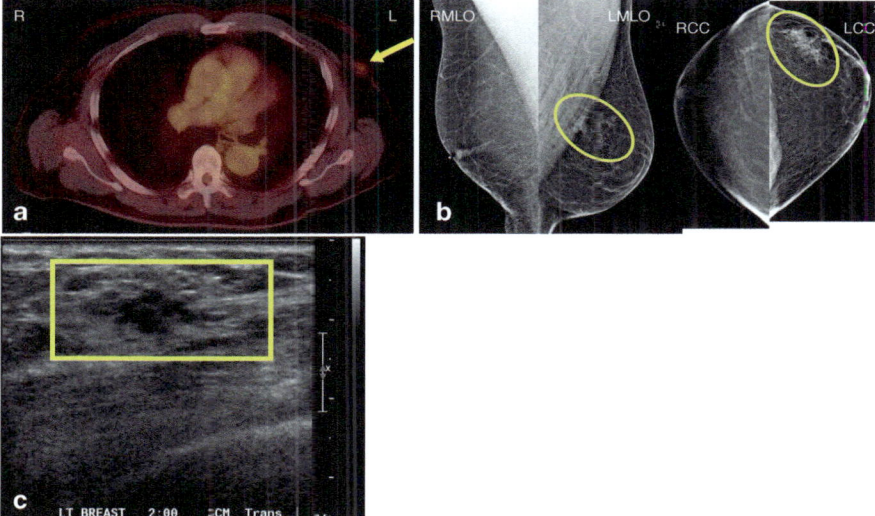

Fig. 13.11 66-year-old man with history of pancreatic adenocarcinoma. Surveillance PET/CT imaging (**a**) revealed focal uptake in the left breast with an SUV_{max} 3.0 (arrow). Bilateral MLO and CC views (**b**) show focal glandular asymmetry in the upper outer left breast (circles) corresponding to the area of concern on the PET scan. Targeted ultrasound (**c**) identifies a focal area of tissue heterogeneity (rectangle). Core biopsy revealed ductal carcinoma in situ (DCIS)

LYMPHOMA

- May be primary to breast or secondary (metastatic to axillary nodes or breast tissue)
- On imaging, either enlarged dense axillary and intramammary nodes or mass with heterogeneous echotexture (Fig. 13.12)
- Percutaneous biopsy must be sent for pathology and flow cytometry to allow for tailored chemotherapy

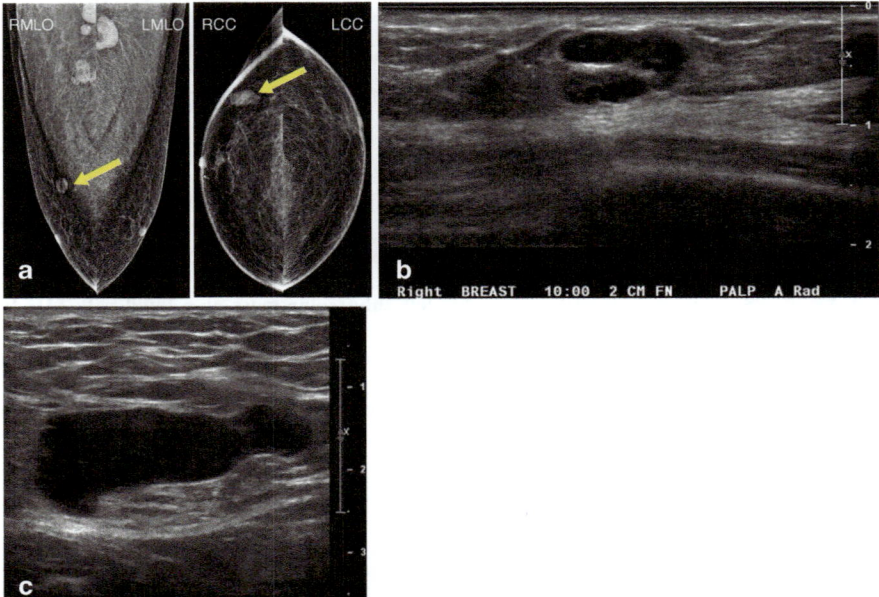

Fig. 13.12 78-year-old man with a palpable right breast lump. Bilateral MLO and CC views (**a**) show a circumscribed mass in the upper outer right breast (arrow) corresponding to the area of concern. Note is also made of small but dense bilateral axillary lymph nodes. Targeted ultrasound revealed a heterogeneous hypoechoic mass at 10:00 (**b**) and an abnormally thickened low axillary lymph node (**c**). Biopsy of the breast mass and axillary node confirmed mantle cell lymphoma

Further Readings

1. Chesebro AL, Rives AF, Shaffer K. Male breast disease: what the radiologist needs to know. Curr Probl Diagn Radiol. 2019;48:482–93.
2. Expert Panel on Breast Imaging, Niell BL, Lourenco AP, et al. ACR Appropriateness Criteria® evaluation of the symptomatic male breast. J Am Coll Radiol. 2018;15:S313–20.
3. Nguyen C, Kettler MD, Swirsky ME, Miller VI, Scott C, Krause R, Hadro JA. Male breast disease: pictorial review with radiologic-pathologic correlation. Radiographics. 2013;33:763–79.
4. Iuanow E, Kettler M, Slanetz PJ. Spectrum of disease in the male breast. Am J Roentgenol. 2011;196:W247–59.

Transgender Patients

14

Priscilla J. Slanetz

TERMINOLOGY

- Transgender—umbrella term for any individual whose gender identity differs from sex assigned at birth
- Transfeminine—identify as female, assigned male at birth
- Transmasculine—identify as male, assigned female at birth

P. J. Slanetz (✉)
Division of Breast Imaging, Department of Radiology, Boston University Medical Center, Boston, MA, USA
e-mail: priscilla.slanetz@bmc.org

© The Author(s), under exclusive license to Springer Nature Switzerland AG 2025
P. J. Slanetz, V. Dialani (eds.), *What Radiology Residents Need to Know: Breast Imaging*, What Radiology Residents Need to Know,
https://doi.org/10.1007/978-3-031-56274-4_14

CLINICAL CONSIDERATIONS

• Gender-affirming therapies include exogenous hormones (antiandrogens and estrogens for transfeminine (Fig. 14.1) and testosterone for transmasculine) and breast surgery (reduction mammoplasty/mastectomy for transmasculine or augmentation with implants (Fig. 14.2a, b), fat grafting or silicone injections (Fig. 14.3a–c) for transfeminine)
• May present with palpable lump (Fig. 14.4), breast pain (Fig. 14.5), nipple discharge (physiologic and pathologic)
   ○ Hormone-induced hyperprolactinemia in transfeminine patients
• Can develop full spectrum of benign and malignant breast disease including fibrocystic changes (Fig. 14.6), fibroadenomas (Fig. 14.7a, b), lipomas, phyllodes, and invasive ductal and lobular cancers (Fig. 14.8a, b)
• Incidence of breast cancer unknown but may develop at younger age

Fig. 14.1 63-year-old transfeminine patient with history of exogenous hormone use for 2 years now presenting with left nipple discharge. Bilateral MLO views reveal retroareolar breast tissue. The discharge was felt to be physiologic

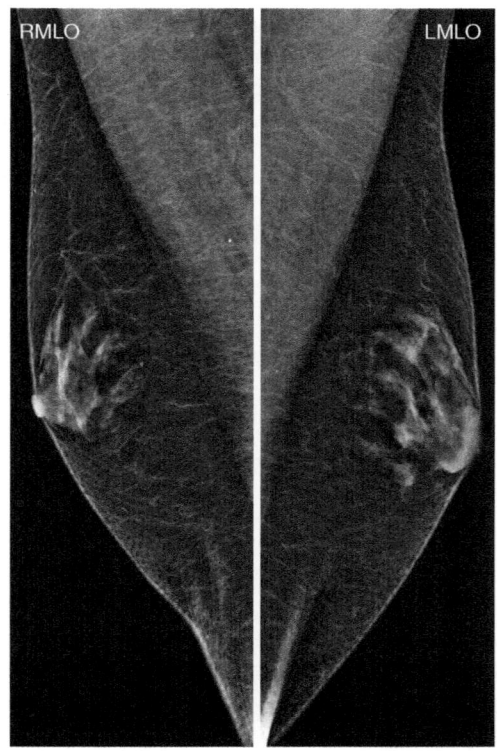

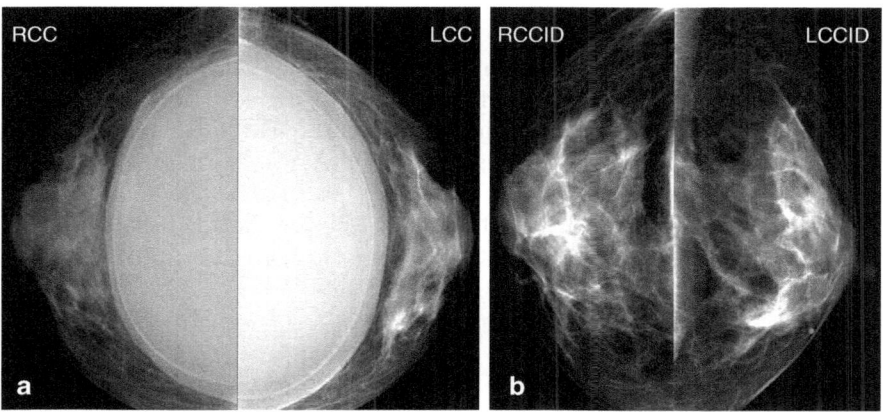

Fig. 14.2 44-year-old transfeminie patient. Bilateral CC (**a**) and implant-displaced CC (**b**) images reveal dense breast tissue and retropectoral silicone implants

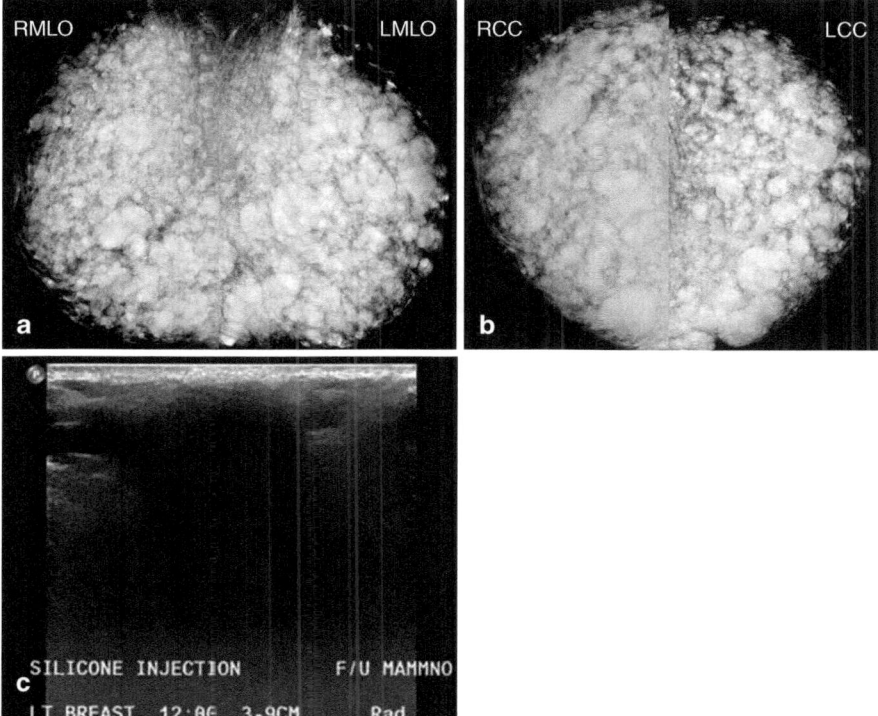

Fig. 14.3 45-year-old transfemirine patient presents with palpable lump at 12:00 in the left breast. Bilateral MLO (**a**) and CC (**b**) views demonstrate diffuse High-density material consistent with free silicone injections. Targeted ultrasound (**c**) reveals a hypoechoic shadowing mass with snowstorm appearance consistent with silicone granuloma

Fig. 14.4 21-year-old transmasculine patient status post bilateral mastectomy now presenting with pain and swelling. Ultrasound revealed a septated fluid collection consistent with a postoperative seroma

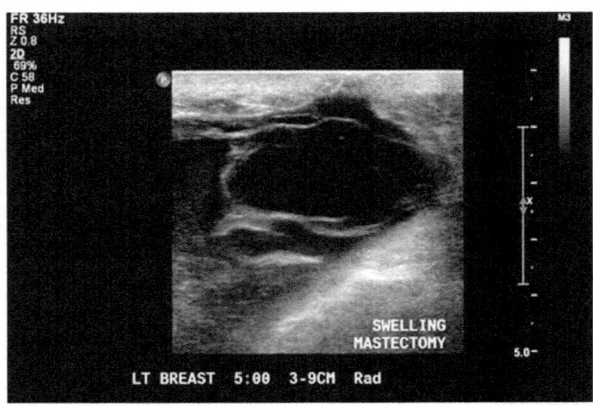

Fig. 14.5 48-year-old transmasculine patient status post reduction mammoplasty now presenting with pain, erythema, and a palpable lump. Targeted ultrasound reveals skin thickening, breast edema, and a complex fluid collection consistent with abscess

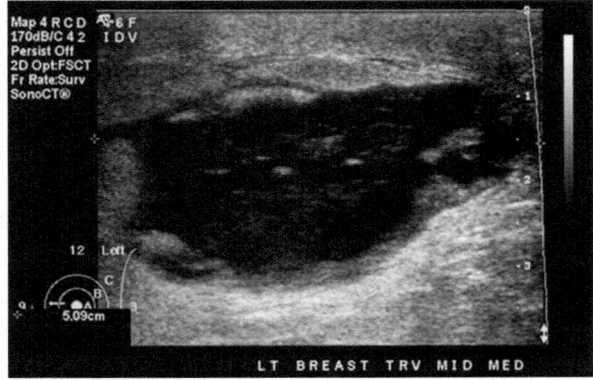

Fig. 14.6 28-year-old transfeminine patient with a palpable tender lump. Ultrasound revealed fibrocystic changes

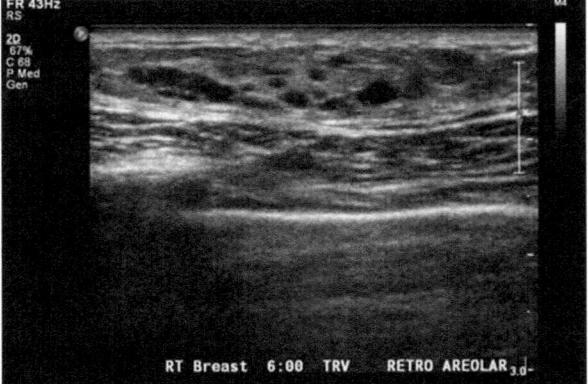

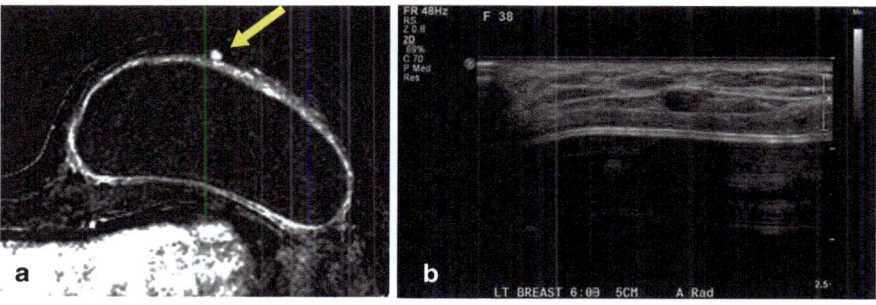

Fig. 14.7 39-year-old high risk transfeminine patient. Screening breast MRI reveals a T2 hyperintense enhancing mass (a; arrow). Targeted ultrasound shows a circumscribed oval mass (b) which subsequently was biopsied and confirmed to represent a fibroadenoma

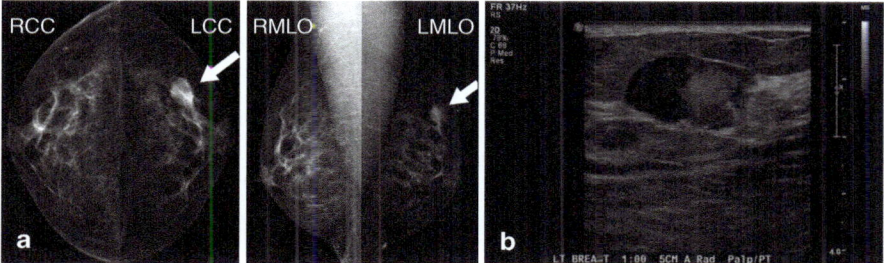

Fig. 14.8 50-year-old transfeminine patient with 5 years of exogenous hormone use presenting with palpable mass in the upper outer left breast. Bilateral CC and MLO (a) views show a circumscribed mass in the upper outer left breast (a; arrows). Targeted ultrasound revealed a mixed solid and cystic mass (b). Biopsy confirmed high-grade invasive ductal cancer

SCREENING

Screening recommendations based on sex assigned at birth, risk factors, and use of exogenous hormones

- Annual screening recommended for:
  - ○ Transfeminine 25–30 years elevated risk, past or current exogenous hormone use ≥ 5 years
  - ○ Transmasculine, ≥ 40 years, reduction mammoplasty or no chest surgery, average risk
- Annual screening may be appropriate for:
  - ○ Transfeminine, ≥ 40 years, average risk, past or current exogenous hormone use ≥ 5 years
  - ○ Transfeminine 25–30 years elevated risk, no or < 5 years exogenous hormone use
- No screening indicated if:
  - ○ Transfeminine, average risk, no or < 5 years exogenous hormone use
  - ○ Transmasculine, bilateral mastectomies

Further Readings

1. ACR Appropriateness Criteria Transgender Breast Cancer Screening. https://acsearch.acr.org/docs/3155692/Narrative/.
2. Parikh U, Mausner E, Chhor CM, et al. Breast imaging in transgender patients: what the radiologist should know. Radiographics. 2019;40:13–27.
3. Phillips J, Fein-Zachary V, Mehta TS, et al. Breast imaging in the transgender patient. Am J Roentgenol. 2014;202:1149–56.

Common Differential Diagnoses in Breast Imaging (in Alphabetical Order)

15

Priscilla J. Slanetz and Anna Rives

Architectural Distortion

Postsurgical change/prior breast reduction
Complex sclerosing lesion/radial scar
Malignancy (DCIS/invasive cancer)
Fat necrosis/trauma
Sclerosing adenosis
Fibromatosis
Granular cell tumor

Axillary Lymphadenopathy, Bilateral

Reactive hyperplasia
Infectious (TB, HIV)
Inflammatory (sarcoidosis, rheumatoid arthritis, SLE)
Lymphoma/leukemia
Metastatic disease

P. J. Slanetz (✉) · A. Rives
Division of Breast Imaging, Department of Radiology, Boston University Medical Center,
Boston, MA, USA
e-mail: priscilla.slanetz@bmc.org; anna.rives@bmc.org

© The Author(s), under exclusive license to Springer Nature Switzerland AG 2025
P. J. Slanetz, V. Dialani (eds.), *What Radiology Residents Need to Know: Breast Imaging*, What Radiology Residents Need to Know,
https://doi.org/10.1007/978-3-031-56274-4_15

Axillary Lymphadenopathy, Unilateral

Reactive hyperplasia
Recent vaccination (esp. COVID-19)
Metastatic disease (breast cancer, melanoma, ovarian cancer)
Unicentric Castleman's disease
Cat-scratch disease
Silicone lymphadenopathy
Inflammatory disease (sarcoidosis)
Lymphoma/leukemia

Axillary Mass

Sebaceous/epidermoid inclusion cyst
Hidradenitis suppurativa
Lymphadenopathy (i.e. reactive, inflammatory, infectious, neoplastic)
Postoperative seroma or lymphocele
Accessory breast tissue
Intramuscular or soft tissue mass

Circumscribed Mass

Skin lesion
Cyst
Fibroadenoma
Hematoma
Papilloma
Oil cyst/fat necrosis
Tubular adenoma
Adenomyoepithelioma
Hamartoma
Phyllodes tumor
Malignancy (papillary, mucinous, medullary carcinomas, malignant phyllodes)
Metastatic disease

Mixed Solid and Cystic Mass

Galactocele
Hematoma
Fat necrosis/oil cyst
Mastitis/breast abscess
Intracystic papilloma

Papillary DCIS/cancer
Necrotic cancer

Cystic Breast Mass

Simple cyst
Complicated cyst
Apocrine metaplasia
Galactocele
Hematoma
Fat necrosis/oil cyst
Mastitis/breast abscess
Intracystic papilloma
Papillary DCIS/cancer
Necrotic cancer

Diffuse Decrease in Breast Density

Weight gain
Chemoprevention (e.g. tamoxifen, aromatase inhibitor)
Tissue involution due to aging

Diffuse Increase in Breast Density

Weight loss
Hormone replacement therapy
Mastitis
Trauma/contusion
Radiation therapy
Edema secondary to lymphatic or venous obstruction
Inflammatory mastitis (SLE, IGM)
Infiltrative malignancy (more often invasive lobular)

Intraductal Mass

Duct ectasia
Chronic inflammatory infiltrates
Blocked duct
Periductal mastitis
Apocrine metaplasia
Papilloma/papillomatosis
Malignancy (DCIS/invasive ductal cancer)

Echogenic Mass

Lipoma/angiolipoma
Hematoma/Contusion
Fat necrosis
Silicone granuloma
Sebaceous or epidermal inclusion cyst
Abscess
Pseudoangiomatous stromal hyperplasia
Galactocele/lactating adenoma
Apocrine metaplasia
Malignancy (invasive ductal or lobular cancer)
Metastasis
Lymphoma
Angiosarcoma

Fat-Containing Mass

Lipoma
Angiolipoma
Hamartoma
Intramammary lymph node
Galactocele
Oil cyst/fat necrosis

Global Asymmetry

Technical (lack of compression, incorrect kV/mAs)
Mastitis
Hormone replacement effect
Infiltrative process (malignancy, recurrence)

Grouped Calcifications

Artifact (ointment/antiperspirant)
Dermal
Fibrocystic change/milk of calcium
Fibroadenoma
Papilloma
Fat necrosis

Sclerosing adenosis
Atypia (ADH, pleomorphic LCIS, ALH)
Breast infarct
Malignancy (DCIS/invasive ductal cancer)

Linear Calcifications

Vascular
Sutural
Secretory/plasma cell mastitis
Filariasis
Malignancy (DCIS/invasive ductal cancer)

Male Breast Lump

Gynecomastia
Sebaceous/epidermoid inclusion cyst
Pseudoangiomatous stromal hyperplasia
Abscess
Hematoma/contusion
Myofibroblastoma
Breast malignancy
Lymphoma

Multiple Circumscribed Masses, Bilateral

Dermal
Cysts
Fibroadenomas
Papillomas/papillomatosis
Neurofibromatosis
Metastasis

Multiple Circumscribed Masses, Unilateral

Cysts
Fibroadenomas
Papillomatosis
Metastasis

New or Increasing Asymmetry (Formerly Developing Asymmetry)

Hematoma/contusion
Hormone replacement effect
Fat necrosis
Pseudoangiomatous stromal hyperplasia
Sarcoidosis/inflammatory disease
Malignancy
Weight loss
Unusual infections (parasitic)

Non-mass Enhancement on MRI

Apocrine metaplasia
Pseudoangiomatous stromal hyperplasia
Radiation effect
Atypia (ADH/FEA)
Radial scar/complex sclerosing lesion
Papilloma
Malignancy (DCIS/invasive cancer)

Segmental Calcifications

Dermal
Secretory/plasma cell mastitis
Fibrocystic change/milk of calcium
Fat necrosis
Sclerosing adenosis
Malignancy (DCIS and invasive ductal cancer)

Segmental Masses

Ductal ectasia
Papillomatosis
Granulomatous mastitis
Malignancy

Skin Thickening, Diffuse

Cellulitis/mastitis
Fluid overload (CHF, renal failure)

Radiation changes
Lymphatic or venous obstruction
Inflammatory breast cancer

Skin Thickening, Focal

Dermatologic condition
Keloid
Cellulitis/mastitis
Radiation-induced sarcoma (often nodular)

Spiculated Mass

Postsurgical change
Complex sclerosing lesion/radial scar
Fat necrosis
Lymphocytic mastitis/mastopathy
Granular cell tumor
Stromal fibrosis
Malignancy

Index